Atlas of
Common
Pain
Syndromes

Additional titles from the frontlines of pain management by Steven D. Waldman, MD, JD

Interventional Pain Management, 2nd Edition   ISBN 0–7216–8748–2

This clinically oriented, practical text offers comprehensive how-to guidance on the full spectrum of pain management. Sixty-two leading experts discuss general topics, cost-effective treatments, possible complications, advances in pain control, and the rapid growth and timely changes affecting the specialty. More than 600 illustrations, and 18 all-new chapters, demonstrate the intricacies of the latest procedures—in crisp detail.

Atlas of Interventional Pain Management   ISBN 0–7216–7577–8

"A nice addition to the pain management physician's library" — Anesthesiology
A reader-friendly "how-to-do-it" approach demonstrates common interventional pain management techniques. Step-by-step full-color illustrations and concise bulleted text explore procedures for all major anatomic sites. You'll also review procedures seldom found in other texts, such as lysis of epidural adhesions (Racz technique), cervical and lumbar subarachnoid neurolytic blocks, and tunneling techniques for one- and two-piece epidural catheters. For each procedure you'll also find potential pitfalls, clinical pearls, and CPT-4 coding.

Atlas of Pain Management Injection Techniques   ISBN 0–7216–8504–8

"A quick reference source on a variety of peripheral injection techniques." — Mayo Clinic Proceedings
Here's outstanding guidence on performing a complete range of clinical injection procedures—from the head and neck to the ankle and foot! Concise step-by-step instructions cover today's best approaches, while 245 crisp illustrations demonstrate relevant anatomy, insertion sites, and nuances of technique. Clinical pearls in each chapter equip you to perform every technique like an expert. **CPT-2000 coding information throughout the text helps you to achieve proper reimbursement.**

Atlas of Uncommon Pain Syndromes   ISBN 0–7216–9372–5

As a companion text to Dr. Waldman's *Common Pain Syndromes*, this all-color atlas examines the diagnosis of unusual, difficult, and untraceable pain problems. Inside you'll find **ICD-9** diagnosis codes, as well as clinical pearls gleaned from years of professional pain management practice. Over 200 specially created **full-color** drawings—many of syndromes not illustrated in other texts—clarify key concepts. **A wealth of radiographs and CT and MRI scans help you to define each unusual disease entity.**

Atlas of
Common
Pain
Syndromes

Steven D. Waldman, MD, JD
Director
    Pain Consortium of Greater Kansas City
    Leawood, Kansas
Clinical Professor of Anesthesiology
    University of Missouri at Kansas City
    School of Medicine
    Kansas City, Missouri

Illustrations by
David A. Rini, MFA, CMI, and Tim Phelps, MS, CMI
The Johns Hopkins University School of Medicine
Department of Art as Applied to Medicine

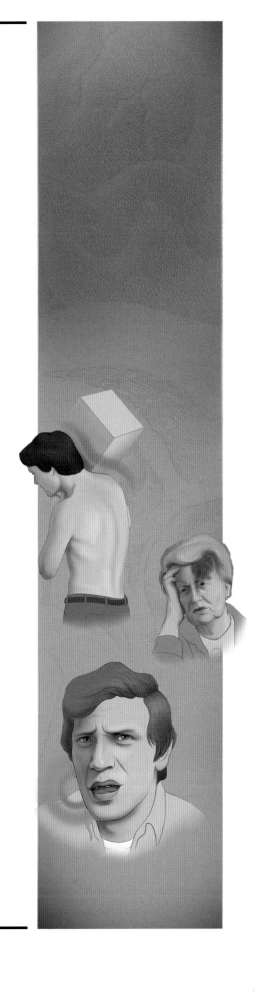

W.B. SAUNDERS COMPANY
An Imprint of Elsevier Science
Philadelphia London New York St. Louis Sydney Toronto

W.B. SAUNDERS COMPANY
An Imprint of Elsevier Science

The Curtis Center
Independence Square West
Philadelphia, Pennsylvania

Library of Congress Cataloging-in-Publication Data

Waldman, Steven D.

Atlas of common pain syndromes / Steven D. Waldman.—1st ed.

p. ; cm.

ISBN 0-7216-9211-7

1. Pain—Atlases. I. Title
[DNLM: 1. Pain—Atlases. 2. Syndrome—Atlases.   WL 17 W164ab 2002]

RB127.W347 2002   616'.0472—dc21   2001042029

Acquisitions Editor: Allan Ross
Developmental Editor: Arlene Chappelle
Production Editor: Edna Dick
Production Manager: Frank Polizzano
Illustration Specialist: Robert Quinn
Book Designer: Steven Stave

The ICD-9 Codes are copyrighted by the World Health Organization and are reproduced in this text with its permission.

ATLAS OF COMMON PAIN SYNDROMES   ISBN 0-7216-9211-7

Printed in China

Last digit is the print number   9   8   7   6   5   4   3   2   1

To my wife Kathy,
Thanks for your intellect, counsel, patience, and most of all your love!

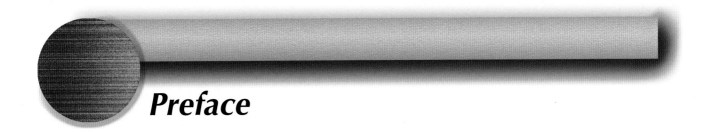

Preface

The *Atlas of Common Pain Syndromes* represents a departure from the previous pain management texts that I have written. Beginning with *Interventional Pain Management,* which is now in its second edition, my previous texts have focused primarily on the treatment of pain. *Common Pain Syndromes* is devoted primarily to the diagnosis of painful conditions. A text with an emphasis on diagnosis helps fill a gap in the current pain management literature and is needed to help round out the skill sets of the various specialties that are now involved in the treatment of pain.

Common Pain Syndromes is a how-to-do-it text. It is designed to be as practical and user-friendly as *Atlas of Interventional Pain Management* and *Atlas of Pain Management Injection Techniques.* Each chapter includes full-color art that illustrates the key signs and symptoms to allow the clinician to easily identify the common pain syndromes encountered in clinical practice.

Pathognomonic physical, laboratory, and radiographic findings are highlighted to help the clinician simplify the diagnostic process. As with the aforementioned Atlases, each chapter contains a Clinical Pearls section which provides the clinician with the most current "tricks of the trade" to enhance patient care. ICD-9 codes for each syndrome are presented to simplify coding and billing.

Recently, pain has been identified as the "fifth vital sign" that must be considered when caring for all patients, no matter what their primary medical complaint. It is hoped that *Common Pain Syndromes* will help the clinician effectively deal with pain by simplifying its diagnosis.

Steven D. Waldman, M.D., J.D.
2001

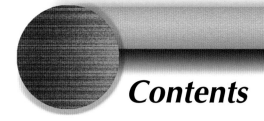

Contents

I Headache Pain Syndromes

1

Acute Herpes Zoster of the First Division of the Trigeminal Nerve

ICD-9 CODE 053.0

THE CLINICAL SYNDROME

Herpes zoster is an infectious disease that is caused by the varicella-zoster virus (VZV), which also is the causative agent of chickenpox (varicella). Primary infection in the nonimmune host manifests itself clinically as the childhood disease chickenpox. It is postulated that during the course of primary infection with VZV, the virus migrates to the dorsal root or cranial ganglia. The virus then remains dormant in the ganglia, producing no clinically evident disease. In some individuals, the virus may reactivate and travel along the sensory pathways of the first division of the trigeminal nerve, producing the pain and skin lesions characteristic of shingles. The reason that reactivation occurs in only some individuals is not fully understood, but it is theorized that a decrease in cell-mediated immunity may play an important role in the evolution of this disease entity by allowing the virus to multiply in the ganglia and spread to the corresponding sensory nerves, producing clinical disease. Patients who are suffering from malignancies (particularly lymphoma), who are receiving immunosuppressive therapy (chemotherapy, steroids, radiation), or who are suffering from chronic diseases are generally debilitated and much more likely than the healthy population to develop acute herpes zoster. These patients all have in common a decreased cell-mediated immune response, which may be the reason for the propensity for shingles to develop. This may also explain why the incidence of shingles increases dramatically in patients older than age 60 and is relatively uncommon in persons younger than age 20.

The first division of the trigeminal nerve is the second most common site for the development of acute herpes zoster after the thoracic dermatomes. Rarely, the virus may attack the geniculate ganglion, resulting in hearing loss, vesicles in the ear, and pain. This constellation of symptoms is called the *Ramsey-Hunt syndrome* and must be distinguished from acute herpes zoster involving the first division of the trigeminal nerve.

SIGNS AND SYMPTOMS

As viral reactivation occurs, ganglionitis and peripheral neuritis cause pain, which is generally localized to the segmental distribution of the first division of the trigeminal nerve. This pain may be accompanied by flulike symptoms and generally progresses from a dull, aching sensation to dysesthetic or neuritic pain in the distribution of the first division of the trigeminal nerve. In most patients, the pain of acute herpes zoster precedes the eruption of rash by 3 to 7 days, often leading to erroneous diagnosis (see Differential Diagnosis). However, in most patients, the clinical diagnosis of shingles is readily made when the characteristic rash appears. Like chickenpox, the rash of herpes zoster appears in crops of macular lesions, which rapidly progress to papules and then to vesicles (Fig. 1–1). As the disease progresses, the vesicles coalesce and crusting occurs. The area affected by the disease can be extremely painful, and the pain tends to be exacerbated by any movement or contact (e.g., with clothing or sheets). As healing takes place, the crusts fall away, leaving pink scars in the distribution of the rash that gradually become hypopigmented and atrophic.

In most patients, the hyperesthesia and pain generally resolve as the skin lesions heal. In some, however, pain may persist beyond lesion healing. This most common and feared complication of acute herpes zoster is called *postherpetic neuralgia*, and the elderly are affected at a higher rate than the general population suffering from acute herpes zoster (Fig. 1–2). The symptoms of postherpetic neuralgia can vary from a mild self-limited problem to a debilitating, constantly burning pain that is exacerbated by light touch, movement, anxiety, and/or temperature change. This unremitting pain may be so severe that it can completely devastate the patient's life, and ultimately it can lead to suicide. It is the desire to avoid this disastrous sequel to a usually benign self-limited disease that dictates the clinician use all possible therapeutic efforts for the patient suffering from acute herpes zoster in the first division of the trigeminal nerve.

TESTING

Although in most instances the diagnosis of acute herpes zoster involving the first division of the trigeminal nerve is easily made on clinical grounds, occasionally, confirmatory testing is required. Such testing may be desirable in patients with other skin lesions that confuse the clinical picture, such as patients with acquired immunodeficiency syndrome who are suffering from Kaposi's sarcoma. In such patients, the diagnosis of acute herpes zoster may be confirmed by obtaining a Tzanck smear from the base of a fresh vesicle that will reveal multinucleated giant cells and eosinophilic inclusions. To differentiate acute herpes zoster from localized herpes simplex infection, the clinician can obtain fluid from a fresh vesicle and submit it for immunofluorescent testing.

DIFFERENTIAL DIAGNOSIS

Careful initial evaluation, including a thorough history and physical examination, is indicated in all patients suffering from acute herpes zoster involving the first division of the trigeminal nerve to rule out occult malignancy or systemic disease that may be responsible for the patient's immunocompromised state. A prompt diagnosis will allow early recognition of changes in clinical status that may presage the development of complications, including myelitis or dissemination of the disease. Other causes of pain in the distribution of the first division of the trigeminal nerve include trigeminal neuralgia, sinus disease, glaucoma, retro-orbital tumors, inflammatory diseases (e.g., Tolosa-Hunt syndrome), and intracranial pathology including tumors.

TREATMENT

The therapeutic challenge of the patient presenting with acute herpes zoster involving the first division of the trigeminal nerve is twofold: (1) the immediate relief of acute pain and symptoms and (2) the prevention of complications, including postherpetic neuralgia. It is the consensus of most pain specialists that the earlier in the natural course of the disease that treatment is initiated, the less likely it is that postherpetic neuralgia will develop in the patient. Furthermore, because the older patient is at highest risk for developing postherpetic neuralgia, early and aggressive treatment of this group of patients is mandatory.

Nerve Blocks

Sympathetic neural blockade with local anesthetic and steroid via stellate ganglion block appears to be the treatment of choice to relieve the symptoms of acute herpes zoster involving the first division of the trigeminal nerve as well as to prevent the occurrence of postherpetic neuralgia. Sympathetic nerve block is thought to achieve these goals by blocking the profound sympathetic stimulation that is a result of the viral inflammation of the nerve and gasserian ganglion. If untreated, this sympathetic hyperactivity can cause ischemia secondary to decreased blood flow of the intraneural capillary bed. If this ischemia is allowed to persist, endoneural edema forms, increasing

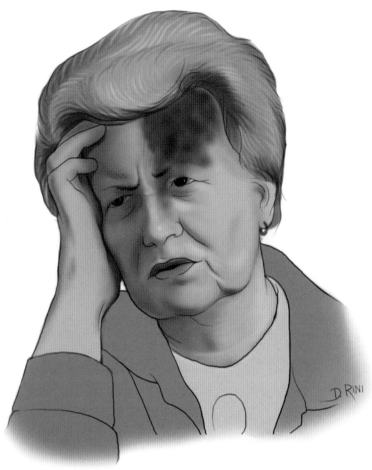

Figure 1–1. The pain of acute herpes zoster of the first division of the trigeminal nerve will often precede onset of the characteristic vesicular rash.

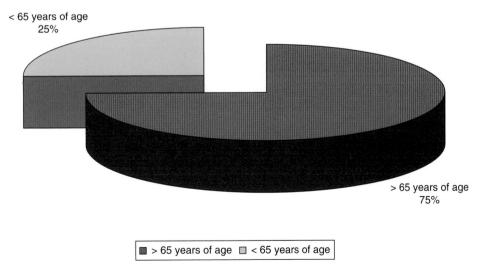

Figure 1–2. Age of patients suffering from acute herpes zoster.

endoneural pressure and causing a further reduction in endoneural blood flow with irreversible nerve damage.

As vesicular crusting occurs, the addition of steroids to the local anesthetic may decrease neural scarring and further decrease the incidence of postherpetic neuralgia. These sympathetic blocks should be continued aggressively until the patient is pain free and should be reimplemented at the return of pain. Failure to use sympathetic neural blockade immediately and aggressively, especially in the elderly, may sentence the patient to a lifetime of suffering from postherpetic neuralgia. Occasionally, some patients suffering from acute herpes zoster involving the first division of the trigeminal nerve may not experience pain relief from stellate ganglion block but will respond to blockade of the trigeminal nerve.

Opioid Analgesics

Opioid analgesics may be useful in relieving the aching pain that is often present during the acute stages of herpes zoster as sympathetic nerve blocks are being implemented. They are less effective in the relief of the neuritic pain that is often present. Careful administration of potent, long-acting narcotic analgesics (e.g., oral morphine elixir or methadone) on a time contingent rather than on an as-needed basis may represent a beneficial adjunct to the pain relief provided by sympathetic neural blockade. Because many patients suffering from acute herpes zoster are elderly or have severe multisystem disease, close monitoring for the potential side effects of potent narcotic analgesics (e.g., confusion or dizziness, which may cause a patient to fall) is warranted. Daily dietary fiber supplementation and milk of magnesia should be started along with opioid analgesics to prevent the side effect of constipation.

Adjuvant Analgesics

The anticonvulsant *gabapentin* represents a first-line treatment in the palliation of neuritic pain of acute herpes zoster involving the first division of the trigeminal nerve. Studies suggest that gabapentin may also help prevent the development of postherpetic neuralgia. Treatment with gabapentin should begin early in the course of the disease, and this drug may be used concurrently with neural blockade, opioid analgesics, and other adjuvant analgesics, including the antidepressant compounds if care is taken to avoid central nervous system side effects. Gabapentin is started at a bedtime dose of 300 mg and is titrated upward in 300-mg increments to a maximum dose of 3600 mg given in divided doses as side effects allow. *Carbamazepine* should be considered in patients suffer-

ing from severe neuritic pain who have failed to respond to nerve blocks and gabapentin. If this drug is used, rigid monitoring for hematologic parameters, especially in patients receiving chemotherapy or radiation therapy, is indicated. Phenytoin may also be beneficial to treat neuritic pain but should not be used in patients with lymphoma because the drug may induce a pseudolymphoma-like state that is difficult to distinguish from the actual lymphoma itself.

Antidepressants may also be useful adjuncts in the initial treatment of the patient suffering from acute herpes zoster. On an acute basis, these drugs will help alleviate the significant sleep disturbance that is commonly seen in this setting. In addition, the antidepressants may be valuable in helping ameliorate the neuritic component of the pain, which is treated less effectively with narcotic analgesics. After several weeks of treatment, the antidepressants may exert a mood-elevating effect that may be desirable in some patients. Care must be taken to observe closely for central nervous system side effects in this patient population. These drugs may cause urinary retention and constipation that may be mistakenly attributed to herpes zoster myelitis.

Antiviral Agents

A limited number of antiviral agents, including famciclovir and acyclovir, have been shown to shorten the course of acute herpes zoster and may help prevent the development of acute herpes zoster. They are probably useful in attenuating the disease in immunosuppressed patients. These antiviral agents can be used in conjunction with the aforementioned treatment modalities. Careful monitoring for side effects is mandatory with the use of these drugs.

Adjunctive Treatments

The application of ice packs to the lesions of acute herpes zoster may provide relief in some patients. Application of heat will increase pain in most patients, presumably because of increased conduction of small fibers, but is beneficial in an occasional patient and may be worth trying if application of cold is ineffective. Transcutaneous electrical nerve stimulation and vibration may also be effective in a limited number of patients. The favorable risk-to-benefit ratio of these modalities makes them reasonable alternatives for patients who cannot or will not undergo sympathetic neural blockade or tolerate pharmacologic interventions.

Topical application of aluminum sulfate as a tepid soak provides excellent drying of the crusting and weeping lesions of acute herpes zoster, and most patients find these soaks soothing. Zinc oxide ointment may also be used as a protective agent, especially during the healing phase when temperature sensitivity is a problem. Disposable diapers can be used as an absorbent padding to protect healing lesions from contact with clothing and sheets.

COMPLICATIONS

In most patients, acute herpes zoster involving the first division of the trigeminal nerve is a self-limited disease. In the elderly and the immunosuppressed, however, complications may occur. Cutaneous and visceral dissemination may range from a mild rash resembling chickenpox to an overwhelming, life-threatening infection in those already suffering from severe multisystem disease. Myelitis may cause bowel, bladder, and lower extremity paresis. Ocular complications from trigeminal nerve involvement may range from severe photophobia to keratitis with loss of sight.

CLINICAL PEARLS

Because the pain of herpes zoster usually precedes the eruption of skin lesions by 5 to 7 days, an erroneous diagnosis of other painful conditions (e.g., trigeminal neuralgia, glaucoma) may be made. In this setting, the astute clinician will advise the patient to call immediately should a rash appear because the diagnosis of acute herpes zoster is a possibility. Some pain specialists believe that in a small number of immunocompetent patients, when reactivation of virus occurs, a rapid immune response may attenuate the natural course of the disease and the characteristic rash of acute herpes zoster may not appear. This pain in the distribution of the first division of the trigeminal nerve without associated rash is called zoster sine herpete and is by necessity a diagnosis of exclusion. Therefore, other causes of head pain must first be ruled out before this diagnosis is invoked.

2

Migraine Headaches

ICD-9 CODE 346.9

THE CLINICAL SYNDROME

Migraine headache is defined as a periodic unilateral headache that may begin in childhood but almost always develops before the age of 30. Attacks may occur with a variable frequency ranging from every few days to once every several months. More frequent migraine headaches are often associated with a phenomenon called *analgesic rebound*. Between 60% and 70% of patients suffering from migraine are female, and many report a family history of migraine headaches. Migraineurs have been described as having a unique personality type characterized by a meticulous, neat, compulsive, and often rigid nature. They tend to be obsessive in their daily routines and often find it hard to cope with the stresses of everyday life. Migraine headaches may be triggered by changes in sleep patterns or diet or by the ingestion of tyramine-containing foods, monosodium glutamate, nitrates, chocolate, or citrus fruits. Changes in endogenous and exogenous hormones such as occur with the use of birth control pills can also trigger migraine headache. Approximately 20% of patients suffering from migraine headache also experience a painless neurologic event before the onset of headache pain that is called *aura*. Aura most often takes the form of visual disturbance but may also present as an alteration in smell or hearing; these are called olfactory and auditory aura, respectively.

CLINICAL SIGNS AND SYMPTOMS

Migraine headache is by definition a unilateral headache. Although with each episode the headache may change sides, the headache is never bilateral. The pain of migraine headache is usually periorbital or retro-orbital. It is pounding in nature, and its inten- sity is severe. The onset-to-peak of migraine headache is rapid, ranging from 20 minutes to 1 hour. In contradistinction to tension-type headache, migraine headache is often associated with systemic symptoms, including nausea and vomiting, photophobia, and sonophobia, as well as alterations in appetite, mood, and libido. Menstruation is also a common trigger of migraine headaches. Migraine that presents without other neurologic symptoms is called *migraine without aura*.

As mentioned, approximately 20% of patients suffering from migraine headache also experience a painless neurologic event before the onset of headache pain called aura. Aura is thought to be the result of ischemia of specific regions of the cerebral cortex. Visual aura will often occur from 30 to 60 minutes before the onset of headache pain and may take the form of blind spots called *scotoma* or a zigzag disruption of the visual field called *fortification spectrum*. Occasionally, migraine patients may lose an entire visual field during aura. Auditory aura most often takes the form of hypersensitivity to sound, but other alterations of hearing, such as sounds perceived as farther away than they are, have also been reported. Olfactory aura may take the form of strong odors of substances that are not actually present or extreme hypersensitivity to otherwise normal odors of items such as coffee or copy machine toner. Migraine headache that is preceded by aura is called *migraine with aura*.

Rare patients who suffer from migraine will experience prolonged neurologic dysfunction associated with their headache pain. Such neurologic dysfunction may last for more than 24 hours and is termed *migraine with prolonged aura*. Although extremely rare, such patients are at risk for the development of permanent neurologic deficit, and risk factors such as hypertension, smoking, and oral contraceptives must be addressed. Even less common than migraine with prolonged aura is *migraine with complex aura*. Patients suffering from migraine with complex aura experience significant neurologic dysfunction associated with their headache pain. This dysfunction may include aphasia or hemiplegia. As with migraine with prolonged aura, patients suffering from migraine with complex aura may develop permanent neurologic deficits.

The patient suffering from all forms of migraine headache will appear systemically ill (Fig. 2–1). Pallor, tremulousness, diaphoresis, and light sensitivity are common physical findings. Tenderness of the temporal artery and associated area may also be present. If aura is present, neurologic examination results will be abnormal; otherwise, the neurologic examination is within normal limits, before, during, and after migraine without aura.

TESTING

There is no specific test for migraine headache. Testing is aimed primarily at identifying occult pathology or other diseases that may mimic migraine headache (see Differential Diagnosis). All patients with a recent onset of headache thought to be migraine should undergo magnetic resonance imaging (MRI) of the brain. If neurologic dysfunction accompanies the patient's headache symptomatology, the MRI should be performed with and without gadolinium contrast medium; magnetic resonance angiography should also be considered. MRI should also be performed in patients with previously stable migraine headache who are experiencing an inexplicable change in headache symptomatology. Screening laboratory testing that includes erythrocyte sedimentation rate, complete blood count, and automated blood chemistry should be performed if the diagnosis of migraine is in question. Ophthalmologic evaluation is indicated in those patients suffering from headache who experience significant ocular symptoms.

DIFFERENTIAL DIAGNOSIS

The diagnosis of migraine headache is usually made on clinical grounds by obtaining a careful targeted headache history. Tension-type headache is often confused with migraine headache, and such confusion leads to illogical treatment plans as the treatments for these two distinct headache syndromes are quite different. Table 2–1 distinguishes migraine headache from tension-type headache and should help clarify the correct diagnosis.

Diseases of the eye, ears, nose, and sinuses may also mimic migraine headache. The targeted history and physical examination combined with appropriate testing should help the astute clinician identify and properly treat underlying diseases of these organ systems. Glaucoma, temporal arteritis, sinusitis, intracranial pathology including chronic subdural hematoma,

tumor, brain abscess, hydrocephalus, and pseudotumor cerebri, and inflammatory conditions including sarcoidosis may all mimic migraine and must be considered when treating the headache patient.

TREATMENT

When deciding how to best treat the patient suffering from migraine, the clinician should consider the frequency and severity of headache, the effect on the patient's lifestyle, the presence of focal or prolonged neurologic disturbances, the results of previous testing and treatment, the history of previous drug abuse or misuse, and the presence of other systemic disease, such as peripheral vascular or coronary artery disease, that might preclude the use of certain treatment modalities.

If the patient's migraine headaches occur infrequently, a trial of abortive therapy may be warranted. However, if headaches occur with greater frequency or cause the patient to miss work or be hospitalized, prophylactic therapy is warranted.

Abortive Therapy

For abortive therapy to be effective in the treatment of migraine headache, it must be initiated at the first sign of headache. This can often be difficult because of the short onset-to-peak of migraine headache coupled with the fact that migraine sufferers often experience nausea and vomiting that may limit the use of oral medications. By altering the route of administration to parenteral or transmucosal, this problem can be avoided.

Abortive medications that can be considered in migraine headache patients include compounds that contain isometheptene mucate (e.g., Midrin), the nonsteroidal anti-inflammatory drug naproxen, ergot alkaloids, the triptans including sumatriptan, and the

Table 2–1. Comparison of Migraine Headache With Tension-Type Headache

	Migraine Headache	Tension-Type Headache
Onset-to-peak	Minutes to 1 hour	Hours to days
Frequency	Rarely more than 1 per week	Often daily or continuous
Location	Temporal	Nuchal or circumferential
Character	Pounding	Aching, pressure, bandlike
Laterality	Always unilateral	Usually bilateral
Aura	May be present	Never present
Nausea and vomiting	Common	Rare
Duration	Usually less than 24 hours	Often for days

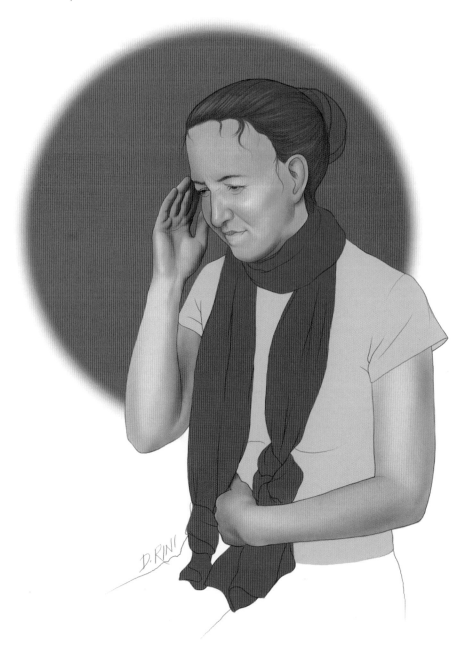

Figure 2-1. Migraine headache is an episodic, unilateral headache which occurs more commonly in females.

intravenous administration of lidocaine combined with antiemetic compounds. The inhalation of 100% oxygen may also abort migraine headache, as well as the use of sphenopalatine ganglion block with local anesthetic. Caffeine-containing preparations, barbiturates, ergotamines, the triptans, and narcotics have a propensity to cause a phenomenon called *analgesic rebound headache*, which may ultimately be more difficult to treat than the patient's original migraine headaches. The ergotamines and triptans should not be used in patients with coexistent peripheral vascular disease, coronary artery disease, or hypertension.

Prophylactic Therapy

For most patients who suffer from migraine headaches, prophylactic therapy represents a better option. The mainstay of the prophylactic therapy of migraine is β-blocking agents. Propranolol and most of the other drugs of this class will help control or decrease the frequency and intensity of migraine headache and help prevent aura. Generally, an 80-mg daily dose of the long-acting formulation is a reasonable starting point for most patients with migraine. Propranolol should not be used in patients with asthma or other reactive airway diseases.

Valproic acid, the calcium channel blockers such as verapamil, clonidine, the tricyclic antidepressants, and the nonsteroidal anti-inflammatory drugs have also been used in the prophylaxis of migraine headache. Each of these drugs has its own profile of advantages and disadvantages, and the clinician should try to pharmacologically tailor a treatment plan that best meets the needs of the individual patient.

COMPLICATIONS

In most patients, migraine headache is a painful but non–limb- or life-threatening disease. However, patients who suffer from migraine with prolonged aura or migraine with complex aura are of risk of the development of permanent neurologic deficit. Such patients are best treated by headache specialists, who are familiar with these unique risks and are better equipped to deal with them. Occasionally, prolonged nausea and vomiting associated with severe migraine headache may result in dehydration necessitating hospitalization and treatment with intravenous fluids.

CLINICAL PEARLS

The most common reason that a patient thought to be suffering from migraine headache does not respond to traditional treatments is that the patient does not have migraine headache but is in fact suffering from tension-type headache, analgesic rebound headache, or a combination. The clinician must be sure the patient is not taking significant doses of over-the-counter headache preparations containing caffeine or other vasoactive drugs such as barbiturates, ergots, or triptans that may cause analgesic rebound headache. Until these drugs are withdrawn, the patient's headache will not improve.

3

Tension-Type Headache

ICD-9 CODE 307.81

THE CLINICAL SYNDROME

Tension-type headache, formerly known as *muscle contraction headache*, is the most common type of headache that afflicts mankind. It can be episodic or chronic, and may or may not be related to muscle contraction. Significant sleep disturbance usually occurs, along with depression and, in some patients, somatization.

The term *tension-type headache* refers to nonvascular headaches, which can be episodic or chronic. Until recently, the condition was known as *muscle contraction headache*. However, because many patients with this disorder have no demonstrable contraction of skeletal muscle associated with their pain, the International Headache Society has returned to use of an earlier name for this constellation of symptoms–*tension-type headache*. Patients with tension-type headaches may be characterized as individuals with multiple unresolved conflicts surrounding work, marriage, social relationships, and psychosexual difficulties. These patients are often depressed, although Minnesota Multiphasic Personality Inventory (MMPI) testing in large groups of tension-type headache patients reveals not only borderline depression but somatization as well. Most researchers believe that, in at least some patients, this somatization takes the form of abnormal muscle contraction and, in others, simply of headache.

SIGNS AND SYMPTOMS

Tension-type headache is usually bilateral but can be unilateral, and often involves the frontal, temporal, and occipital regions (Fig. 3–1). It may present as a bandlike nonpulsatile ache or tightness in the aforementioned anatomic areas. There often is associated neck symptomatology. Tension-type headache evolves over a period of hours or days and then tends to remain constant without progressive symptomatology. There is no aura associated with this headache. Significant sleep disturbance is usually present. This may manifest itself as difficulty in falling asleep, frequent awakening at night, or early awakening. These headaches most frequently occur between 4 and 8 AM and between 4 and 8 PM. Although both sexes are affected, females predominate. There is no hereditary pattern to tension-type headache, but it may occur in family clusters as children mimic and learn the pain behavior of their parents.

The triggering event for acute episodic tension-type headache is invariably either physical or psychological stress. This may take the form of a fight with a coworker or spouse, or an exceptionally heavy workload. Physical stress such as a long drive, working with the neck in a strained position, acute cervical spine injury due to whiplash, or prolonged exposure to the glare from a cathode ray tube may also precipitate a headache. A worsening of preexisting degenerative cervical spine conditions, such as cervical spondylosis, can also trigger a tension-type headache. The pathology responsible for the development of tension-type headache can also produce temporomandibular joint dysfunction.

TESTING

There is no specific test for tension-type headache. Testing is aimed primarily at identifying occult pathology or other diseases that may mimic tension-type headaches (see Differential Diagnosis). All patients with the recent onset of headache thought to be tension type should undergo magnetic resonance imaging of the brain and, if significant occipital or nuchal symptoms are present, of the cervical spine. Magnetic resonance imaging should also be performed in patients with previously stable tension-type headaches who have experienced a recent change in headache symptomatology. Screening laboratory testing consisting of complete blood count, erythrocyte

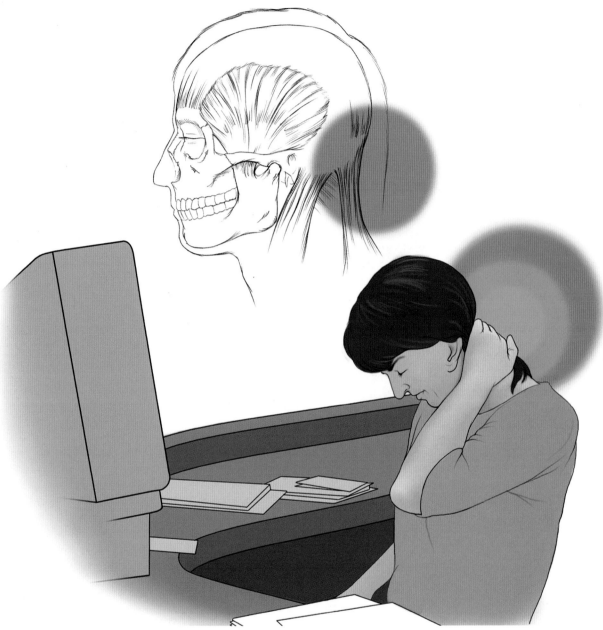

Figure 3–1. Mental and physical stress will often be the precipitating factors in tension-type headaches.

sedimentation rate, and automated blood chemistry testing should be performed if the diagnosis of tension-type headache is in question.

DIFFERENTIAL DIAGNOSIS

Tension-type headache is usually diagnosed on clinical grounds by obtaining a careful targeted headache history. Despite their obvious differences, tension-type headache is often incorrectly diagnosed as migraine headache. Such misdiagnosis leads to illogical treatment plans and poor control of headache symptomatology. Table 3–1 helps distinguish tension-type headache from migraine headache and should aid the clinician in making the correct diagnosis.

Diseases of the cervical spine and surrounding soft tissues may also mimic tension-type headache. Arnold-Chiari malformations may also present clinically as tension-type headache but will be easily identified on imaging of the cervical spine. Occasionally, frontal sinusitis can also be confused with tension-type headache, although individuals with acute frontal sinusitis appear systemically ill. Temporal arteritis, chronic subdural hematoma, and other intracranial pathology such as tumor may be incorrectly diagnosed as tension-type headache.

TREATMENT

Abortive Treatment

In determining treatment, the physician must consider the frequency and severity of headaches, how the headaches affect the patient's lifestyle, the results of any previous therapy, and previous drug misuse and abuse. If the patient suffers from an attack of tension-type headache only once every 1 or 2 months, the condition can often be managed through teaching the patient to reduce or avoid stress. Analgesics or nonsteroidal anti-inflammatory drugs (NSAIDs) can provide symptomatic relief during acute attacks. Combination analgesic drugs used concomitantly with barbiturates and/or narcotic analgesics have no place in the management of headache patients. The risk of abuse and dependence more than outweighs any theoretical benefit. The physician should also avoid an abortive treatment approach in patients with a prior history of drug misuse or abuse. Many abortive drugs, including simple analgesics and NSAIDs, can produce serious consequences if abused.

Table 3–1. Comparison of Tension-Type Headache With Migraine Headache

	Tension-Type Headache	Migraine Headache
Onset-to-peak	Hours to days	Minutes to 1 hour
Frequency	Often daily or continuous	Rarely more than one per week
Localization	Nuchal or circumferential	Temporal
Character	Aching, pressure, bandlike	Pounding
Laterality	Usually	Usually bilateral
Aura	Never present	May be present
Nausea and vomiting	Rare	Common
Duration	Often for days	Usually less than 24 hours

Prophylactic Treatment

If the headaches occur more frequently than once every 1 or 2 months or are of such severity that the patient repeatedly misses work or social engagements, the following prophylactic therapy is indicated.

Antidepressants

These are generally the drugs of choice for prophylactic treatment of headaches. The antidepressants not only help decrease the frequency and intensity of tension-type headaches but also normalize sleep patterns and treat underlying depression. Patients should be educated about the potential side effects of sedation, dry mouth, blurred vision, constipation, and urinary retention that may be experienced when using this class of drugs. They should also be told that relief of headache pain generally takes 3 to 4 weeks. However, the normalization of sleep that occurs immediately may be enough to noticeably improve the headache symptomatology.

Amitriptyline, started at a single bedtime dose of 25 mg, is a reasonable initial choice. The dose may be increased in 25-mg increments as side effects allow. Other drugs that can be considered if the patient does not tolerate the sedation and anticholinergic effects of amitriptyline include trazodone (75 to 300 mg at bedtime) or fluoxetine (20 to 40 mg at lunch time). Because of the sedating nature of these drugs (with the exception of fluoxetine), they must be used with caution in the elderly or in patients who are at risk for falling. Care should also be exercised when using these drugs in patients prone to cardiac arrhythmia because these drugs may be arrhythmogenic. Simple analgesics or the longer-acting NSAIDs may be used with the antidepressant compounds to treat exacerbations of headache pain.

Biofeedback

Monitored relaxation training combined with patient education about coping strategies and stress reduction techniques may be of value in the motivated tension-type headache sufferer. Appropriate patient selection is of paramount importance if good results are to be achieved. If the patient is significantly depressed at the time of initiation of therapy, it may be beneficial to treat the depression before trying biofeedback. The use of biofeedback may allow the patient to control the headache while at the same time avoiding the side effects of medications.

Cervical Steroid Epidural Nerve Blocks

Multiple studies have demonstrated the efficacy of cervical steroid epidural nerve blocks (CSENBs) in providing long-term relief of tension-type headache in a group of patients for whom all treatment modalities failed. CSENBs may be used early in the course of treatment while waiting for the antidepressant compounds to become effective. CSENBs may be performed on a daily to weekly basis as clinical symptoms dictate.

COMPLICATIONS AND PITFALLS

A small number of patients with tension-type headache have major depression or uncontrolled anxiety states in addition to chemical dependence on narcotic analgesics, barbiturates, minor tranquilizers, and, occasionally, alcohol. Attempts to treat these patients in the outpatient setting is a disappointing and frustrating experience. Inpatient treatment in a specialized headache unit or psychiatric setting will result in more rapid amelioration of the underlying and coexisting problems and allow concurrent treatment of headaches. Monoamine oxidase inhibitors can often reduce the frequency and severity of tension-type headaches in this subset of patients. Phenelzine, at a dosage of 15 mg three times daily, is usually effective. After 2 to 3 weeks, the dosage is tapered downward to an appropriate maintenance dose of 5 to 10 mg three times daily. Monoamine oxidase inhibitors can produce life-threatening hypertensive crises if special diets are not followed or if the patient combines these drugs with some commonly used prescription or over-the-counter medications. Therefore, their use should be limited to highly reliable and compliant patients. Physicians prescribing this potentially dangerous group of drugs should be well versed in how to use them safely.

CLINICAL PEARLS

Although tension-type (muscle contraction) headache occurs frequently, it is commonly misdiagnosed as migraine headache. By obtaining a targeted headache history and performing a targeted physical examination, the physician can make a diagnosis with a high degree of certainty. The avoidance of addicting medications coupled with the appropriate use of pharmacologic and nonpharmacologic therapies should result in excellent palliation and long-term control of pain in the vast majority of patients suffering from this headache syndrome.

4

Cluster Headache

THE CLINICAL SYNDROME

Cluster headache derives its name from the pattern by which cluster headaches occur, namely, the headaches occur in clusters followed by headache-free remission periods. Unlike other common headache disorders that affect primarily females, cluster headache happens much more commonly in males at a ratio of 5:1. Much less common than tension-type headache or migraine headache, cluster headache is thought to affect approximately 0.5% of the male population. Cluster headache is most often confused with migraine by clinicians unfamiliar with the headache syndrome. A careful, targeted headache history will allow the clinician to easily distinguish these two distinct headache types (Table 4–1).

The onset of cluster headache occurs in the late third or early fourth decade of life, in contradistinction to migraine, which almost always manifests itself by the early second decade. Unlike migraine, cluster headache does not appear to run in families and cluster sufferers do not experience aura. Attacks of cluster headache will generally occur approximately 90 minutes after the patient falls asleep. This association with sleep is reportedly maintained when a shift worker changes to and from nighttime to daytime hours of sleep. Cluster headache also appears to follow a distinct chronobiological pattern that coincides with the seasonal change in the length of day. This results in an increased frequency of cluster headaches in the spring and fall.

During a cluster period, attacks occur two or three times a day and last for 45 minutes to 1 hour. Cluster periods usually last for 8 to 12 weeks, interrupted by remission periods of less than 2 years. In rare patients, the remission periods become shorter and shorter and the frequency may increase up to 10-fold. This situation is termed *chronic cluster headache* and differs from the more common episodic cluster headache described earlier.

SIGNS AND SYMPTOMS

Cluster headache is characterized as a unilateral headache that is retro-orbital and temporal in location. The pain has a deep burning or boring quality. Physical findings during an attack of cluster headache may include Horner's syndrome, consisting of ptosis, abnormal pupil constriction, facial flushing, and conjunctival injection. Additionally, profuse lacrimation and rhinorrhea are often present. The ocular changes may become permanent with repeated attacks. Peau d'orange skin over the malar region, deeply furrowed and glabellar folds, and telangiectasia may be observed (Fig. 4–1).

Attacks of cluster headache may be provoked by small amounts of alcohol, nitrates, histamines, and other vasoactive substances and occasionally by high altitude. When the attack is in progress, the patient may not be able to lie still and may pace or rock back and forth in a chair. This behavior contrasts with that characterizing other headache syndromes, during which patients seeking relief will lie down in a dark, quiet room.

Table 4–1. Comparison of Cluster Headache With Migraine Headache

	Cluster Headache	Migraine Headache
Gender	Male 5:1	Female 2:1
Age of onset	Late 30s to early 40s	Menarche to early 20s
Family history	No	Yes
Aura	Never	Yes 20% of time
Chronobiological pattern	Yes	No
Onset-to-peak	Seconds to minutes	Minutes to hours
Frequency	Two or three per day	Once a week
Duration	45 minutes	Hours

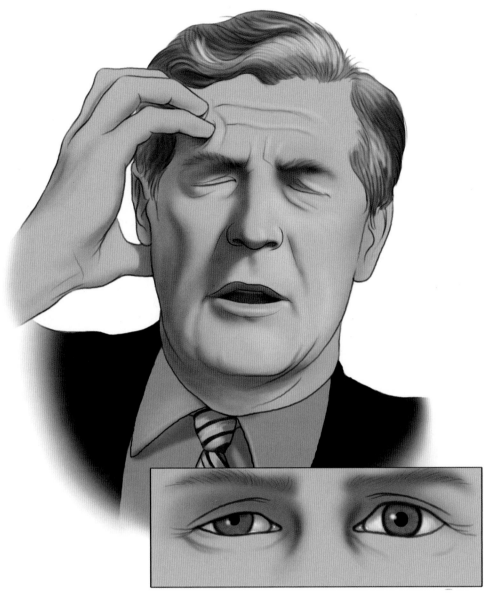

Figure 4–1. Horner's syndrome may be present during acute attacks of cluster headache.

The pain of cluster headache is said to be among the worst pain from which mankind suffers. Because of the severity of pain associated with cluster headaches, the clinician must watch closely for medication overuse or misuse. Suicides have been associated with prolonged, unrelieved attacks of cluster headaches.

TESTING

There is no specific test for cluster headache. Testing is aimed primarily at identifying occult pathology or other diseases that may mimic cluster headache (see Differential Diagnosis). All patients with a recent onset of headache thought to be cluster should undergo magnetic resonance imaging (MRI) of the brain. If neurologic dysfunction accompanies the patient's headache symptomatology, MRI should be performed with and without gadolinium contrast medium; magnetic resonance angiography should also be considered. MRI should also be performed in patients with previously stable cluster headache who are experiencing an inexplicable change in headache symptomatology. Screening laboratory testing including erythrocyte sedimentation rate, complete blood count, and automated blood chemistry should be performed if the diagnosis of cluster is in question. Ophthalmologic evaluation including measurement of intraocular pressures is indicated in those patients suffering with headache who experience significant ocular symptoms.

DIFFERENTIAL DIAGNOSIS

Cluster headache is usually made on clinical grounds by obtaining a careful, targeted headache history. Migraine headache is often confused with cluster headache, and such confusion leads to illogical treatment plans as the treatments of these two distinct headache syndromes are quite different. Table 4–1 distinguishes cluster headache from migraine headache and should help to clarify the correct diagnosis.

Diseases of the eyes, ears, nose, and sinuses may also mimic cluster headache. The targeted history and physical examination combined with appropriate testing should help the astute clinician identify and properly treat underlying diseases of these organ systems. Glaucoma, temporal arteritis, sinusitis, intracranial pathology including chronic subdural hematoma, tumor, brain abscess, hydrocephalus, and pseudotumor cerebri, and inflammatory conditions including sarcoidosis may all mimic cluster and must be considered when treating the headache patient.

TREATMENT

In contradistinction to migraine headache, in which most patients experience improvement with the implementation of therapy with β-blockers, patients suffering from cluster headache will usually require more individualized therapy. A reasonable starting place in the treatment of cluster headache is to begin treatment with prednisone combined with daily sphenopalatine ganglion blocks with local anesthetic. A reasonable starting dose of prednisone would be 80 mg given in divided doses tapered by 10 mg per dose per day. If headaches are not rapidly brought under control, inhalation of 100% oxygen via close-fitting mask is added.

If headaches persist and the diagnosis of cluster headache is not in question, a trial of lithium carbonate may be considered. It should be noted that the therapeutic window of lithium carbonate is small and this drug should be used with caution. A starting dose of 300 mg at bedtime may be increased after 48 hours to 300 mg twice a day. If no side effects are noted, after 48 hours the dose may again be increased to 300 mg three times a day. The patient should be continued at this dosage level for a total of 10 days, and the drug should then be tapered downward over a 1-week period. Other medications that can be considered if these treatments are ineffective include methysergide and sumatriptan and sumatriptan-like drugs.

In rare patients suffering from cluster headaches, the aforementioned treatments are ineffective. In this setting, given the severity of pain and the risk of suicide, more aggressive treatment is indicated. Destruction of the gasserian ganglion either by injection of glycerol or by radiofrequency lesioning may be a reasonable next step.

COMPLICATIONS

The major risk to patients suffering from uncontrolled cluster headaches is that patients may become despondent due to the unremitting severe pain and commit suicide. This is a real risk, and should the clinician have difficulty gaining control of the patient's cluster headaches, hospitalization should be considered.

CLINICAL PEARLS

Cluster headache represents one of the most painful conditions encountered in clinical practice and must be viewed as a true pain emergency. In general, cluster headache is harder to treat than migraine headache and requires more individualized therapy. Given the severity of the pain associated with cluster headache, multiple modalities should be used early in the course of an episode of cluster headache.

Because of the characteristic nature of these headaches, the clinician should beware of patients presenting with a classic history of cluster headache who request narcotic analgesics.

5

Analgesic Rebound Headache

ICD-9 CODE 784.0

THE CLINICAL SYNDROME

Analgesic rebound headache is a recently identified headache syndrome that occurs commonly in headache sufferers who overuse abortive medications to treat their headache symptomatology. The overuse of these abortive medications will result in increasingly frequent headaches that become unresponsive to both abortive and prophylactic medications. Over a period of weeks, the patient's episodic migraine or tension-type headache becomes more frequent and transforms into a chronic daily headache. This daily headache becomes increasingly unresponsive to analgesics and other headache medications, and patients will note an exacerbation of headache symptomatology if abortive or prophylactic analgesic medications are missed or delayed (Fig. 5–1). Analgesic rebound headache is probably underdiagnosed by healthcare professionals, and its frequency is on the rise due to the heavy advertising by pharmaceutical companies of over-the-counter headache medications containing caffeine.

SIGNS AND SYMPTOMS

Clinically, analgesic rebound headache presents as a transformed migraine or tension-type headache and may assume the characteristics of both of these common headache types, blurring their distinctive features and making correct diagnosis difficult. Common to all analgesic rebound headaches is the excessive use of the following medications (summarized in Table 5–1): simple analgesics, such as acetaminophen; sinus medications, including simple analgesics; combinations of aspirin, caffeine, and butalbital, such as Fiorinal; nonsteroidal anti-inflammatory drugs; opioid analgesics; ergotamines; and the triptans, such as sumatriptan. As with migraine and tension-type headache, the physical examination will most often be within normal limits.

TESTING

There is no specific test for analgesic rebound headache. Testing is aimed primarily at identifying occult pathology or other diseases that may mimic tension-type or migraine headaches (see Differential Diagnosis). All patients with the recent onset of chronic daily headache thought to be analgesic rebound headache should undergo magnetic resonance imaging of the brain and, if significant occipital or nuchal symptoms are present, of the cervical spine. Magnetic resonance imaging should also be performed in patients with previously stable tension-type or migraine headaches who have experienced a recent change in headache symptomatology. Screening laboratory testing consisting of complete blood count, erythrocyte sedimentation rate, and automated blood chemistry testing should be performed if the diagnosis of analgesic rebound headache is in question.

Table 5–1. Drugs Implicated in Analgesic Rebound Headache

Simple analgesics
Nonsteroidal anti-inflammatory drugs
Opioid analgesics
Sinus medications
Ergotamines
Combination headache medications that include butalbital
The triptans (e.g., sumatriptan)

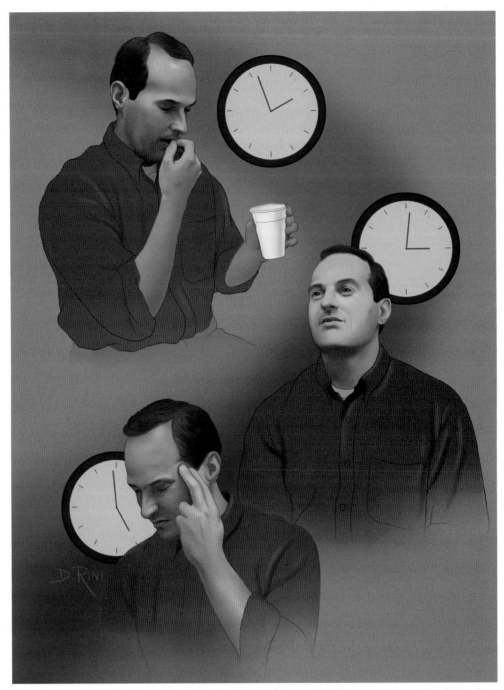

Figure 5-1. The classic temporal relationship of abortive medication intake to onset and relief of analgesic rebound headache.

DIFFERENTIAL DIAGNOSIS

Analgesic rebound headache is usually diagnosed on clinical grounds by obtaining a careful, targeted headache history. Because analgesic rebound headache assumes many of the characteristics of the underlying primary headache, diagnosis can be confusing at best if a careful medication history with specific questioning regarding the intake of over-the-counter headache medications and analgesics is not obtained. Any change in a previously stable headache pattern needs to be taken seriously and should not automatically be attributed to analgesic overuse without careful reevaluation of the patient.

TREATMENT

Treatment of analgesic rebound headache is the discontinuation of the overused or abused drugs and complete abstention from them for a period of at least 3 months. Many patients cannot tolerate outpatient discontinuation of these medications and will ultimately require hospitalization in a specialized inpatient headache unit. If outpatient discontinuation of the offending medications is considered, the following should be carefully explained to the patient:

■ Their headaches and associated symptoms will get worse before they get better.
■ Any use, no matter how small, of the offending medication will result in continued analgesic rebound headaches.
■ The patient may not self-medicate with over-the-counter drugs.

■ The significant overuse of opioids or combination medications containing butalbital or ergotamine will result in physical dependence, and their discontinuation must be done only under the supervision of a physician familiar with the treatment of physical dependencies.
■ If the patient follows the physician's orders regarding discontinuation of the offending medications, he or she can expect the headaches to improve.

COMPLICATIONS AND PITFALLS

Patients who overuse or abuse medications, including opioids, ergotamines, and/or butalbital, will develop physical dependence on these medications. Abrupt cessation of these medications will result in a drug abstinence syndrome that can be life threatening if not properly treated. Most of these patients will require inpatient tapering in a controlled setting to safely deal with this problem.

CLINICAL PEARLS

Analgesic rebound headache occurs much more commonly than was previously thought. The occurrence of analgesic rebound headache is a direct result of the overprescribing of abortive headache medications in patients for whom they are inappropriate. When in doubt, the clinician will be better served by avoiding the abortive medications altogether and treating most headache sufferers prophylactically.

6

Occipital Neuralgia

ICD-9 729.2

THE CLINICAL SYNDROME

Occipital neuralgia is usually the result of blunt trauma to the greater and lesser occipital nerves. Repetitive microtrauma from working with the neck hyperextended (e.g., painting ceilings) or working for prolonged periods with computer monitors whose focal point is too high, causing extension of the cervical spine, may also cause occipital neuralgia. The pain of occipital neuralgia is characterized as persistent pain at the base of the skull with occasional sudden shock-like paresthesias in the distribution of the greater and lesser occipital nerves. Tension-type headache, which is much more common than occipital neuralgia, will occasionally mimic the pain of occipital neuralgia.

SIGNS AND SYMPTOMS

The greater occipital nerve arises from fibers of the dorsal primary ramus of the second cervical nerve and, to a lesser extent, fibers from the third cervical nerve. The greater occipital nerve pierces the fascia just below the superior nuchal ridge along with the occipital artery. It supplies the medial portion of the posterior scalp as far anterior as the vertex (Fig. 6-1).

The lesser occipital nerve arises from the ventral primary rami of the second and third cervical nerves. The lesser occipital nerve passes superiorly along the posterior border of the sternocleidomastoid muscle, dividing into cutaneous branches that innervate the lateral portion of the posterior scalp and the cranial surface of the pinna of the ear (see Fig. 6-1).

The patient suffering from occipital neuralgia will experience neuritic pain in the distribution of the greater and lesser occipital nerves when the nerves are palpated at the level of the nuchal ridge. Some patients can elicit pain with rotation or lateral bending of the cervical spine.

TESTING

There is no specific test for occipital neuralgia. Testing is aimed primarily at identifying occult pathology or other diseases that may mimic occipital neuralgia (see Differential Diagnosis). All patients with the recent onset of headache thought to be occipital neuralgia should undergo magnetic resonance imaging of the brain and cervical spine. Magnetic resonance imaging should also be performed in patients with previously stable occipital neuralgia who have experienced a recent change in headache symptomatology. Screening laboratory testing consisting of complete blood count, erythrocyte sedimentation rate, and automated blood chemistry testing should be performed if the diagnosis of occipital neuralgia is in question.

Neural blockade of the greater and lesser occipital nerves can serve as a diagnostic maneuver to help confirm the diagnosis and to distinguish it from tension-type headache. The greater and lesser occipital nerves can easily be blocked at the nuchal ridge (Fig. 6-2).

DIFFERENTIAL DIAGNOSIS

Occipital neuralgia is an infrequent cause of headaches and rarely occurs in the absence of trauma to the greater and lesser occipital nerves. More often, the patient with headaches involving the occipital region is in fact suffering from tension-type headaches. Tension-type headaches will not respond to occipital nerve blocks but are very amenable to treatment with antidepressant compounds such as amitriptyline in conjunction with cervical steroid epidural nerve blocks. Therefore, the clinician should reconsider the diagnosis of occipital neuralgia in those patients whose symptoms are consistent with occipital neuralgia but who fail to respond to greater and lesser occipital nerve blocks.

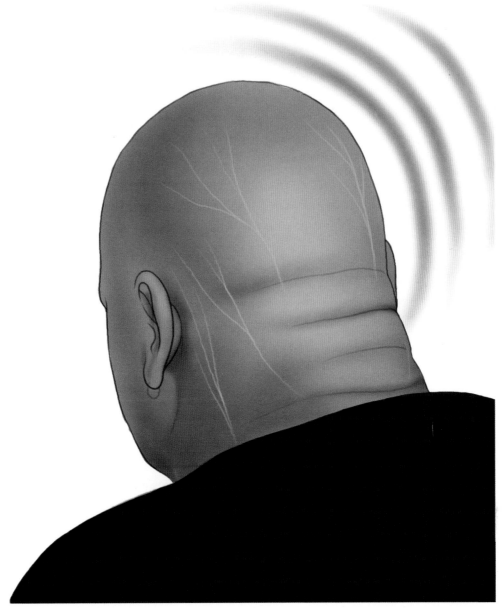

Figure 6–1. Occipital neuralgia is caused by trauma to the greater and lesser occipital nerves.

TREATMENT

The treatment of occipital neuralgia consists primarily of neural blockade with local anesthetic and steroid combined with the judicious use of nonsteroidal anti-inflammatory drugs, muscle relaxants, tricyclic antidepressants, and physical therapy. Neural blockade of the greater and lesser occipital nerves is carried out using the following technique: The patient is placed in a sitting position with the cervical spine flexed and the forehead on a padded bedside table. A total of 8 ml of local anesthetic is drawn up in a 12-ml sterile syringe. When occipital neuralgia or other painful conditions involving the greater and lesser occipital nerves is treated, a total of 80 mg of methylprednisolone acetate steroid is added to the local anesthetic with the first block and 40 mg of depot steroid is added with subsequent blocks.

The occipital artery is then palpated at the level of the superior nuchal ridge. After preparation of the skin with antiseptic solution, a 22-gauge 1½-inch needle is inserted just medial to the artery and is advanced perpendicularly until the needle approaches the periosteum of the underlying occipital bone. Paresthesias may be elicited, and the patient should be warned of such. The needle is then redirected superiorly, and after gentle aspiration, 5 ml of solution is injected in a fanlike distribution with care being taken to avoid the foramen magnum, which is located medially (see Fig. 6–2).

The lesser occipital nerve and a number of superficial branches of the greater occipital nerve are then blocked by directing the needle laterally and slightly inferiorly. After gentle aspiration, an additional 3 to 4 ml of solution is injected (see Fig. 6–2).

COMPLICATIONS AND PITFALLS

The scalp is highly vascular, and this coupled with the fact that both the greater and lesser occipital nerves are in close proximity to arteries means that the clinician should carefully calculate the total milligram dosage of local anesthetic that may be safely given, especially if bilateral nerve blocks are being performed. This vascularity and proximity to the arterial supply give rise to an increased incidence of post-block ecchymosis and hematoma formation. These complications can be decreased if manual pressure is applied to the area of the block immediately after injection. Application of cold packs for a 20-minute period after the block will also decrease the amount of postprocedural pain and bleeding the patient may experience. Care must be taken to avoid inadvertent needle placement into the foramen magnum, as the subarachnoid administration of local anesthetic in this region will result in an immediate total spinal anesthesia.

As with other headache syndromes, the clinician must be sure that the diagnosis is correct and that there is no coexistent intracranial pathology or diseases of the cervical spine that may be erroneously attributed to occipital neuralgia.

CLINICAL PEARLS

The most common reason that greater and lesser occipital nerve blocks fail to relieve headache pain is that the headache syndrome being treated has been misdiagnosed as occipital neuralgia. Any patient with headaches that are so severe as to require neural blockade as part of the treatment plan should undergo magnetic resonance imaging of the head to rule out unsuspected intracranial pathology. Furthermore, cervical spine radiographs should be considered to rule out congenital abnormalities such as Arnold-Chiari malformations that may be the hidden cause of the patient's occipital headaches.

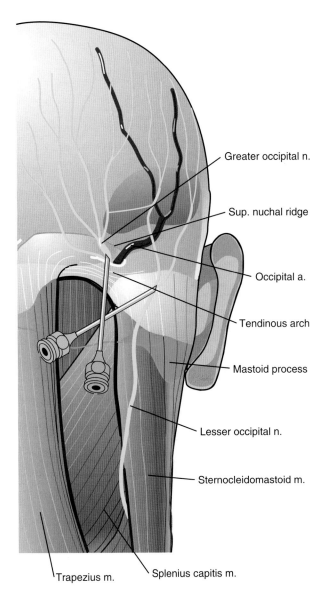

Greater occipital n.

Sup. nuchal ridge

Occipital a.

Tendinous arch

Mastoid process

Lesser occipital n.

Sternocleidomastoid m.

Trapezius m.

Splenius capitis m.

Figure 6–2. Proper needle placement for greater and lesser occipital nerve block. (From Waldman SD: Atlas of Interventional Pain Management. Philadelphia, WB Saunders, 1998, p 21.)

II Facial Pain Syndromes

7

Trigeminal Neuralgia

ICD-9 350-1

THE CLINICAL SYNDROME

Trigeminal neuralgia occurs in many patients because of tortuous blood vessels that compress the trigeminal root as it exits the brain stem. Acoustic neuromas, cholesteatomas, aneurysms, angiomas, and bony abnormalities may also lead to the compression of nerve. The severity of pain produced by trigeminal neuralgia can be rivaled only by that of cluster headache. Uncontrolled pain has been associated with suicide and therefore should be treated as an emergency. Attacks can be triggered by daily activities involving contact with the face such as brushing the teeth, shaving, and washing. Pain can be controlled with medication in most patients. About 2% to 3% of patients experiencing trigeminal neuralgia also have multiple sclerosis. Trigeminal neuralgia is also called *tic douloureux.*

SIGNS AND SYMPTOMS

Trigeminal neuralgia is an episodic pain afflicting the areas of the face supplied by the trigeminal nerve. The pain is unilateral in 97% of cases reported. When it does occur bilaterally, it is in the same division of the nerve. The second or third division of the nerve is affected in the majority of patients, with the first division affected less than 5% of the time (Fig. 7–1). The pain develops on the right side of the face in unilateral disease 57% of the time. The pain is characterized by paroxysms of electric shocklike pain lasting from several seconds to less than 2 minutes. The progression from onset to peak is essentially instantaneous.

The patient with trigeminal neuralgia will go to great lengths to avoid any contact with trigger areas.

Persons with other types of facial pain, such as temporomandibular joint dysfunction, tend to constantly rub the affected area or apply heat or cold to it. Patients with uncontrolled trigeminal neuralgia frequently require hospitalization for rapid control of pain. Between attacks, the patient is relatively pain free. A dull ache remaining after the intense pain subsides may indicate persistent compression of the nerve by a structural lesion. This disease is almost never seen in persons under 30 unless it is associated with multiple sclerosis.

The patient with trigeminal neuralgia will often have severe and, at times, even suicidal depression with high levels of superimposed anxiety during acute attacks. Both of these problems may by exacerbated by the sleep deprivation that often occurs during episodes of pain. Patients with coexisting multiple sclerosis may exhibit the euphoric dementia characteristic of that disease. Physicians should reassure persons with trigeminal neuralgia that the pain can almost always be controlled.

TESTING

All patients with a new diagnosis of trigeminal neuralgia should undergo magnetic resonance imaging of the brain and brain stem with and without gadolinium contrast medium to rule out posterior fossa or brain stem lesions and demyelinating disease (Fig. 7–2). Magnetic resonance angiography is also useful in confirming vascular compression of the trigeminal nerve by aberrant blood vessels (Fig. 7–3). Additional imaging of the sinuses should be considered if a question of occult or coexisting sinus disease is entertained. If the first division of the trigeminal nerve is affected, ophthalmologic evaluation to measure intraocular pressure and to rule out intraocular pathology is indicated. Screening laboratory testing consisting of complete blood count, erythrocyte sedimentation rate, and automated blood chemistry test-

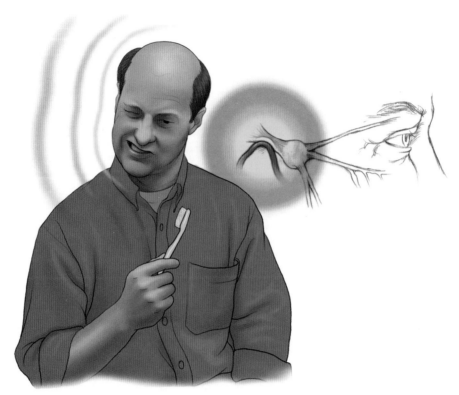

Figure 7–1. Paroxysms of pain triggered by brushing of teeth.

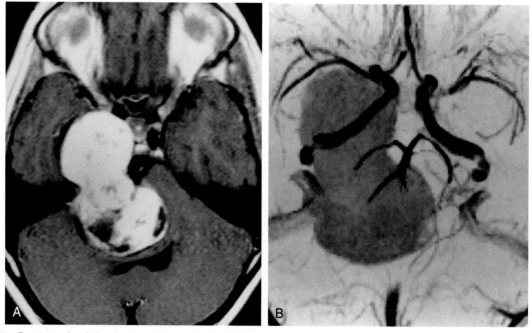

Figure 7–2. Cystic and solid schwannoma of the right trigeminal nerve and ganglion. *A,* Axial enhanced image showing a dumbbell-shaped tumor extending across the incisura from the posterior fossa into the medial portion of the right middle fossa. Note the heterogeneous enhancement of the tumor, suggesting areas of decreased cellularity and cystic change and a more solid component. *B,* Axial magnetic resonance angiogram performed after the magnetic resonance examination showing near-homogeneous enhancement of the tumor because of the delay in imaging. Note the exquisite demonstration of the tumor in the skull base, including the displaced right petrous carotid artery. (From Stark DD, Bradley WG Jr: Magnetic Resonance Imaging, Vol. III, 3rd ed. St. Louis, Mosby, 1999, p 1218.)

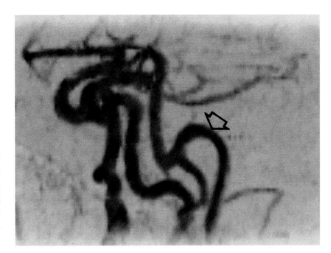

Figure 7–3. Vascular compression of the left fifth nerve in a 69-year-old man with tic douloureux. Three-dimensional time-of-flight magnetic resonance angiogram demonstrates that the compressive lesion is the markedly dominant right vertebral artery, which extends cephalad into the left CPA cistern (*open arrowhead*). (From Stark DD, Bradley WG Jr: Magnetic Resonance Imaging, Vol. III, 3rd ed. St. Louis, Mosby, 1999, p 1214.)

ing should be performed if the diagnosis of trigeminal neuralgia is in question. A complete blood count will be required as a baseline before starting treatment with carbamazepine (see Treatment).

DIFFERENTIAL DIAGNOSIS

Trigeminal neuralgia is generally a straightforward clinical diagnosis that can be made of the basis of a targeted history and physical examination. Diseases of the eye, ears, nose, throat, and teeth may all mimic trigeminal neuralgia or may coexist and confuse the diagnosis. Atypical facial pain is sometimes confused with trigeminal neuralgia but can be distinguished by the character of pain, which is dull and aching compared with the pain of trigeminal neuralgia, which is sharp and neuritic in nature. Additionally, the pain of trigeminal neuralgia occurs in the distribution of the divisions of the trigeminal nerve, whereas the pain of atypical facial pain does not follow any specific nerve distribution. Multiple sclerosis should be considered in all patients who present with trigeminal neuralgia before the fifth decade of life.

TREATMENT

Drug Therapy

Carbamazepine

This drug is considered first-line treatment for trigeminal neuralgia. In fact, rapid response to this drug essentially confirms a clinical diagnosis of trigeminal neuralgia. Despite the safety and efficacy of carbamazepine compared with other treatments for trigeminal neuralgia, much confusion and unfounded anxiety surround its use. This medication, which may be the patient's best chance for pain control, is sometimes discontinued because of laboratory abnormalities er-

roneously attributed to it. Therefore, baseline screening laboratory measures, consisting of a complete blood count, urinalysis, and automated chemistry profile, should be obtained before starting the drug.

Carbamazepine should be started slowly if the pain is not out of control, with a starting dose of 100 to 200 mg at bedtime for two nights. The patient should be cautioned regarding side effects, including dizziness, sedation, confusion, and rash. The drug is increased in 100- to 200-mg increments, given in equally divided doses over 2 days, as side effects allow until pain relief is obtained or a total dose of 1200 mg daily is reached. Careful monitoring of laboratory parameters is mandatory to avoid the rare possibility of life-threatening blood dyscrasia. *At the first sign of blood count abnormality or rash, this drug should be discontinued.* Failure to monitor patients started on carbamazepine can be disastrous because aplastic anemia can occur. When pain relief is obtained, the patient should be kept at that dosage of carbamazepine for at least 6 months before tapering of this medication is considered. The patient should be informed that under no circumstances should the dosage of drug be changed or the drug refilled or discontinued without the physician's knowledge.

Gabapentin

In the uncommon event that carbamazepine does not adequately control a patient's pain, gabapentin may be considered. As with carbamazepine, baseline blood tests should be obtained before starting therapy. Start with 300 mg of gabapentin at bedtime for two nights, and caution the patient about potential side effects, including dizziness, sedation, confusion, and rash. The drug is then increased in 300-mg increments, given in equally divided doses over 2 days, as side effects allow until pain relief is obtained or a total dose of 2400 mg daily is reached. At this point, if the patient has experienced partial relief of pain, blood values are measured and the drug is carefully titrated upward using 100-mg tablets. Rarely will more than 3600 mg daily be required.

Baclofen

This drug has been reported to be of value in some patients who fail to obtain relief from the aforementioned medications. Baseline laboratory tests should also be obtained before starting baclofen. Start with a 10-mg dose at bedtime for two nights, and caution the patient about potential adverse effects, which are the same as those of carbamazepine and gabapentin. The drug is increased in 10-mg increments, given in equally divided doses over 7 days as side effects allow, until pain relief is obtained or a total dose of 80 mg daily is reached. This drug has significant hepatic and central nervous system side effects, including weakness and sedation. As with carbamazepine, careful monitoring of laboratory values is indicated during the initial use of this drug.

In treating individuals with any of these drugs, the physician should make the patient aware that premature tapering or discontinuation of the medication may lead to the recurrence of pain and that it will be more difficult to control pain thereafter.

Invasive Therapy

Trigeminal Nerve Block

The use of trigeminal nerve block with local anesthetic and steroid serves as an excellent adjunct to drug treatment of trigeminal neuralgia. This technique rapidly relieves pain while medications are being titrated to effective levels. The initial block is carried out with preservative-free bupivacaine combined with methylprednisolone. Subsequent daily nerve blocks are carried out in a similar manner, substituting a lower dose of methylprednisolone. This approach may also be used to obtain control of breakthrough pain.

Retrogasserian Injection of Glycerol

The injection of small quantities of glycerol into the area of the gasserian ganglion has been shown to provide long-term relief for patients suffering from trigeminal neuralgia who have not responded to optimal trials of therapy. This procedure should be performed only by a physician well versed in the problems and pitfalls associated with neurodestructive procedures.

Radiofrequency Destruction of the Gasserian Ganglion

The destruction of the gasserian ganglion can be carried out by creating a radiofrequency lesion under biplanar fluoroscopic guidance. This procedure is reserved for patients who have failed all the treatments previously discussed for intractable trigeminal neuralgia and are not candidates for microvascular decompression of the trigeminal root.

Microvascular Decompression of the Trigeminal Root

This technique, which is also called *Janetta's procedure*, is the major neurosurgical procedure of choice for intractable trigeminal neuralgia. It is based on the theory that trigeminal neuralgia is in fact a compressive mononeuropathy. The operation consists of identifying the trigeminal root close to the brain stem and isolating the offending compressing blood vessel. A sponge is then interposed between the vessel and nerve, relieving the compression and thus the pain.

COMPLICATIONS AND PITFALLS

The pain of trigeminal neuralgia is among the most severe pain that mankind suffers from and thus must be considered a medical emergency. The uncontrolled pain of trigeminal neuralgia has led to suicide, and strong consideration should be given to the hospitalization of such patients. Between attacks of trigeminal neuralgia, the patient is relatively pain free. If a dull ache remains after the intense pain subsides, this is highly suggestive of a persistent compression of the nerve by a structural lesion such as a brain stem tumor or schwannoma. Trigeminal neuralgia is almost never seen in persons younger than 30 unless it is associated with multiple sclerosis, and all such patients should undergo magnetic resonance imaging with sequences designed to identify demyelinating disease.

CLINICAL PEARLS

Trigeminal nerve block with local anesthetic and steroid represents an excellent stopgap measure for patients suffering the uncontrolled pain of trigeminal neuralgia while waiting for pharmacologic treatments to take effect. This technique may allow the clinician to gain rapid control of pain and allow the patient to maintain adequate oral hydration and nutrition and to avoid hospitalization.

Temporomandibular Joint Dysfunction

ICD-9 524.60

THE CLINICAL SYNDROME

Temporomandibular joint dysfunction (TMD) (also known as *myofascial pain dysfunction of the muscles of mastication*) is characterized by pain in the joint itself that radiates into the mandible, ear, neck, and tonsillar pillars (Fig. 8–1). Headache often accompanies the pain of TMD and is clinically indistinguishable from the pain of tension-type headache. Stress often is the precipitating or exacerbating factor in the development of TMD. Dental malocclusion may play a role in the evolution of TMD. Internal derangement and arthritis of the temporomandibular joint may present as clicking or grating when the joint is opened and closed. Untreated, the patient may experience increasing pain in the aforementioned areas and limitation of jaw movement and opening.

SIGNS AND SYMPTOMS

The temporomandibular joint is a true joint that is divided into an upper and a lower synovial cavity by a fibrous articular disk. Internal derangement of this disk may result in pain and TMD, but extracapsular causes of temporomandibular joint pain are much more common. The joint space between the mandibular condyle and the glenoid fossa of the zygoma may be injected with small amounts of local anesthetic and steroid. The temporomandibular joint is innervated by branches of the mandibular nerve. The muscles involved in TMD often include the temporalis, masseter, external pterygoid, and internal pterygoid and may include the trapezius and sternocleidomastoid. Trigger points may be identified when palpating these muscles. Crepitus on range of motion of the joint is suggestive of arthritis rather than of dysfunc-

tion of myofascial origin. A history of bruxism and/or jaw clenching is often present.

TESTING

Radiographs of the temporomandibular joint are usually within normal limits in patients suffering from TMD but may be useful to help identify inflammatory or degenerative arthritis of the joint. Magnetic resonance imaging of the joint will help the clinician to identify derangement of the disk as well as other abnormalities of the joint itself. Complete blood count, erythrocyte sedimentation rate, and antinuclear antibody testing are indicated if inflammatory arthritis or temporal arteritis is suspected. Injection of the joint with small amounts of local anesthetic will serve as a diagnostic maneuver to help determine if the temporomandibular joint is in fact the source of the patient's pain (Fig. 8–2).

DIFFERENTIAL DIAGNOSIS

The clinical symptomatology of TMD may often be confused with pain of dental or sinus origin or may be characterized as atypical facial pain. Careful questioning and physical examination will usually allow the clinician to help separate these overlapping pain syndromes. Tumors of the zygoma and mandible as well as retropharyngeal tumors may produce ill-defined pain that may be attributed to TMD, and these potentially life-threatening diseases must be carefully searched for in any patient with facial pain. Reflex sympathetic dystrophy of the face should also be considered in any patient presenting with ill-defined facial pain after trauma, infection, or central nervous system injury. The pain of TMD is dull and aching in character, whereas the pain of reflex sympathetic dystrophy of the face is burning in nature with significant allodynia often present. Stellate ganglion block may help distinguish the two pain syndromes, because the pain of reflex sympathetic dystrophy of the face readily responds to this sympathetic nerve block, whereas the pain of TMD does not. In addition, the pain of TMD must be distinguished from the pain of jaw claudication associated with temporal arteritis.

TREATMENT

The mainstay of TMD is the combination of pharmacologic treatment with tricyclic antidepressants, physical modalities such as oral orthotic devices and physical therapy, and intra-articular injection of the joint with small amounts of local anesthetic and steroid. Antidepressant compounds such as nortriptyline at a single bedtime dose of 25 mg will help normalize sleep disturbance and treat underlying myofascial pain syndrome. Orthotic devices help the patient avoid jaw clenching and bruxism, which may exacerbate the clinical syndrome. Intra-articular injection is useful to provide palliation of acute pain to allow physical therapy as well as to treat joint arthritis that may contribute to the patient's pain symptomatology and joint dysfunction. Rarely, surgical treatment of the displaced intra-articular disk is required to restore the joint to normal function and to reduce pain.

For intra-articular injection of the temporomandibular joint, the patient is placed in the supine position with the cervical spine in the neutral position. The temporomandibular joint is identified by asking the patient to open and close the mouth several times and palpating the area just anterior and slightly inferior to the acoustic auditory meatus. After the joint is identified, the patient is asked to hold his or her mouth in neutral position.

A total of 0.5 ml of local anesthetic is drawn up in a 3-ml sterile syringe. In treating TMD, internal derangement of the temporomandibular joint, arthritis pain of the temporomandibular joint, or other painful conditions involving the temporomandibular joint, a total of 20 mg of methylprednisolone is added to the local anesthetic with the first block and 10 mg of methylprednisolone is added to the local anesthetic with subsequent blocks. After the skin overlying the temporomandibular joint is prepared with antiseptic solution, a 25-gauge, 1-inch styleted needle is inserted just below the zygomatic arch directly in the middle of the joint space. The needle is advanced approxi-

mately ¼ to ¾ inch in a plane perpendicular to the skull until a pop is felt, indicating that the joint space has been entered (see Fig. 8–2). After careful aspiration, 1 ml of solution is slowly injected. Injection of the joint may be repeated in 5- to 7-day intervals if the symptoms persist.

COMPLICATIONS AND PITFALLS

This anatomic region is highly vascular. This vascularity and proximity to major blood vessels also give rise to an increased incidence of postblock ecchymosis and hematoma formation, and the patient should be warned of this. Despite the vascularity of the anatomic region, this technique can safely be performed in the presence of anticoagulation by using a 25- or 27-gauge needle, albeit at increased risk of hematoma, if the clinical situation dictates a favorable risk-to-benefit ratio. These complications can be decreased if manual pressure is applied to the area of the block immediately after injection. Application of cold packs for a 20-minute period after the block will also decrease the amount of postprocedural pain and bleeding that the patient may experience. Additional side effects that occur with sufficient frequency include inadvertent block of the facial nerve with associated facial weakness. When this occurs, protection of the cornea with sterile ophthalmic lubricant and patching is mandatory.

CLINICAL PEARLS

Pain from TMD requires careful evaluation to design an appropriate treatment plan. Infection and inflammatory causes including collagen vascular diseases must first be ruled out. When temporomandibular joint pain occurs in older patients, the pain must be distinguished from the jaw claudication associated with temporal arteritis. Stress and anxiety often accompany TMD, and these factors must be addressed and managed. The myofascial pain component of TMD is best treated with the tricyclic antidepressant compounds, such as amitriptyline. Dental malocclusion and nighttime bruxism should be treated with an acrylic bite appliance. Narcotic analgesics and benzodiazepines should be avoided in patients suffering from TMD.

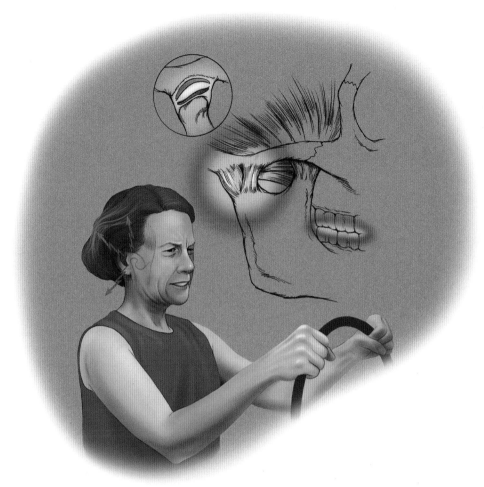

Figure 8-1. Stress is often a trigger for TMD.

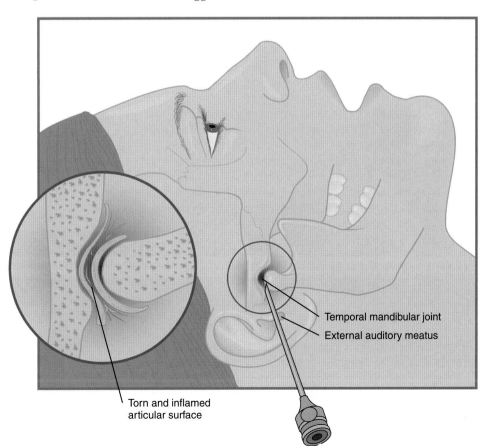

Temporal mandibular joint

External auditory meatus

Torn and inflamed articular surface

Figure 8-2. Correct needle placement for injections of the temporomandibular joint. (From Waldman SD: Atlas of Pain Management Injection Techniques. Philadelphia, WB Saunders, 2000, p 5.)

9

Atypical Facial Pain

ICD-9 350.2

THE CLINICAL SYNDROME

Atypical facial pain (also known as *atypical facial neuralgia*) is a term used to describe a heterogeneous group of pain syndromes that share in common the fact that the patient is suffering from facial pain that cannot be classified as trigeminal neuralgia. The pain is continuous but may vary in intensity. It is almost always unilateral and can be characterized as aching or cramping rather than shocklike neuritic pain typical of trigeminal neuralgia. The vast majority of patients suffering from atypical facial pain are female. The distribution of pain is in the distribution of the trigeminal nerve but invariably overlaps divisions of the nerve (Fig. 9–1).

Headache often accompanies the pain of atypical facial pain and is clinically indistinguishable from the pain of tension-type headache. Stress is often the precipitating or exacerbating factor in the development of atypical facial pain. Depression and sleep disturbance are also present in a significant number of patients suffering from atypical facial pain. A history of facial trauma, infection, or tumor of the head and neck may be elicited in some patients with atypical facial pain, but in most cases, no precipitating event can be identified.

SIGNS AND SYMPTOMS

Table 9–1 compares atypical facial pain with trigeminal neuralgia. Unlike trigeminal neuralgia, which is characterized by sudden paroxysms of neuritic shocklike pain, the pain of atypical facial pain is constant and of a dull, aching quality, but it may vary in intensity. The pain of trigeminal neuralgia is always within the distribution of a division of the trigeminal

nerve, whereas the pain of atypical facial pain will invariably overlap these divisional boundaries. The trigger areas that are characteristic of trigeminal neuralgia are absent in patients suffering from atypical facial pain.

TESTING

Radiographs of the head are usually within normal limits in patients suffering from atypical facial pain but may be useful to help identify tumor or bony abnormality. Magnetic resonance imaging of the brain and sinuses will help the clinician to identify intracranial pathology including tumor, sinus disease, and infection. Complete blood count, erythrocyte sedimentation rate, and antinuclear antibody testing are indicated if inflammatory arthritis or temporal arteritis is suspected. Injection of the temporomandibular joint with small amounts of local anesthetic will serve as a diagnostic maneuver to help determine if the temporomandibular joint is in fact the source of the patient's pain. Magnetic resonance imaging of the cervical spine is also indicated if the patient is exper-

Table 9–1. Comparison of Trigeminal Neuralgia With Atypical Facial Pain

	Trigeminal Neuralgia	Atypical Facial Pain
Temporal pattern of pain	Sudden and intermittent	Constant
Character of pain	Shocklike and neuritic	Dull, cramping, and aching
Pain-free intervals	Usual	Rare
Distribution of pain	In division of trigeminal nerve	Overlaps division of trigeminal nerve
Trigger areas	Present	Absent
Underlying psychopathology	Rare	Common

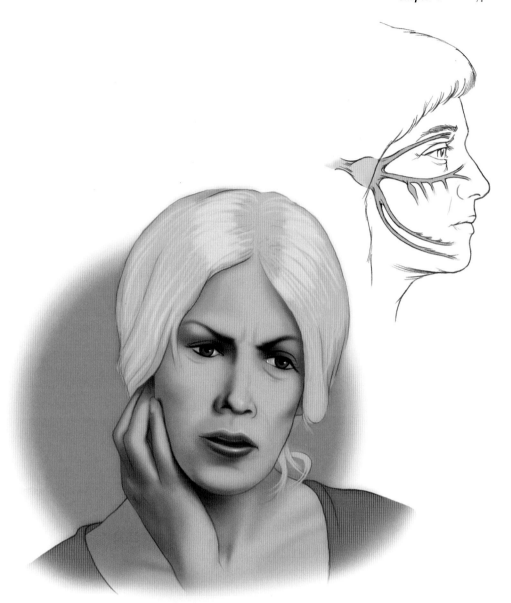

Figure 9-1. Patients with atypical facial pain will often rub the affected area; those with trigeminal neuralgia will not.

iencing significant occipital or nuchal pain symptomatology.

DIFFERENTIAL DIAGNOSIS

The clinical symptomatology of atypical facial pain may often be confused with pain of dental or sinus origin or may be erroneously characterized as trigeminal neuralgia. Careful questioning and physical examination will usually allow the clinician to distinguish these overlapping pain syndromes. Tumors of the zygoma and mandible as well as posterior fossa tumors and retropharyngeal tumors may produce ill-defined pain that may be attributed to atypical facial pain, and these potentially life-threatening diseases must be carefully searched for in any patient with facial pain. Reflex sympathetic dystrophy of the face should also be considered in any patient presenting with ill-defined facial pain after trauma, infection, or central nervous system injury. The pain of atypical facial pain is dull and aching in character, whereas the pain of reflex sympathetic dystrophy of the face is burning in nature with significant allodynia often present. Stellate ganglion block may help distinguish the two pain syndromes, as the pain of reflex sympathetic dystrophy of the face readily responds to this sympathetic nerve block, whereas atypical facial pain does not. The pain of atypical facial pain must be distinguished from the pain of jaw claudication associated with temporal arteritis.

TREATMENT

The mainstay of atypical facial pain is the combination of pharmacologic treatment with tricyclic antidepressants and physical modalities such as oral orthotic devices and physical therapy. Trigeminal nerve block and intra-articular injection of the temporomandibular joint with small amounts of local anesthetic and steroid may also be of value. Antidepressant compounds such as nortriptyline at a single bedtime dose of 25 mg will help normalize sleep disturbance and treat underlying myofascial pain syndrome. Orthotic devices help the patient avoid jaw clenching and bruxism, which may exacerbate the clinical syndrome. Management of underlying depression and anxiety is mandatory if the clinician hopes to help relieve the symptoms of atypical facial pain.

COMPLICATIONS AND PITFALLS

The major pitfall when caring for patients thought to suffer from atypical facial pain is the failure to accurately diagnose underlying pathology responsible for the patient's pain. It must be remembered that atypical facial pain is essentially a diagnosis of exclusion. If trigeminal nerve block or intra-articular injection of the temporomandibular joint is being considered as part of the treatment plan for a patient suffering from atypical facial pain, it must be remembered that this anatomic region is highly vascular. This vascularity and proximity to major blood vessels also give rise to an increased incidence of postblock ecchymosis and hematoma formation, and the patient should be warned of this.

CLINICAL PEARLS

Atypical facial pain requires careful evaluation to design an appropriate treatment plan. Infection and inflammatory causes including collagen vascular diseases must first be ruled out. When temporomandibular joint pain occurs in older patients, the pain must be distinguished from the jaw claudication associated with temporal arteritis. Stress and anxiety often accompany atypical facial pain, and these factors must be addressed and treated. The myofascial pain component of atypical facial pain is best treated with the tricyclic antidepressant compounds such as amitriptyline. Dental malocclusion and nighttime bruxism should be treated with an acrylic bite appliance. Narcotic analgesics and benzodiazepines should be avoided in patients suffering from atypical facial pain.

10

Reflex Sympathetic Dystrophy of the Face

ICD-9 337.20

THE CLINICAL SYNDROME

Reflex sympathetic dystrophy (RSD) is an infrequent cause of face and neck pain. Although the symptom complex in this disorder is relatively constant from patient to patient, the diagnosis is often missed. This diagnosis is overlooked despite the fact that RSD of the face and neck presents in a manner that closely parallels its presentation in the upper or lower extremity. This difficulty in diagnosis often results in extensive diagnostic and therapeutic endeavors in an effort to palliate the patient's pain. The common denominator in all patients suffering from RSD of the face is trauma to tissue. This trauma may take the form of actual injury to the soft tissues, dentition, or bones of the face; infection; cancer; arthritis; or insults to the central nervous system or cranial nerves.

SIGNS AND SYMPTOMS

The hallmark of RSD of the face is pain that is burning in nature (Fig. 10–1). The pain is frequently associated with cutaneous or mucosal allodynia and does not follow the path of either cranial or peripheral nerves. Trigger areas, especially in the oral mucosa, are common, as are trophic skin and mucosal changes in the area affected by the RSD. Sudomotor and vasomotor changes may also be identified but are often less obvious than in patients suffering from RSD of the extremities. Often, patients suffering from RSD of the face will have evidence of previous dental extractions that were performed in an effort to provide the patient with pain relief. Patients suffering from RSD of the face frequently experience significant sleep disturbance and depression.

TESTING

Although there is no specific test for RSD, a presumptive diagnosis of RSD of the face can be made if the patient experiences significant pain relief after stellate ganglion block with local anesthetic. It should be noted that given the diverse nature of tissue injury that can cause RSD of the face, the clinician must assiduously search for occult pathology that may mimic or coexist with the RSD. Testing is aimed primarily at identifying occult pathology or other diseases that may mimic RSD of the face (see Differential Diagnosis). All patients with a presumptive diagnosis of RSD of the face should undergo magnetic resonance imaging of the brain and, if significant occipital or nuchal symptoms are present, of the cervical spine. Screening laboratory testing consisting of complete blood count, erythrocyte sedimentation rate, and automated blood chemistry testing should be performed to rule out infection or other inflammatory causes of tissue injury that may serve as the nidus for the RSD.

DIFFERENTIAL DIAGNOSIS

The clinical symptomatology of RSD of the face may often be confused with pain of dental or sinus origin or may be erroneously characterized as atypical facial pain or trigeminal neuralgia (Table 10–1). Careful questioning and physical examination will usually allow the clinician to distinguish these overlapping pain syndromes. Tumors of the zygoma and mandible as well as posterior fossa tumors and retropharyngeal tumors may produce ill-defined pain that may be attributed to RSD of the face, and these potentially life-threatening diseases must be carefully searched for in any patient with facial pain. The pain of atypical facial pain is constant and dull and aching in character, whereas the pain of trigeminal neuralgia is intermittent and shocklike in nature. Stellate gan-

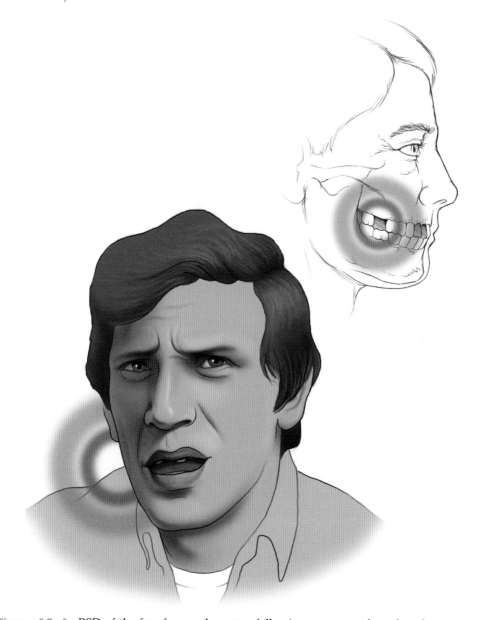

Figure 10–1. RSD of the face frequently occurs following trauma such as dental extractions.

Table 10-1. Differential Diagnosis

	Trigeminal Neuralgia	**Atypical Facial Pain**	**Reflex Sympathetic Dystrophy of the Face**
Temporal pattern of pain	Sudden and intermittent	Constant	Constant
Character of pain	Shocklike and neuritic	Dull, cramping, and aching	Burning with allodynia
Pain-free intervals	Usual	Rare	Rare
Distribution of pain	In division of trigeminal nerve	Overlaps division of trigeminal nerve	Overlaps division of trigeminal nerve
Trigger areas	Present	Absent	Present
Underlying psychopathology	Rare	Common	Common
Trophic skin changes	Absent	Absent	Present
Sudomotor and vasomotor changes	Absent	Absent	Often present

glion block may help distinguish it from these two pain syndromes, as the pain of RSD of the face readily responds to this sympathetic nerve block, whereas atypical facial pain does not. The pain of RSD of the face must be distinguished from the pain of jaw claudication associated with temporal arteritis.

TREATMENT

The successful treatment of RSD of the face requires two phases. First, any nidus of tissue trauma that is contributing to the ongoing sympathetic dysfunction responsible for the symptoms of RSD of the face must be identified and removed. Second, interruption of the sympathetic innervation of the face via stellate ganglion block with local anesthetic must be implemented. This may require daily stellate ganglion block for a significant period of time. Occupational therapy consisting of tactile desensitization of the affected skin may also be of value. Underlying depression and sleep disturbance are best treated with a tricyclic antidepressant such as nortriptyline given as a single bedtime dose of 25 mg. Gabapentin may help palliate any component of neuritic pain. Opioid analgesics and benzodiazepines should be avoided to prevent iatrogenic chemical dependence.

COMPLICATIONS AND SIDE EFFECTS

The main complications associated with RSD of the face are the problems associated with any chronic painful condition that is frequently incorrectly diagnosed. Chemical dependence, depression, and multiple failed therapeutic endeavors and procedures are the rule rather than the exception. Stellate ganglion block is a safe and effective pain management technique, but it is not without side effects and risks.

CLINICAL PEARLS

The key to recognizing RSD of the face is a high index of clinical suspicion. RSD should be suspected in any patient who has pain associated with antecedent trauma or pain that is burning or allodynic in nature. Once the syndrome is recognized, blockade of the sympathetic nerves subserving the painful area will confirm the diagnosis. Once confirmed, repeated sympathetic blockade, combined with adjunctive therapies, will in most cases result in pain relief. The frequency and number of sympathetic blocks recommended to treat sympathetic dystrophies vary among pain practitioners; however, it is our belief that early aggressive neural blockade allows for more rapid resolution of both pain and disability.

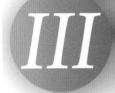

III Neck and Brachial Plexus Pain Syndromes

11

Cervical Facet Syndrome

ICD-9 724.5

THE CLINICAL SYNDROME

Cervical facet syndrome is a constellation of symptoms consisting of neck, head, shoulder, and proximal upper extremity pain that radiates in a nondermatomal pattern. The pain is dull and ill defined in character. It may be unilateral or bilateral and is thought to be the result of pathology of the facet joint. The pain of cervical facet syndrome is exacerbated by flexion, extension, and lateral bending of the cervical spine. It is often worse in the morning after physical activity. Each facet joint receives innervation from two spinal levels. Each joint receives fibers from the dorsal ramus at the same level as the vertebra as well as fibers from the dorsal ramus of the vertebra above. This fact has clinical import in that it provides an explanation for the ill-defined nature of facet-mediated pain and explains why the dorsal nerve from the vertebra above the offending level must often also be blocked to provide complete pain relief.

SIGNS AND SYMPTOMS

Most patients with cervical facet syndrome have tenderness to deep palpation of the cervical paraspinous musculature. Spasm of these muscles may also be present. The patient will exhibit decreased range of motion of the cervical spine and will usually complain of pain on flexion, extension, rotation, and lateral bending of the cervical spine. There will be no motor or sensory deficit unless there is coexisting radiculopathy, plexopathy, or entrapment neuropathy.

If the C1-2 facet joints are involved, the pain will be referred to the posterior auricular and occipital region. If the C2-3 facet joints are involved, the pain may radiate to the forehead and eyes. Pain emanating from the C3-4 facet joints will be referred superiorly to the suboccipital region and inferiorly to the posterolateral neck, with pain from the C4-5 facet joints radiating to the base of the neck. Pain from the C5-6 joints is referred to the shoulders and intrascapular region, with pain from the C6-7 facet joints radiating to the supraspinous and infraspinous fossae (Fig. 11-1).

TESTING

As patients enter the fifth decade of life, almost all of them will exhibit some degree of abnormality of the facet joints of the cervical spine on plain radiographs (Fig. 11-2). The clinical import of the findings has long been debated by pain specialists, but it was not until the advent of computed tomography scanning and magnetic resonance imaging (MRI) that the relationship of these abnormal facet joints to the cervical nerve roots and other surrounding anatomic structures was clearly understood. However, any data gleaned from these sophisticated imaging techniques can provide only a presumptive diagnosis to guide the clinician. To prove that in fact a specific facet joint is contributing to the patient's pain, a diagnostic intra-articular injection of that joint with local anesthetic is required.

DIFFERENTIAL DIAGNOSIS

Cervical facet syndrome is a diagnosis of exclusion that is supported by a combination of clinical history, physical examination, radiography, and MRI and by intra-articular injection of the suspect facet joints. Pain syndromes that may mimic cervical facet syndrome include cervicalgia, cervical bursitis, cervical fibromyositis, inflammatory arthritis, and disorders of the cervical spinal cord, roots, plexus, and nerves. MRI of the cervical spine should be carried out on all patients suspected of suffering from cervical facet syn-

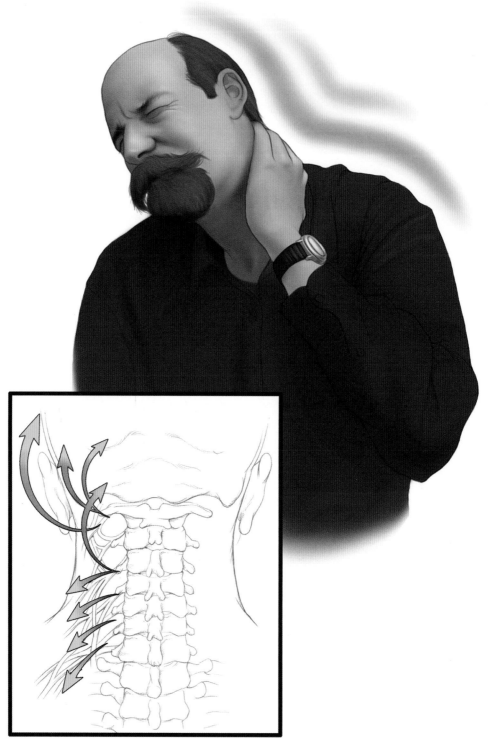

Figure 11-1. The pain of cervical facet syndrome is made worse by flexion, extension, and lateral bending of the cervical spine.

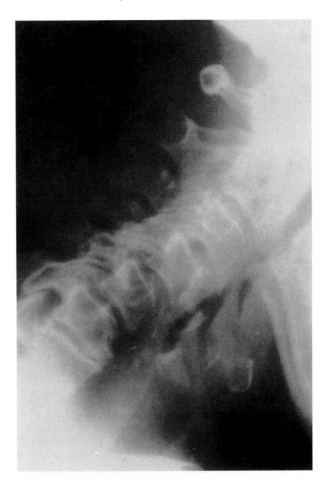

Figure 11–2. Lateral view of the cervical spine showing osteo-arthritis of the apophyseal joints of the upper cervical spine. There is a resultant subluxation of C-4 on C-5. There also is degenerative disk disease present at C5-6 and C6-7. There is associated osteophyte formation at C6-7, and there is subluxation of C-5 on C-6. (From Brower AC, Flemming DJ: Arthritis in Black and White, 2nd ed. Philadelpia, WB Saunders, 1997, p 290.)

drome. Screening laboratory testing consisting of complete blood count, erythrocyte sedimentation rate, antinuclear antibody testing, HLA B-27 antigen screening, and automated blood chemistry testing should be performed if the diagnosis of cervical facet syndrome is in question to help rule out other causes of the patient's pain.

TREATMENT

Cervical facet syndrome is best treated with a multi-modality approach. Physical therapy including heat modalities and deep sedative massage, combined with nonsteroidal anti-inflammatory drugs and skeletal muscle relaxants, represents a reasonable starting point. The addition of cervical facet blocks is a logical next step. For symptomatic relief, blockade of the medial branch of the dorsal ramus or intra-articular injection of the facet joint with local anesthetic and steroid has been shown to be extremely effective in the treatment of cervical facet syndrome. Underlying sleep disturbance and depression are best treated with a tricyclic antidepressant compound such as nortriptyline, which can be started at a single bedtime dose of 25 mg.

SIDE EFFECTS AND COMPLICATIONS

The proximity to the spinal cord and exiting nerve roots makes it imperative that cervical facet block be carried out only by those well versed in the regional anatomy and experienced in performing interventional pain management techniques. The proximity to the vertebral artery combined with the vascular nature of this anatomic region makes the potential for intravascular injection high. The injection of even small amounts of local anesthetic into the vertebral arteries will result in seizures. Given the proximity of the brain and brain stem, ataxia after cervical facet block due to vascular uptake of local anesthetic is not an uncommon occurrence. Many patients will also complain of a transient increase in headache and cervicalgia after injection of the joint.

CLINICAL PEARLS

Cervical facet syndrome is a common cause of neck, occipital, shoulder, and upper extremity pain. It is often confused with cervicalgia and cervical fibromyositis. Diagnostic intra-articular facet block will help confirm the diagnosis. The clinician must take care to rule out diseases of the cervical spinal cord, such as syringomyelia, that may initially present in a manner similar to cervical facet syndrome. Ankylosis spondylitis may also present as cervical facet syndrome and must be correctly identified in order to avoid ongoing joint damage and functional disability.

Cervical facet block is often combined with atlanto-occipital block when treating pain in the aforementioned areas. Although neither joint is a true facet joint in the anatomic sense of the word, the block is analogous to the facet joint block technique used commonly by pain practitioners and may be viewed as such. Many pain specialists believe that these techniques are currently underutilized in the treatment of "post-whiplash" cervicalgia and cervicogenic headaches. These specialists believe that both techniques should be considered when cervical epidural nerve blocks and/or occipital nerve blocks fail to provide palliation of these headache and neck pain syndromes.

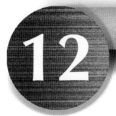

Cervical Radiculopathy

ICD-9 724.3

THE CLINICAL SYNDROME

Cervical radiculopathy is a constellation of symptoms consisting of neurogenic neck and upper extremity pain emanating from the cervical nerve roots. In addition to the pain, the patient with cervical radiculopathy may experience associated numbness, weakness, and loss of reflexes. The causes of cervical radiculopathy include herniated disk, foraminal stenosis, tumor, osteophyte formation, and, rarely, infection.

SIGNS AND SYMPTOMS

The patient suffering from cervical radiculopathy will complain of pain, numbness, tingling, and paresthesias in the distribution of the affected nerve root or roots (Table 12–1). Patients may also note weakness and lack of coordination in the affected extremity. Muscle spasms and neck pain as well as pain referred into the trapezius and intrascapular region are common (Fig. 12–1). Decreased sensation, weakness, and reflex changes are demonstrated on physical examination. Patients with C-7 radiculopathy will commonly place the hand of the affected extremity on top of their head to obtain relief (see Fig. 12–1). Oc-

casionally, a patient suffering from cervical radiculopathy will experience compression of the cervical spinal cord, resulting in myelopathy. Cervical myelopathy is most commonly due to midline herniated cervical disk, spinal stenosis, tumor, or, rarely, infection. Patients suffering from cervical myelopathy will experience lower extremity weakness and bowel and bladder symptomatology. This represents a neurosurgical emergency and should be treated as such.

TESTING

Magnetic resonance imaging (MRI) of the cervical spine will provide the clinician with the best information regarding the cervical spine and its contents (Fig. 12–2). MRI is highly accurate and will help identify abnormalities that may put the patient at risk for the development of cervical myelopathy. In patients who cannot undergo MRI, such as patients with a pacemaker, computed tomography or myelography is a reasonable second choice. Radionucleotide bone scanning and plain radiography are indicated if fractures or bony abnormalities such as metastatic disease are being considered.

Although these tests provide the clinician with useful neuroanatomic information, electromyography and nerve conduction velocity testing will provide the clinician with neurophysiologic information that can delineate the actual status of each individual nerve root and the brachial plexus. Screening laboratory testing consisting of complete blood count, erythrocyte sedi-

Table 12–1. Clinical Features of Cervical Radiculopathy

Cervical Root	Pain	Sensory Changes	Weakness	Reflex Changes
C-5 root	Neck, shoulder, and anterolateral arm	Numbness in deltoid area	Deltoid and biceps	Biceps reflex
C-6 root	Neck, shoulder, and lateral aspect of arm	Dorsolateral aspect of thumb and index finger	Biceps, wrist extensors, and pollicus longus	Brachioradialis reflex
C-7 root	Neck, shoulder, lateral aspect of arm, and dorsal forearm	Index and middle finger and dorsum of hand	Triceps	Triceps reflex

mentation rate, and automated blood chemistry testing should be performed if the diagnosis of cervical radiculopathy is in question.

DIFFERENTIAL DIAGNOSIS

Cervical radiculopathy is a clinical diagnosis that is supported by a combination of clinical history, physical examination, radiography, and MRI. Pain syndromes that may mimic cervical radiculopathy include cervicalgia, cervical bursitis, cervical fibromyositis, inflammatory arthritis, and disorders of the cervical spinal cord, roots, plexus, and nerves. MRI of the cervical spine should be carried out on all patients suspected of suffering from cervical radiculopathy. Screening laboratory testing consisting of complete blood count, erythrocyte sedimentation rate, antinuclear antibody testing, HLA B-27 antigen screening, and automated blood chemistry testing should be performed if the diagnosis of cervical radiculopathy is in question to help rule out other causes of the patient's pain.

TREATMENT

Cervical radiculopathy is best treated with a multi-modality approach. Physical therapy including heat modalities and deep sedative massage, combined with nonsteroidal anti-inflammatory drugs and skeletal muscle relaxants, represents a reasonable starting point. The addition of cervical steroid epidural nerve blocks is a logical next step. Cervical epidural blocks with local anesthetic and steroid has been shown to be extremely effective in the treatment of cervical radiculopathy. Underlying sleep disturbance and depression are best treated with a tricyclic antidepressant compound such as nortriptyline, which can be started at a single bedtime dose of 25 mg.

COMPLICATIONS AND SIDE EFFECTS

A failure to accurately diagnose cervical radiculopathy may put the patient at risk for the development of cervical myelopathy, which if untreated may progress to quadriparesis or quadriplegia. Electromyography will help to distinguish plexopathy from radiculopathy and to identify coexistent entrapment neuropathy such as carpal tunnel syndrome that confuses the diagnosis.

CLINICAL PEARLS

Carpal tunnel syndrome should also be differentiated from cervical radiculopathy involving the cervical nerve roots, which may at times mimic median nerve compression. Furthermore, it should be remembered that cervical radiculopathy and median nerve entrapment may coexist in the "double crush" syndrome. The double crush syndrome is seen most commonly with median nerve entrapment at the wrist or with carpal tunnel syndrome.

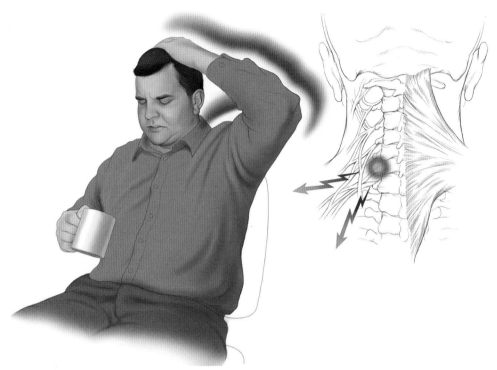

Figure 12–1. Patients with C-7 radiculopathy will often place the hand of the affected extremity on the head to obtain relief.

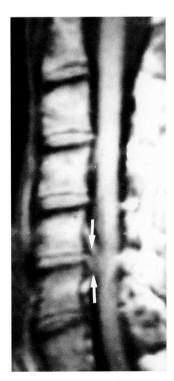

Figure 12–2. Disk herniation at C5-6 level. Sagittal T1-weighted spin-echo image showing a herniated fragment (*arrows*) extending below the disk space level. (From Stark DD, Bradley WG Jr: Magnetic Resonance Imaging, Vol. III, 3rd ed. St. Louis, Mosby, 1999, p 1848.)

13

Fibromyalgia of the Cervical Musculature

ICD-9 729.1

THE CLINICAL SYNDROME

Fibromyalgia of the cervical spine is one of the most common painful conditions encountered in clinical practice. Fibromyalgia is a chronic pain syndrome that affects a focal or regional portion of the body. The sine qua non of fibromyalgia of the cervical spine is the finding of myofascial trigger points on physical examination. Although these trigger points are generally localized to the cervical paraspinous musculature, trapezius, and other muscles of the neck, the pain of fibromyalgia of the cervical spine is often referred to other areas. This referred pain is often misdiagnosed or attributed to other organ systems, leading to extensive evaluations and ineffective treatment.

The trigger point is the pathognomonic lesion of fibromyalgia pain and is thought to be the result of microtrauma to the affected muscles. Stimulation of the myofascial trigger point will reproduce or exacerbate the patient's pain. Often, stiffness and fatigue will coexist with the pain of fibromyalgia of the cervical spine, increasing the functional disability associated with this disease and complicating its treatment. Fibromyalgia of the cervical spine may occur as a primary disease state or may occur in conjunction with other painful conditions, including radiculopathy and chronic regional pain syndromes. Psychological or behavioral abnormalities including depression frequently coexist with the muscle abnormalities associated with fibromyalgia of the cervical spine. Treatment of these psychological and behavioral abnormalities must be an integral part of any successful treatment plan for fibromyalgia of the cervical spine.

Although the exact etiology of fibromyalgia of the cervical spine remains unknown, tissue trauma seems to be the common denominator. Acute trauma to muscle as a result of overstretching will commonly result in the development of fibromyalgia of the cervical spine. More subtle injury to muscle in the form of repetitive microtrauma can also result in the development of fibromyalgia of the cervical spine, as can damage to muscle fibers from exposure to extreme heat or cold. Extreme overuse or other coexistent disease processes such as radiculopathy may also result in the development of fibromyalgia of the cervical spines.

In addition to tissue trauma, a variety of other factors seem to predispose the patient to the development of fibromyalgia of the cervical spine. The weekend athlete who subjects his or her body to unaccustomed physical activity may often develop fibromyalgia of the cervical spine. Poor posture while sitting at a computer keyboard or while watching television has also been implicated as a predisposing factor to the development of fibromyalgia of the cervical spine. Previous injuries may result in abnormal muscle function and predispose to the subsequent development of fibromyalgia of the cervical spine. All of these predisposing factors may be intensified if the patient also suffers from poor nutritional status or coexisting psychological or behavioral abnormalities, including depression.

SIGNS AND SYMPTOMS

The sine qua non of fibromyalgia of the cervical spine is the identification of myofascial trigger points. The trigger point is the pathologic lesion of fibromyalgia of the cervical spine and is characterized by a local point of exquisite tenderness in affected muscle. Mechanical stimulation of the trigger point by palpation or stretching will produce not only intense local pain but also referred pain. In addition to this local and referred pain, there will often be an involuntary withdrawal of the stimulated muscle that is called a *jump sign* (Fig. 13–1). This jump sign is also

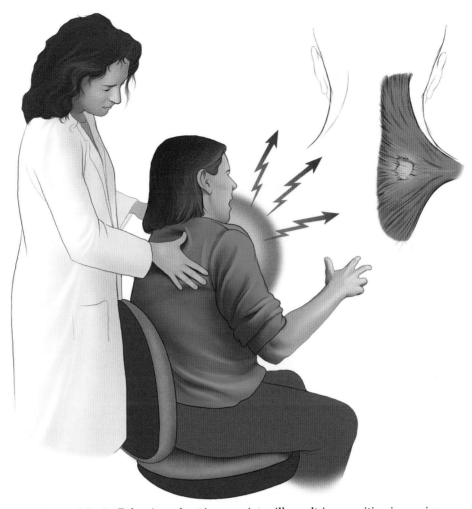

Figure 13–1. Palpation of a trigger point will result in a positive jump sign.

characteristic of fibromyalgia of the cervical spine, as is stiffness of the neck, pain of range of motion of the cervical spine, and pain referred into the upper extremities in a nondermatomal pattern.

Although the patterns of referred pain have been well studied and occur in a characteristic pattern, this referred pain is often misdiagnosed and attributed to diseases of organ systems in the distribution of the referred pain. This often leads to extensive evaluation and ineffective treatments. Taut bands of muscle fibers are often identified when myofascial trigger points are palpated. Despite this consistent physical finding in patients suffering from fibromyalgia of the cervical spine, the pathophysiology of the myofascial trigger point remains elusive, although many theories have been advanced. Common to all of these theories is the belief that trigger points are the result of microtrauma to the affected muscle. This microtrauma may occur as a single injury to the affected muscle or may occur as the result of repetitive microtrauma or as the result of chronic deconditioning of the agonist and antagonist muscle unit.

TESTING

The exact pathophysiologic processes responsible for the development of fibromyalgia of the cervical spine remain elusive. Biopsies of clinically identified trigger points have not revealed consistently abnormal histology. The muscle hosting the trigger points has been alternatively described as "moth eaten" or as containing "waxy degeneration." Increased plasma myoglobin has been reported in some patients with fibromyalgia of the cervical spine, but this finding has not been reproduced by other investigators. Electrodiagnostic testing of patients suffering from fibromyalgia of the cervical spine has revealed an increase in muscle tension in some patients. Again, this finding has not been reproducible. However, regardless of the pathophysiology of fibromyalgia of the cervical spine, there is little doubt that the clinical findings of trigger points in the cervical paraspinous muscles and associated jump sign exist in combination with a clinically recognizable constellation of symptoms that are consistently diagnosed as fibromyalgia of the cervical spine by clinicians.

The diagnosis of fibromyalgia of the cervical spine is made on the basis of clinical findings rather than on specific diagnostic laboratory, electrodiagnostic, or radiographic testing. For this reason, a targeted history and physical examination with a systematic search for trigger points and identification of a positive jump sign must be carried out on every patient suspected of suffering from fibromyalgia of the cervical spine. Because of the lack of objective diagnostic testing, the clinician must also rule out other coexisting disease processes that may mimic fibromyalgia of the cervical spine, including primary inflammatory muscle disease and collagen vascular disease. The judicious use of electrodiagnostic and radiographic testing will also help identify coexisting pathology such as herniated nucleus propulsus and rotator cuff tears. The clinician must also identify coexisting psychological and behavioral abnormalities that may mask or exacerbate the symptoms associated with fibromyalgia of the cervical spine and other coexisting pathologic processes.

DIFFERENTIAL DIAGNOSIS

The diagnosis of fibromyalgia of the cervical spine is made on the basis of clinical findings rather than specific diagnostic laboratory, electrodiagnostic, or radiographic testing. For this reason, a targeted history and physical examination with a systematic search for trigger points and identification of a positive jump sign must be carried out on every patient suspected of suffering from fibromyalgia of the cervical spine. Because of the lack of objective diagnostic testing, the clinician must also rule out other coexisting disease processes that may mimic fibromyalgia of the cervical spine, including primary inflammatory muscle disease, multiple sclerosis, and collagen vascular disease. The judicious use of electrodiagnostic and radiographic testing will also help identify coexisting pathology such as herniated nucleus propulsus and rotator cuff tears. The clinician must also identify coexisting psychological and behavioral abnormalities that may mask or exacerbate the symptoms associated with fibromyalgia of the cervical spine and other coexisting pathologic processes.

TREATMENT

The treatment of fibromyalgia of the cervical spine involves the use of techniques that will help eliminate the trigger point that may serve as the source of the perpetuation of this painful condition. It is hoped that interruption of the pain cycle by the elimination of trigger points will allow the patient to experience prolonged relief. The mechanism of action of each of the above modalities is poorly understood, and thus an element of trial and error in developing a treatment plan is the expected norm.

Because underlying depression and a substrate of anxiety are present in many patients suffering from fibromyalgia of the cervical spine, the inclusion of antidepressant compounds as an integral part of most treatment plans represents a reasonable choice.

In addition to this treatment modality, a variety of adjuvant methods are available for the treatment of fibromyalgia of the cervical spine. The therapeutic use of heat and cold is often combined with trigger point injections and antidepressant compounds to effect pain relief. Some patients will experience decreased pain with the application of transcutaneous nerve stimulation or electrical stimulation to fatigue affected muscles. Although not currently approved by the Food and Drug Administration, the injection of minute quantities of botulinum toxin, type A directly into trigger points has gained favor in the treatment of persistent fibromyalgia of the cervical spine in patients who have not responded to traditional treatment modalities.

SIDE EFFECTS AND COMPLICATIONS

Trigger point injections are an extremely safe procedure if careful attention is paid to the clinically relevant anatomy in the areas to be injected. Care must be taken to use sterile technique to avoid infection as well as to use universal precautions to avoid risk to the operator. Most side effects of trigger point injection are related to needle-induced trauma to the injection site and underlying tissues. The incidence of ecchymosis and hematoma formation can be decreased if pressure is placed on the injection site immediately after trigger point injection. The avoidance of overly long needles will help decrease the incidence of trauma to underlying structures. Special care must be taken to avoid pneumothorax when injecting trigger points in proximity to the underlying pleural space.

CLINICAL PEARLS

Fibromyalgia of the cervical spine is a common disorder that commonly coexists with a variety of somatic and psychological disorders. Fibromyalgia of the cervical spine is often misdiagnosed. In patients suspected of suffering from fibromyalgia of the cervical spine, a careful evaluation to identify underlying disease processes is mandatory.

Treatment is focused on blocking the myofascial trigger and achieving prolonged relaxation of the affected muscle. Conservative therapy consisting of treatment with the antidepressant compounds and trigger point injections with local anesthetic or saline is the starting point for the treatment of fibromyalgia of the cervical spine. Adjunct therapies, including physical therapy, therapeutic heat and cold, transcutaneous nerve stimulation, and electrical stimulation, can be used on a case-by-case basis. For patients who do not respond to these traditional measures, consideration should be given to the use of botulinum toxin, type A, which has been shown to be a safe and effective treatment for this disorder.

14

Cervical Strain

ICD-9 CODE 847.0

THE CLINICAL SYNDROME

Acute cervical strain is a constellation of symptoms consisting of nonradicular neck pain that radiates in a nondermatomal pattern into the shoulders and intrascapular region. Headaches often accompany the symptoms of cervical strain. The trapezius is often affected, with resultant spasm and limitation in range of motion of the cervical spine. Cervical strain is usually the result of trauma to the cervical spine and associated soft tissues but may occur without an obvious inciting incident. The pathologic lesions responsible for this clinical syndrome may emanate from the soft tissues, facet joints, and/or intervertebral disks.

SIGNS AND SYMPTOMS

Neck pain is the hallmark of cervical strain. It may begin in the occipital region and radiate in a nondermatomal pattern into the shoulders and intrascapular region (Fig. 14–1). The pain of cervical strain is often exacerbated by movement of the cervical spine and shoulders. Headaches often occur along with the aforementioned symptoms and may worsen with emotional stress. Sleep disturbance is common, as is difficulty in concentrating on simple tasks. Depression may occur with prolonged symptomatology.

On physical examination, there is tenderness on palpation, and spasm of the paraspinous musculature and trapezius is often present. Decreased range of motion is invariably present, with pain increasing with this maneuver. The neurologic examination of the upper extremities is within normal limits despite the frequent complaint of upper extremity pain.

TESTING

There is no specific test for cervical strain. Testing is aimed primarily at identifying occult pathology or other diseases that may mimic cervical strain (see Differential Diagnosis). Plain radiographs will help delineate bony abnormality of the cervical spine, including arthritis, fracture, congenital abnormalities (e.g., Arnold-Chiari malformation), and tumor. Straightening of the lordotic curve will frequently be noted. All patients with the recent onset of cervical strain should undergo magnetic resonance imaging (MRI) of the cervical spine and, if significant occipital or headache symptoms are present, of the brain. Screening laboratory testing consisting of complete blood count, erythrocyte sedimentation rate, antinuclear antibody testing, and automated blood chemistry testing should be performed to rule out occult inflammatory arthritis, infection, and tumor.

DIFFERENTIAL DIAGNOSIS

Cervical strain is a clinical diagnosis that is supported by a combination of clinical history, physical examination, radiography, and MRI. Pain syndromes that may mimic cervical strain include cervical bursitis, cervical fibromyositis, inflammatory arthritis, and disorders of the cervical spinal cord, roots, plexus, and nerves. MRI of the cervical spine should be carried out on all patients suspected of suffering from cervical strain. Screening laboratory testing consisting of complete blood count, erythrocyte sedimentation rate, antinuclear antibody testing, HLA B-27 antigen screening, and automated blood chemistry testing should be performed if the diagnosis of cervical strain is in question to help rule out other causes of the patient's pain.

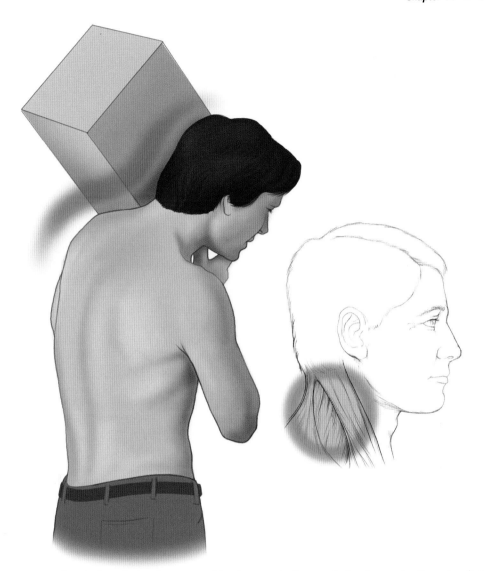

Figure 14–1. Cervical strain is often caused by trauma to the cervical spine and adjacent soft tissue.

TREATMENT

Cervical strain is best treated with a multimodality approach. Physical therapy including heat modalities and deep sedative massage, combined with nonsteroidal anti-inflammatory drugs and skeletal muscle relaxants, represent a reasonable starting point. The addition of cervical epidural nerve blocks and occasionally cervical facet blocks is a reasonable next step. For symptomatic relief, cervical epidural block and/or blockade of the medial branch of the dorsal ramus or intra-articular injection of the facet joint with local anesthetic and steroid has been shown to be extremely effective in the treatment of cervical strain. Underlying sleep disturbance and depression are best treated with a tricyclic antidepressant compound such as nortriptyline, which can be started at a single bedtime dose of 25 mg.

SIDE EFFECTS AND COMPLICATIONS

The proximity to the spinal cord and exiting nerve roots makes it imperative that cervical epidural block and cervical facet block be carried out only by those well versed in the regional anatomy and experienced in performing interventional pain management techniques. The proximity to the vertebral artery combined with the vascular nature of this anatomic region makes the potential for intravascular injection high. The injection of even small amounts of local anesthetic into the vertebral arteries will result in seizures. Given the proximity of the brain and brain stem, ataxia after cervical facet block due to vascular uptake of local anesthetic is not an uncommon occurrence. Many patients will also complain of a transient increase in headache and cervicalgia after injection of the cervical facet joints.

CLINICAL PEARLS

Cervical strain is a common cause of neck, occipital, shoulder, and upper extremity pain. It is often confused with cervical radiculopathy and cervical fibromyositis. The clinician must take care to rule out diseases of the cervical spinal cord, such as syringomyelia, that may initially present in a manner similar to cervical strain. Ankylosis spondylitis may also present as cervical strain and must be correctly identified to the patient to avoid ongoing joint damage and functional disability.

Cervical facet block is often combined with atlanto-occipital block when treating pain in the areas discussed. Although neither joint is a true facet joint in the anatomic sense of the word, the block is analogous to the facet joint block technique used commonly by pain practitioners and may be viewed as such. Many pain specialists believe that these techniques are underused in the treatment of "post-whiplash" cervicalgia and cervicogenic headaches. These specialists think that both techniques should be considered when cervical epidural nerve blocks and/or occipital nerve blocks fail to provide palliation of these headache and neck pain syndromes.

15

Brachial Plexopathy

ICD-9 353.0

THE CLINICAL SYNDROME

There are numerous causes of the clinical syndrome called brachial plexopathy. In common to all of them is the constellation of symptoms consisting of neurogenic pain and associated weakness that radiates into the supraclavicular region and upper extremity. More common causes of brachial plexopathy include compression of the plexus by cervical ribs or abnormal muscles (e.g., thoracic outlet syndrome), invasion of the plexus by tumor (e.g., Pancoast's syndrome), direct trauma to the plexus (e.g., stretch injuries and avulsions), inflammatory causes (e.g., Parsonage-Turner syndrome), and postradiation plexopathy (Fig. 15–1).

SIGNS AND SYMPTOMS

Patients suffering from brachial plexopathy will complain of pain radiating to the supraclavicular region and upper extremity. The pain is neuritic in character and may take on a deep, boring quality with invasion of the plexus by tumor. Movement of the neck and shoulder will exacerbate the pain, and patients suffering from brachial plexopathy will often avoid such movements in an effort to palliate the pain. Frozen shoulder often results and may confuse the diagnosis. If thoracic outlet syndrome is suspected, Adson's test may be performed (Fig. 15–2). A positive test is indicated if the radial pulse disappears with neck extended and the head turned toward the affected side. It must be noted that this test is nonspecific and treatment decisions should not be based on this finding alone (see Testing). If the patient presents with severe pain that is shortly followed by profound weakness, brachial plexitis should be considered and can be confirmed with electromyography.

TESTING

All patients presenting with brachial plexopathy, especially without a clear history of antecedent trauma, must undergo magnetic resonance imaging (MRI) of the cervical spine and the brachial plexus. Computed tomography scanning is a reasonable second choice if MRI is contraindicated. Electromyography and nerve conduction velocity testing are extremely sensitive, and the skilled electromyographer can help delineate the specific portion of the plexus that is abnormal. If an inflammatory basis for the plexopathy is suspected, serial electromyography is indicated. If Pancoast's tumor or other tumors of the brachial plexus are suspected, chest x-rays with apical lordotic views may be helpful. Screening laboratory testing consisting of complete blood count, erythrocyte sedimentation rate, antinuclear antibody testing, and automated blood chemistry testing should be performed if the diagnosis of brachial plexopathy is in question to help rule out other causes of the patient's pain.

DIFFERENTIAL DIAGNOSIS

Diseases of the cervical spinal cord, bony cervical spine, and disk can mimic brachial plexopathy. Appropriate testing including MRI and electromyography will help sort out the myriad possibilities, but the clinician should also be aware that more than one pathologic process may exist and contribute to the patient's symptomatology. Syringomyelia, tumors of the cervical spinal cord, and tumors of the cervical nerve roots as they exit the spinal cord (e.g., schwannomas) can be of insidious onset and quite difficult to diagnosis. Pancoast's tumor should be high on the list of diagnostic possibilities in all patients presenting with brachial plexopathy in the absence of clear antecedent trauma, especially if there is a past history of tobacco abuse. Lateral herniated cervical disk, meta-

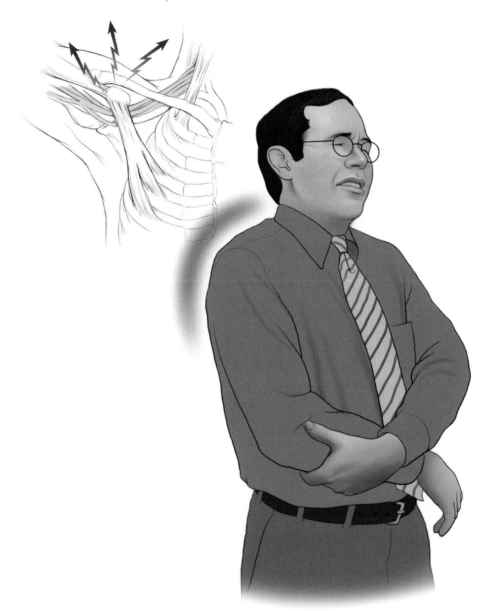

Figure 15–1. The pain of brachial plexopathy radiates from the shoulder and supraclavicular region into the affected upper extremity.

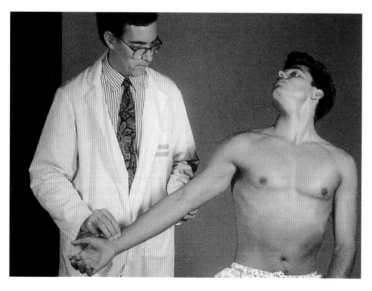

Figure 15–2. The Adson maneuver. The patient inhales deeply, extends the neck fully, and turns the head to the side being examined. This tests for compression in the scalene triangle and is positive if there is a diminution in the radial pulse and reproduction of the patient's symptoms. (From Klippel JH, Dieppe PA: Rheumatology, 2nd ed. London, Mosby, 1998.)

static tumor, or cervical spondylosis, which result in significant nerve root compression, may also present as a brachial plexopathy. Rarely, infection involving the apex of the lung may compress and irritate the plexus.

TREATMENT

Drug Therapy

Gabapentin

Gabapentin is the first-line treatment for the neuritic pain of brachial plexopathy to be considered. Start with a 300-mg dose of gabapentin at bedtime for two nights, and caution the patient about potential side effects, including dizziness, sedation, confusion, and rash. The drug is then increased in 300-mg increments, given in equally divided doses over 2 days, as side effects allow until pain relief is obtained or a total dose of 2400 mg daily is reached. At this point, if the patient has experienced partial relief of pain, blood values are measured and the drug is carefully titrated upward using 100 mg tablets. Rarely will more than 3600 mg daily be required.

Carbamazepine

This drug is useful in those patients suffering from brachial plexopathy who do not experience pain relief with gabapentin. Despite the safety and efficacy of carbamazepine compared with other treatments for brachial plexopathy, much confusion and unfounded anxiety surround its use. This medication, which may be the patient's best chance for pain control, is sometimes discontinued due to laboratory abnormalities erroneously attributed to it. Therefore, baseline screening laboratory values, consisting of a complete blood count, urinalysis, and automated chemistry profile, should be obtained before starting the drug.

Carbamazepine should be started slowly if the pain is not out of control at a starting dose of 100 to 200 mg at bedtime for two nights. The patient should be cautioned regarding side effects, including dizziness, sedation, confusion, and rash. The drug is increased in 100- to 200-mg increments, given in equally divided doses over 2 days, as side effects allow until pain relief is obtained or a total dose of 1200 mg daily is reached. Careful monitoring of laboratory parameters is mandatory to avoid the rare possibility of life-threatening blood dyscrasia. At the first sign of blood count abnormality or rash, this drug should be discontinued. Failure to monitor patients started on carbamazepine can be disastrous because aplastic anemia can occur. When pain relief is obtained, the patient should be kept at that dosage of carbamazepine

for at least 6 months before tapering of this medication is considered. The patient should be informed that under no circumstances should the dosage of drug be changed or the drug refilled or discontinued without the physician's knowledge.

Baclofen

This drug has been reported to be of value in some patients who fail to obtain relief from the aforementioned medications. Baseline laboratory tests should also be obtained before starting baclofen. Start with a 10-mg dose at bedtime for 2 nights, and caution the patient about potential adverse effects, which are the same as those of carbamazepine and gabapentin. The drug is increased in 10-mg increments, given in equally divided doses over 7 days as side effects allow, until pain relief is obtained or a total dose of 80 mg daily is reached. This drug has significant hepatic and central nervous system side effects, including weakness and sedation. As with carbamazepine, careful monitoring of laboratory values is indicated during the initial use of this drug.

In treating individuals with any of the drugs discussed, the physician should make the patient aware that premature tapering or discontinuation of the medication may lead to the recurrence of pain and that it will be more difficult to control pain thereafter.

Invasive Therapy

Brachial Plexus Block

The use of brachial plexus block with local anesthetic and steroid serves as an excellent adjunct to drug treatment of brachial plexopathy. This technique rapidly relieves pain while medications are being titrated to effective levels. The initial block is carried out with preservative-free bupivacaine combined with methylprednisolone. Subsequent daily nerve blocks are carried out in a similar manner with substitution of a lower dose of methylprednisolone. This approach may also be used to obtain control of breakthrough pain.

Radiofrequency Destruction of the Brachial Plexus

The destruction of the brachial plexus can be carried out by creating a radiofrequency lesion under biplanar fluoroscopic guidance. This procedure is reserved for patients for whom all of the aforementioned treatments for brachial plexopathy have failed and whose pain is secondary to tumor or avulsion of the brachial plexus.

Dorsal Root Entry Zone Lesioning (DREZ)

This technique, which is called DREZ lesioning, is the neurosurgical procedure of choice for intractable brachial plexopathy in those patients for whom all of the aforementioned treatments for brachial plexopathy have failed and whose pain is secondary to tumor or avulsion of the brachial plexus. This is a major neurosurgical procedure and carries significant risks.

Physical Modalities

The use of physical and occupational therapy to maintain function and to help palliate pain is a crucial part of the treatment plan for patients suffering from brachial plexopathy. Shoulder abnormalities, including subluxation and adhesive capsulitis, must be aggressively searched for and treated. Occupation therapy to assist in activities of daily living is also important to avoid further deterioration of function.

COMPLICATIONS AND PITFALLS

The pain of brachial plexopathy is difficult to treat. It responds poorly to opioid analgesics and may respond poorly to the medications discussed.

The uncontrolled pain of brachial plexopathy has led to suicide, and strong consideration should be given to the hospitalization of such patients. Correct diagnosis is crucial to successfully treat the pain and dysfunction associated with brachial plexopathy as stretch injuries and contusions of the plexus may respond with time, but plexopathy secondary to tumor or avulsion of the cervical roots will require aggressive treatment.

CLINICAL PEARLS

Brachial plexus block with local anesthetic and steroid represents an excellent stopgap measure for patients suffering the uncontrolled pain of brachial plexopathy while waiting for pharmacologic treatments to take effect. As mentioned, correct diagnosis is paramount to allow the clinician to design a logical treatment plan for patients suffering from brachial plexopathy.

16

Pancoast's Tumor Syndrome

ICD-9 CODE 162.3

THE CLINICAL SYNDROME

Pancoast's tumor syndrome is the result of local growth of tumor from the apex of the lung directly into the brachial plexus. Such tumors usually involve the first and second thoracic nerves as well as the eighth cervical nerve, producing a classic clinical syndrome consisting of severe arm pain and, in some patients, Horner's syndrome (Fig. 16–1). Destruction of the first and second ribs is also common. Diagnosis is usually delayed, and patients are often erroneously treated for cervical radiculopathy or primary shoulder pathology until the diagnosis becomes clear.

SIGNS AND SYMPTOMS

Patients suffering from Pancoast's tumor syndrome will complain of pain radiating to the supraclavicular region and upper extremity. Initially, the lower portion of the brachial plexus is involved as the tumor growth is from below, causing pain in the upper thoracic and lower cervical dermatomes. The pain is neuritic in character and may take on a deep, boring quality with invasion of the brachial plexus by tumor. Movement of the neck and shoulder will exacerbate the pain, and patients suffering from brachial plexopathy will often avoid such movements in an effort to palliate the pain. Frozen shoulder often results and may confuse the diagnosis. As the disease progresses, Horner's syndrome may occur.

TESTING

All patients presenting with brachial plexopathy, especially without a clear history of antecedent

trauma, must undergo magnetic resonance imaging (MRI) of the cervical spine and the brachial plexus (Fig. 16–2). Computed tomography is a reasonable second choice if MRI is contraindicated. Electromyography and nerve conduction velocity testing are extremely sensitive, and the skilled electromyographer can help delineate the specific portion of the plexus that is abnormal. All patients with a significant smoking history in whom Pancoast's tumor or other tumors of the brachial plexus are suspected should undergo chest radiography with apical lordotic views or computed tomography scanning through the apex of the lung. Screening laboratory testing consisting of complete blood count, erythrocyte sedimentation rate, antinuclear antibody testing, and automated blood chemistry testing should be performed if the diagnosis of brachial plexopathy is in question to help rule out other causes of the patient's pain.

DIFFERENTIAL DIAGNOSIS

Diseases of the cervical spinal cord, bony cervical spine, and disk can mimic the brachial plexopathy associated with Pancoast's tumor syndrome. Appropriate testing including MRI and electromyography will help sort out the myriad possibilities, but the clinician should also be aware that more than one pathologic process may exist and contribute to the patient's symptomatology. Syringomyelia, tumors of the cervical spinal cord, and tumors of the cervical nerve roots as they exit the spinal cord (e.g., schwannomas) can be of insidious onset and quite difficult to diagnose. Pancoast's tumor should be high on the list of diagnostic possibilities in all patients presenting with brachial plexopathy in the absence of clear antecedent trauma, especially if there is a past history of tobacco abuse. Lateral herniated cervical disk, metastatic tumor, or cervical spondylosis, which result in significant nerve root compression, may also present as a brachial plexopathy. Rarely, infection involving the apex of the lung may compress and irritate the plexus.

TREATMENT

The primary treatment of Pancoast's tumor syndrome should be aimed at the tumor itself. Based on the cell type and extent of involvement, chemotherapy and radiation therapy may be indicated. Primary surgical treatment of tumors involving the brachial plexus is difficult, and the results are disappointing.

Drug Therapy

Opioid Analgesics

The mainstay of the treatment of pain associated with Pancoast's tumor syndrome is the opioid analgesics. Although as a general rule neuropathic pain responds poorly to opioid analgesics, given the severity of pain and lack of options available to treat the pain of Pancoast's tumor syndrome, a trial of opioid analgesics is warranted. The use of a short-acting potent opioid such as oxycodone is a reasonable starting point. Immediate-release morphine or methadone can also be considered. These drugs can be used in combination with nonsteroidal anti-inflammatory drugs and the adjuvant analgesics described here.

Gabapentin

Gabapentin is the first-line treatment for the neuritic pain of Pancoast's tumor syndrome. Start with 300-mg dose of gabapentin at bedtime for two nights, and caution the patient about potential side effects, including dizziness, sedation, confusion, and rash. The drug is then increased in 300-mg increments, given in equally divided doses over 2 days, as side effects allow until pain relief is obtained or a total dose of 2400 mg daily is reached. At this point, if the patient has experienced partial relief of pain, blood values are measured, and the drug is carefully titrated upward using 100-mg tablets. Rarely will more than 3600 mg daily be required.

Carbamazepine

This drug is useful in those patients suffering from Pancoast's tumor syndrome who do not experience pain relief with gabapentin. Despite the safety and efficacy of carbamazepine compared with other treatments for brachial plexopathy, much confusion and unfounded anxiety surround its use. This medication, which may be the patient's best chance for pain control, is sometimes discontinued due to laboratory ab-

normalities erroneously attributed to it. Therefore, baseline screening laboratory values, consisting of a complete blood count, urinalysis, and automated chemistry profile, should be obtained before starting the drug.

Carbamazepine should be started slowly if the pain is not out of control at a starting dose of 100 to 200 mg at bedtime for two nights. The patient should be cautioned regarding side effects, including dizziness, sedation, confusion, and rash. The drug is increased in 100- to 200-mg increments, given in equally divided doses over 2 days, as side effects allow until pain relief is obtained or a total dose of 1200 mg daily is reached. Careful monitoring of laboratory parameters is mandatory to avoid the rare possibility of life-threatening blood dyscrasia. At the first sign of blood count abnormality or rash, this drug should be discontinued. Failure to monitor patients started on carbamazepine can be disastrous, as aplastic anemia can occur. When pain relief is obtained, the patient should be kept at that dosage of carbamazepine for at least 6 months before tapering of this medication is considered. The patient should be informed that under no circumstances should the dosage of drug be changed or the drug refilled or discontinued without the physician's knowledge.

Baclofen

This drug has been reported to be of value in some patients who fail to obtain relief from the other medications mentioned. Baseline laboratory tests should also be obtained before starting baclofen. Start with a 10-mg dose at bedtime for two nights, and caution the patient about potential adverse effects, which are the same as those of carbamazepine and gabapentin. The drug is increased in 10-mg increments, given in equally divided doses over 7 days as side effects allow, until pain relief is obtained or a total dose of 80 mg daily is reached. This drug has significant hepatic and central nervous system side effects, including weakness and sedation. As with carbamazepine, careful monitoring of laboratory values is indicated during the initial use of this drug.

Invasive Therapy

Brachial Plexus Block

The use of brachial plexus block with local anesthetic and steroid serves as an excellent adjunct to drug treatment of Pancoast's tumor syndrome. This technique rapidly relieves pain while medications are being titrated to effective levels. The initial block is carried out with preservative-free bupivacaine combined with methylprednisolone. Subsequent daily

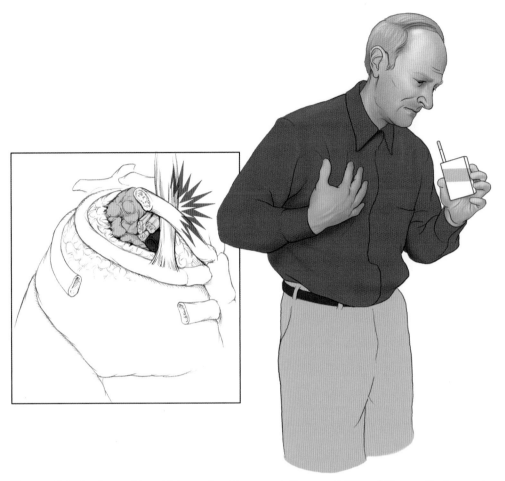

Figure 16–1. A smoking history should suggest the possibility of Pancoast's tumor in patients suffering from shoulder and upper extremity pain.

Figure 16–2. Pancoast's tumor (adenocarcinoma) with infiltration of the brachial plexus. A 65-year-old man complained of severe pain in the shoulder radiating to the elbow, medial side of the forearm, and the fourth and fifth fingers in an ulnar nerve distribution. Screening coronal T1-weighted image shows the brachial plexus from the region of the roots (*long arrows*) to the region of the trunks and divisions, where there is tumor invasion (*short arrow*) and loss of fat planes on the left. (From Stark DD, Bradley WG Jr: Magnetic Resonance Imaging, 3rd ed. St. Louis, Mosby, 1999, p 1824.)

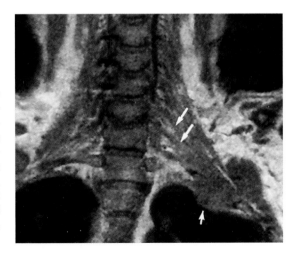

nerve blocks are carried out in a similar manner with the substitution of a lower dose of methylprednisolone. This approach may also be used to obtain control of breakthrough pain.

Radiofrequency Destruction of the Brachial Plexus

The destruction of the brachial plexus can be carried out by creating a radiofrequency lesion under biplanar fluoroscopic guidance. This procedure is reserved for patients for whom all of the aforementioned treatments for Pancoast's tumor syndrome have failed.

Dorsal Root Entry Zone Lesioning (DREZ)

This technique, which is called DREZ lesioning, is the neurosurgical procedure of choice for intractable brachial plexopathy associated with Pancoast's tumor in those patients in whom all other treatments for brachial plexopathy have failed. This is a major neurosurgical procedure and carries significant risks.

Other Neurosurgical Options

The pain of Pancoast's tumor syndrome is notoriously difficult to treat. Cordotomy, deep brain stimulation, and thalamotomy have all been tried in such patients with varying degrees of success.

Physical Modalities

The use of physical and occupational therapy to maintain function and to help palliate pain is a cru-cial part of the treatment plan for patients suffering from Pancoast's tumor syndrome. Shoulder abnormalities, including subluxation and adhesive capsulitis, must be aggressively searched for and treated. Occupational therapy to assist in activities of daily living is also important to avoid further deterioration of function.

COMPLICATIONS AND PITFALLS

The pain of Pancoast's tumor syndrome is difficult to treat. It responds poorly to opioid analgesics and may respond poorly to the aforementioned medications.

The uncontrolled pain of Pancoast's tumor syndrome has led to suicide, and strong consideration should be given to the hospitalization of such patients. Correct diagnosis is crucial to successfully treat the pain and dysfunction associated with brachial plexopathy, as stretch injuries and contusions of the plexus may respond with time, but plexopathy secondary to tumor or avulsion of the cervical roots will require aggressive treatment.

CLINICAL PEARLS

Brachial plexus block with local anesthetic and steroid represents an excellent stopgap measure for patients suffering the uncontrolled pain of brachial plexopathy while waiting for pharmacologic treatments to take effect. As mentioned, correct diagnosis is paramount to allow the clinician to design a logical treatment plan for patients suffering from brachial plexopathy.

17

Thoracic Outlet Syndrome

ICD-9 CODE 353.0

THE CLINICAL SYNDROME

Thoracic outlet syndrome is the name given to a constellation of signs and symptoms including paresthesias and aching pain of the neck, shoulder, and arm that are thought to be due to compression of the brachial plexus and subclavian artery and vein as they exit the space between the shoulder girdle and the first rib or congenitally abnormal structures such as cervical ribs (Fig. 17–1). Either one or all of the structures may be compressed, giving the syndrome a varied clinical expression. Thoracic outlet syndrome is seen most commonly in women between 25 and 50 years of age. The subject of significant debate, the diagnosis and treatment of thoracic outlet syndrome remain controversial.

SIGNS AND SYMPTOMS

Although the symptoms of thoracic outlet syndrome vary, compression of neural structures accounts for most clinical symptomatology. Paresthesias of the upper extremity radiating into the distribution of the ulnar nerve may be misdiagnosed as tardy ulnar palsy. Aching and incoordination of the affected extremity are also common findings. If vascular compression exists, edema or discoloration of the arm may be noted, and in rare instances, venous or arterial thrombosis may occur.

Rarely, the symptoms of thoracic outlet syndrome can be caused by arterial aneurysm, and auscultation of the supraclavicular region will reveal a bruit.

Provocation of the symptoms of thoracic outlet syndrome may be elicited by a variety of maneuvers, including the Adson test and the elevated arm stress test. The Adson test is carried out by palpating the radial pulse on the affected side with the patient's neck extended and the head turned toward the affected side. A diminished pulse is suggestive of thoracic outlet syndrome. The elevated arm stress test is performed by having the patient hold his or her arms over the head and open and close the hands. A patient without thoracic outlet syndrome can perform this maneuver for approximately 3 minutes, whereas patients suffering from thoracic outlet syndrome will experience the onset of symptoms within 30 seconds.

TESTING

Plain radiographs of the cervical spine should be performed on all patients suspected of suffering from thoracic outlet syndrome. Careful review for congenital abnormalities such as cervical ribs or overly elongated transverse processes should be carried out. Patients should also undergo chest radiography with apical lordotic views to rule out Pancoast's tumor. Magnetic resonance imaging (MRI) of the cervical spine is indicated to rule out lesions of the cervical spinal cord and exiting nerve roots. If a diagnosis is still in doubt, MRI of the brachial plexus is also indicated to rule out occult pathology, including primary tumors of the plexus. Screening laboratory testing consisting of complete blood count, erythrocyte sedimentation rate, antinuclear antibody testing, and automated blood chemistry testing should be performed if the diagnosis of brachial plexopathy is in question to help rule out other causes of the patient's pain.

DIFFERENTIAL DIAGNOSIS

Diseases of the cervical spinal cord, the bony cervical spine, and disk can mimic brachial plexopathy. Appropriate testing, including MRI and electromyography, will help sort out the myriad possibilities, but the clinician should also be aware that more than one pathologic process may coexist and contribute to the patient's symptomatology. Syringomyelia, tumors of the cervical spinal cord, and tumors of the cervical nerve roots as they exit the spinal cord (e.g., Schwannomas) can be of insidious onset and quite difficult to diagnose. Pancoast's tumor should be high on the list of diagnostic possibilities in all patients presenting with brachial plexopathy in the absence of clear antecedent trauma, especially if there is a past history of tobacco abuse. Lateral herniated cervical disk, metastatic tumor, or cervical spondylosis, which result in significant nerve root compression, may also present as a brachial plexopathy. Rarely, infection involving the apex of the lung may compress and irritate the plexus.

TREATMENT

Physical Modalities

The primary treatment for patients suffering from thoracic outlet syndrome is the rational use of physical therapy to maintain function and to help palliate pain. Shoulder abnormalities, including subluxation and adhesive capsulitis, must be aggressively searched for and treated. Occupation therapy to assist in activities of daily living is also important to avoid further deterioration of function.

Drug Therapy

Gabapentin

Gabapentin is the first-line pharmacologic treatment for the neuritic pain of thoracic outlet syndrome. Start with a 300-mg dose of gabapentin at bedtime for 2 nights and caution the patient about potential side effects, including dizziness, sedation, confusion, and rash. The drug is then increased in 300-mg increments, given in equally divided doses over 2 days, as side effects allow until pain relief is obtained or a total dosage of 2400 mg/day is reached. At this point, if the patient has experienced partial relief of pain, blood values are measured and the drug is carefully titrated upward using 100-mg tablets. Rarely will more than 3600 mg/day be required.

Carbamazepine

This drug is useful in those patients suffering from thoracic outlet syndrome who do not experience pain relief with gabapentin. Despite the safety and efficacy of carbamazepine compared with other treatments for thoracic outlet syndrome, much confusion and unfounded anxiety surround its use. This medication, which may be the patient's best chance for pain control, is sometimes discontinued due to laboratory abnormalities erroneously attributed to it. Therefore, baseline screening laboratory values, consisting of a complete blood count, urinalysis, and automated chemistry profile, should be obtained before starting the drug.

Carbamazepine should be started slowly if the pain is not out of control. The starting dose is 100 to 200 mg at bedtime for 2 nights, and the patient should be cautioned regarding side effects, including dizziness, sedation, confusion, and rash. The drug is increased in 100- to 200-mg increments, given in equally divided doses over 2 days, as side effects allow until pain relief is obtained or a total dosage of 1200 mg/day is reached. Careful monitoring of laboratory parameters is mandatory to avoid the rare possibility of life-threatening blood dyscrasia. At the first sign of blood count abnormality or rash, this drug should be discontinued. Failure to monitor patients started on carbamazepine can be disastrous because aplastic anemia can occur. When pain relief is obtained, the patient should be kept at that dosage of carbamazepine for at least 6 months before considering tapering of this medication. The patient should be informed that under no circumstances should the dosage of drug be changed or the drug refilled or discontinued without the physician's knowledge.

Baclofen

This drug has been reported to be of value in some patients who fail to obtain relief with gabapentin and carbamazepine. Baseline laboratory tests should also be obtained before starting baclofen. Start with a 10-mg dose at bedtime for 2 nights, and caution the patient about potential adverse effects, which are the same as those of carbamazepine and gabapentin. The drug is increased in 10-mg increments, given in equally divided doses over 7 days as side effects allow, until pain relief is obtained or a total dosage of 80 mg/day is reached. This drug has significant hepatic and central nervous system side effects, including weakness and sedation. As with carbamazepine, careful monitoring of laboratory values is indicated during the initial use of this drug.

In treating individuals with any of these drugs, the physician should make the patient aware that premature tapering or discontinuation of the medication may lead to the recurrence of pain and that it will be more difficult to control pain thereafter.

Invasive Therapy

Brachial Plexus Block

The use of brachial plexus block with local anesthetic and steroid serves as an excellent adjunct to

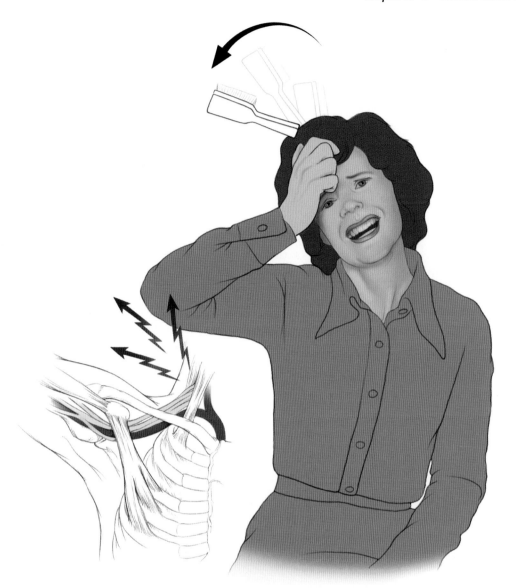

Figure 17–1. Compression of the brachial plexus results in pain and weakness of the affected upper extremity.

drug treatment of thoracic outlet syndrome. This technique rapidly relieves pain while medications are being titrated to effective levels. The initial block is carried out with preservative-free bupivacaine combined with methylprednisolone. Subsequent daily nerve blocks are carried out in a similar manner, substituting a lower dose of methylprednisolone. This approach may also be used to obtain control of breakthrough pain.

Surgical Treatment

In the absence of demonstrable pathology (e.g., a cervical rib), the outcome of surgical treatment for thoracic outlet syndrome is dismal regardless of the surgical technique chosen. In patients with a clear etiology for their symptoms for whom all attempts at conservative therapy have failed, the judicious use of surgical treatment may be a reasonable last step.

COMPLICATIONS AND PITFALLS

The pain and dysfunction of thoracic outlet syndrome are difficult to treat. Physical therapy should be included as a primary treatment in any well-thought-out treatment plan. In general, the pain of thoracic outlet syndrome responds poorly to opioid analgesics, and these drugs should be avoided. The careful use of adjuvant analgesics may help palliate the pain and allow the patient to participate in physical therapy. Correct diagnosis is crucial to successfully treat the pain and dysfunction associated with thoracic outlet syndrome, as stretch injuries and contusions of the plexus may respond with time, but plexopathy secondary to tumor or avulsion of the cervical roots requires aggressive treatment.

CLINICAL PEARLS

Brachial plexus block with local anesthetic and steroid represents an excellent stopgap measure for patients suffering from the uncontrolled pain of thoracic outlet syndrome while waiting for pharmacologic treatments to take effect. As mentioned, correct diagnosis is paramount to allow the clinician to design a logical treatment plan for patients suffering from thoracic outlet syndrome.

IV

Shoulder Pain Syndromes

18
Degenerative Arthritis of the Shoulder

ICD-9 CODE 715.91

THE CLINICAL SYNDROME

The shoulder joint is susceptible to the development of arthritis from a variety of conditions that have in common the ability to damage the joint cartilage. Osteoarthritis is the most common cause of shoulder pain and functional disability. It may occur after seemingly minor trauma or may be the result of repeated microtrauma. Pain around the shoulder and upper arm that is worse with activity will be present in most patients suffering from osteoarthritis of the shoulder. Difficulty in sleeping is also common, as is progressive loss of motion (Fig. 18–1).

SIGNS AND SYMPTOMS

The majority of patients presenting with shoulder pain secondary to osteoarthritis, rotator cuff arthropathy, and post-traumatic arthritis pain will present with the complaint of pain that is localized around the shoulder and upper arm. Activity makes the pain worse, with rest and heat providing some relief. The pain is constant and characterized as aching in nature. The pain may interfere with sleep. Some patients will complain of a grating or popping sensation with use of the joint, and crepitus may be present on physical examination.

In addition the pain, patients suffering from arthritis of the shoulder joint will often experience a gradual decrease in functional ability with decreasing shoulder range of motion, making simple everyday tasks such as hair combing, fastening a brassiere, or reaching overhead quite difficult. With continued disuse, muscle wasting may occur and a frozen shoulder may develop.

TESTING

Plain radiographs are indicated in all patients who present with shoulder pain (Fig. 18–2). Based on the patient's clinical presentation, additional testing, including complete blood count, sedimentation rate, and antinuclear antibody testing, may be indicated. Magnetic resonance imaging of the shoulder is indicated if rotator cuff tear is suspected. Radionucleotide bone scan is indicated if metastatic disease or primary tumor involving the shoulder is being considered.

DIFFERENTIAL DIAGNOSIS

Osteoarthritis of the joint is the most common form of arthritis that results in shoulder joint pain. However, rheumatoid arthritis, post-traumatic arthritis, and rotator cuff tear arthropathy are also common causes of shoulder pain secondary to arthritis. Less common causes of arthritis-induced shoulder pain include the collagen vascular diseases, infection, villonodular synovitis, and Lyme disease. Acute infectious arthritis will usually be accompanied by significant systemic symptoms, including fever and malaise, and should be easily recognized by the astute clinician and treated appropriately with culture and antibiotics, rather than injection therapy. The collagen vascular diseases will generally present as a polyarthropathy rather than as a monoarthropathy limited to the shoulder joint, although shoulder pain secondary to collagen vascular disease responds exceedingly well to the intra-articular injection technique described here.

TREATMENT

Initial treatment of the pain and functional disability associated with osteoarthritis of the shoulder should include a combination of the nonsteroidal anti-inflammatory drugs or cyclooxygenase-2 inhibitors and physical therapy. The local application of heat and cold may also be beneficial. For patients who do not respond to these treatment modalities, an intra-articular injection of local anesthetic and steroid may be a reasonable next step.

Intra-articular injection of the shoulder is performed by placing the patient in the supine position and preparing with antiseptic solution the skin overlying the shoulder, subacromial region, and joint space. A sterile syringe containing 2.0 mL of 0.25% preservative-free bupivacaine and 40 mg methylprednisolone is attached to a 1½-inch 25-gauge needle using strict aseptic technique. With strict aseptic technique, the midpoint of the acromion is identified, and at a point approximately 1 inch below the midpoint, the shoulder joint space is identified. The needle is then carefully advanced through the skin and subcutaneous tissues through the joint capsule into the joint (see Fig. 18–2). If bone is encountered, the needle is withdrawn into the subcutaneous tissues and redirected superiorly and slightly more medial. After entering of the joint space, the contents of the syringe are gently injected. There should be little resistance to injection. If resistance is encountered, the needle is probably in a ligament or tendon and should be advanced slightly into the joint space until the injection proceeds without significant resistance. The needle is then removed, and a sterile pressure dressing and ice pack are placed at the injection site.

SIDE EFFECTS AND COMPLICATIONS

The major complication of intra-articular injection of the shoulder is infection. This complication should be exceedingly rare if strict aseptic technique is followed. Approximately 25% of patients will complain of a transient increase in pain after intra-articular injection of the shoulder joint and should be warned of such.

CLINICAL PEARLS

Osteoarthritis of the shoulder is a common complaint encountered in clinical practice. It must be separated from other causes of shoulder pain, including rotator cuff tears. Intra-articular injection of the shoulder is extremely effective in the treatment of pain secondary to the aforementioned causes of arthritis of the shoulder joint. Coexistent bursitis and tendinitis may also contribute to shoulder pain and may require additional treatment with more localized injection of local anesthetic and methylprednisolone acetate steroid. This technique is a safe procedure if careful attention is paid to the clinically relevant anatomy in the areas to be injected. Care must be taken to use sterile technique to avoid infection, and to use universal precautions to avoid risk to the operator. The incidence of ecchymosis and hematoma formation can be decreased if pressure is placed on the injection site immediately after injection. The use of physical modalities including local heat as well as gentle range of motion exercises should be introduced several days after the patient undergoes this injection technique for shoulder pain. Vigorous exercises should be avoided because they will exacerbate the patient's symptomatology. Simple analgesics and nonsteroidal anti-inflammatory drugs or a cyclooxygenase-2 inhibitor may be used concurrently with this injection technique.

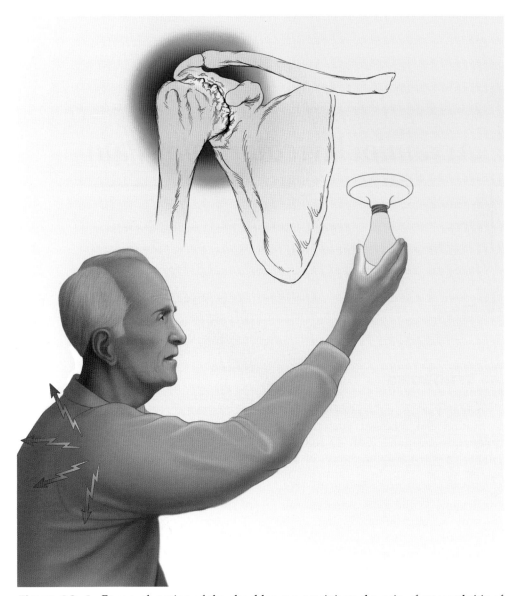

Figure 18–1. Range of motion of the shoulder can precipitate the pain of osteoarthritis of the shoulder.

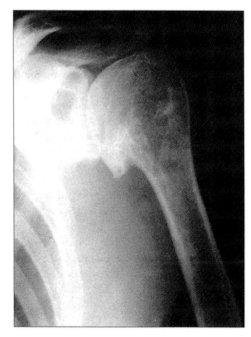

Figure 18–2. Osteoarthritis of the shoulder. The radiograph shows all the features of a "hypertrophic" form of osteoarthritis of the glenohumeral joint, with joint space narrowing, subchondral sclerosis, large cysts in the glenoid, and the massive inferior osteophytosis that is characteristic of this condition. (From Klippel JH, Dieppe PA: Rheumatology, 2nd ed. London, Mosby, 1998.)

19 Acromioclavicular Joint Pain

ICD-9 CODE 719.41

THE CLINICAL SYNDROME

The acromioclavicular joint is vulnerable to injury from both acute trauma and repeated microtrauma. Acute injuries frequently take the form of falls directly onto the shoulder when playing sports or falling from bicycles. Repeated strain from throwing injuries or working with the arm raised across the body may also result in trauma to the joint. After trauma, the joint may become acutely inflamed, and if the condition becomes chronic, arthritis of the acromioclavicular joint may develop.

SIGNS AND SYMPTOMS

The patient suffering from acromioclavicular joint dysfunction will frequently complain of pain when reaching across the chest (Fig. 19–1). Often, the patient will be unable to sleep on the affected shoulder and may complain of a grinding sensation in the joint, especially on first awakening. Physical examination may reveal enlargement or swelling of the joint with tenderness to palpation. Downward traction or passive adduction of the affected shoulder may cause increased pain. If there is disruption of the ligaments of the acromioclavicular joint, these maneuvers may reveal joint instability.

TESTING

Plain radiographs of the joint may reveal narrowing or sclerosis of the joint consistent with osteoarthritis. Magnetic resonance imaging is indicated if disruption of the ligaments is suspected. The injection technique described here will serve as both a diagnos-

tic and therapeutic maneuver. If polyarthritis is present, screening laboratory testing, consisting of a complete blood count, erythrocyte sedimentation rate, and antinuclear antibody testing, should be performed.

DIFFERENTIAL DIAGNOSIS

Osteoarthritis of the acromioclavicular joint is a frequent cause of shoulder pain. This is usually the result of trauma. However, rheumatoid arthritis and rotator cuff tear arthropathy are also common causes of shoulder pain that may mimic the pain of acromioclavicular joint pain and confuse the diagnosis. Less common causes of arthritis-induced shoulder pain include the collagen vascular diseases, infection, and Lyme disease. Acute infectious arthritis will usually be accompanied by significant systemic symptoms, including fever and malaise, and should be easily recognized by the astute clinician and treated appropriately with culture and antibiotics rather than with injection therapy. The collagen vascular diseases will generally present as a polyarthropathy rather than as monoarthropathy limited to the shoulder joint, although shoulder pain secondary to collagen vascular disease responds exceedingly well to the intra-articular injection technique described here.

TREATMENT

Initial treatment of the pain and functional disability associated with acromioclavicular joint pain should include a combination of the nonsteroidal anti-inflammatory drugs or cyclooxygenase-2 inhibitors and physical therapy. The local application of heat and cold may also be beneficial. For patients who do not respond to these treatment modalities, an intra-articular injection of local anesthetic and steroid may be a reasonable next step.

Intra-articular injection of the acromioclavicular

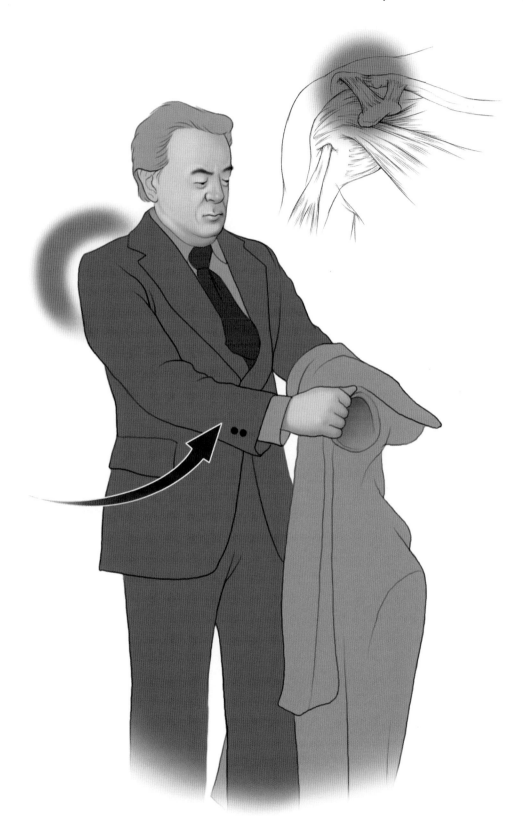

Figure 19–1. The pain of acromioclavicular joint dysfunction is made worse by reaching across the chest.

joint is performed by placing the patient in the supine position and preparing with antiseptic solution the skin overlying the superior shoulder and distal clavicle. A sterile syringe containing 1.0 mL of 0.25% preservative-free bupivacaine and 40 mg methylprednisolone is attached to a 1½-inch 25-gauge needle using strict aseptic technique. With strict aseptic technique, the top of the acromion is identified, and at a point approximately 1 inch medially, the acromioclavicular joint space is identified. The needle is then carefully advanced through the skin and subcutaneous tissues through the joint capsule into the joint (Fig. 19–2). If bone is encountered, the needle is withdrawn into the subcutaneous tissues and redirected slightly more medially. After the joint space is entered, the contents of the syringe are gently injected. There should be some resistance to injection because the joint space is small and the joint capsule is dense. If significant resistance is encountered, the needle is probably in a ligament and should be advanced slightly into the joint space until the injection proceeds with only limited resistance. If no resistance is encountered on injection, the joint space is probably not intact and magnetic resonance imaging is recommended. The needle is then removed, and a sterile pressure dressing and ice pack are placed at the injection site.

SIDE EFFECTS AND COMPLICATIONS

The major complication of intra-articular injection of the acromioclavicular joint is infection. This complication should be exceedingly rare if strict aseptic technique is followed. Approximately 25% of patients will complain of a transient increase in pain after intra-articular injection of the shoulder joint and should be warned in advance of such.

CLINICAL PEARLS

This injection technique is extremely effective in the treatment of pain secondary to the aforementioned causes of arthritis of the acromioclavicular joint. Coexistent bursitis and tendinitis may also contribute to shoulder pain and may require additional treatment with more localized injection of local anesthetic and methylprednisolone acetate steroid. This technique is a safe procedure if careful attention is paid to the clinically relevant anatomy in the areas to be injected. Care must be taken to use sterile technique to avoid infection, as well as the use of universal precautions to avoid risk to the operator. The incidence of ecchymosis and hematoma formation can be decreased if pressure is placed on the injection site immediately after injection. The use of physical modalities including local heat as well as gentle range of motion exercises should be introduced several days after the patient undergoes this injection technique for shoulder pain. Vigorous exercises should be avoided because they will exacerbate the patient's symptomatology. Simple analgesics and nonsteroidal anti-inflammatory drugs or a cyclooxygenase-2 inhibitor may be used concurrently with this injection technique.

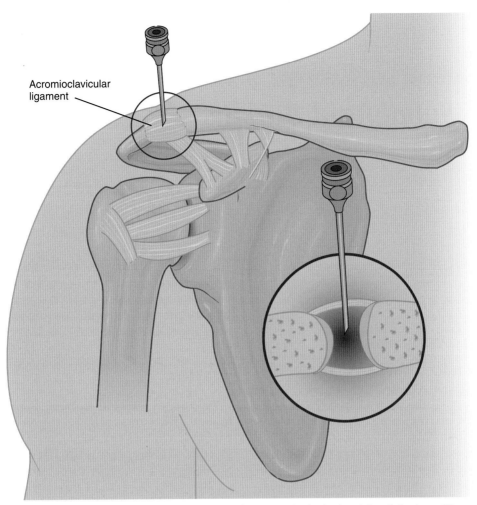

Acromioclavicular
ligament

Figure 19–2. Proper needle placement for acromioclavicular joint injection. (From Waldman SD: Atlas of Pain Management Injection Techniques. Philadelphia, WB Saunders, 2000, p 41.)

20

Subdeltoid Bursitis

ICD-9 CODE 726.19

THE CLINICAL SYNDROME

The subdeltoid bursa is vulnerable to injury from both acute trauma and repeated microtrauma. Acute injuries frequently take the form of direct trauma to the shoulder when playing sports or falling from bicycles. Repeated strain from throwing injuries, bowling, carrying a heavy briefcase, working with the arm raised across the body, rotator cuff injuries, or repetitive motion associated with assembly line work may result in inflammation of the subdeltoid bursa. The subdeltoid bursa lies primarily under the acromion extending laterally between the deltoid muscle and joint capsule under the deltoid muscle. It may exist as a single bursal sac or in some patients as a multisegmented series of sacs that may be loculated in nature. If the inflammation of the subdeltoid bursa becomes chronic, calcification of the bursa may occur.

The patient suffering from subdeltoid bursitis will frequently complain of pain with any movement of the shoulder but especially with abduction. The pain is localized to the subdeltoid area with referred pain often noted at the insertion of the deltoid at the deltoid tuberosity on the upper third of the humerus (Fig. 20–1). Often, the patient will be unable to sleep on the affected shoulder and may complain of a sharp, catching sensation when abducting the shoulder, especially on first awakening.

SIGNS AND SYMPTOMS

Physical examination may reveal point tenderness over the acromion, and occasionally swelling of the bursa will give the affected deltoid muscle an edematous feel. Passive elevation and medial rotation of the affected shoulder will reproduce the pain, as will re-sisted abduction and lateral rotation. Sudden release of resistance during this maneuver will markedly increase the pain. Rotator cuff tear may mimic or coexist with subdeltoid bursitis and may confuse the diagnosis (See Differential Diagnosis).

TESTING

Plain radiographs of the shoulder may reveal calcification of the bursa and associated structures consistent with chronic inflammation. Magnetic resonance imaging is indicated if tendinitis, partial disruption of the ligaments, or rotator cuff tear is considered. Based on the patient's clinical presentation, additional testing, including complete blood count, sedimentation rate, and antinuclear antibody testing, may be indicated. Magnetic resonance imaging of the shoulder is indicated if rotator cuff tear is suspected. Radionucleotide bone scan is indicated if metastatic disease or primary tumor involving the shoulder is being considered. The injection technique described here will serve as both a diagnostic and therapeutic maneuver.

DIFFERENTIAL DIAGNOSIS

Subdeltoid bursitis is one of the most common causes of shoulder joint pain. Osteoarthritis, rheumatoid arthritis, post-traumatic arthritis, and rotator cuff tear arthropathy are also common causes of shoulder pain that may coexist with subdeltoid bursitis. Less common causes of arthritis-induced shoulder pain include the collagen vascular diseases, infection, villonodular synovitis, and Lyme disease. Acute infectious arthritis will usually be accompanied by significant systemic symptoms, including fever and malaise, and should be easily recognized by the astute clinician and treated appropriately with culture and antibiotics, rather than with injection therapy. The collagen vascular diseases will generally present as a polyarthropathy rather than as a monoarthropathy limited

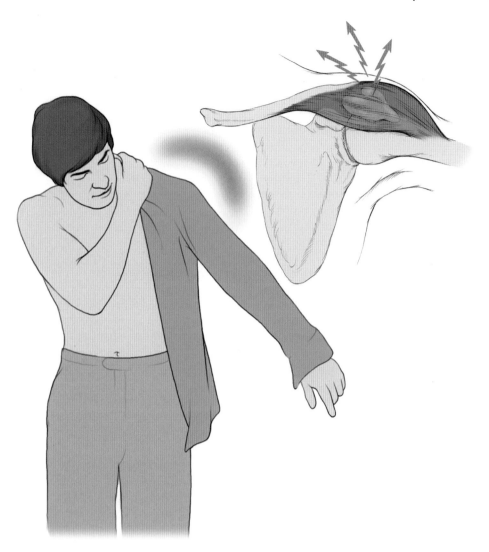

Figure 20–1. Abduction of the shoulder will exacerbate the pain of subdeltoid bursitis.

to the shoulder joint, although shoulder pain secondary to collagen vascular disease responds exceedingly well to the injection technique described here.

TREATMENT

Initial treatment of the pain and functional disability associated with osteoarthritis of the shoulder should include a combination of the nonsteroidal anti-inflammatory drugs or cyclooxygenase-2 inhibitors and physical therapy. The local application of heat and cold may also be beneficial. For patients who do not respond to these treatment modalities, an injection of local anesthetic and steroid into the subdeltoid bursa may be a reasonable next step.

Injection into the subdeltoid bursa is performed by placing the patient in the supine position. Proper preparation with antiseptic solution of the skin overlying the superior shoulder, acromion, and distal clavicle is carried out. A sterile syringe containing 4.0 mL of 0.25% preservative-free bupivacaine and 40 mg methylprednisolone is attached to a 1½-inch 25-gauge needle using strict aseptic technique. With strict aseptic technique, the lateral edge of the acromion is identified, and at the midpoint of the lateral edge, the injection site is identified. At this point, the needle is carefully advanced in a slightly cephalad trajectory through the skin and subcutaneous tissues beneath the acromion capsule into the bursa (Fig. 20–2). If bone is encountered, the needle is withdrawn into the subcutaneous tissues and redirected slightly more inferiorly. After entering the bursa, the contents of the syringe are gently injected while the needle is slowly withdrawn. There should be minimal resistance to injection unless calcification of the bursal sac is present. Calcification of the bursal sac will be identified as a resistance to needle advancement with an associated gritty feel. Significant calcific bursitis may ultimately require surgical excision to effect complete relief of symptoms. The needle is then removed, and a sterile pressure dressing and ice pack are placed at the injection site.

SIDE EFFECTS AND COMPLICATIONS

The major complication of injection of the subdeltoid bursa is infection. This complication should be exceedingly rare if strict aseptic technique is followed. Approximately 25% of patients will complain of a transient increase in pain after injection of the subdeltoid bursa and should be warned of such.

CLINICAL PEARLS

This injection technique is extremely effective in the treatment of pain secondary to subdeltoid bursitis. Coexistent arthritis and tendinitis may also contribute to shoulder pain and may require additional treatment with more localized injection of local anesthetic and methylprednisolone acetate steroid. This technique is a safe procedure if careful attention is paid to the clinically relevant anatomy in the areas to be injected. Care must be taken to use sterile technique to avoid infection as well as universal precautions to avoid risk to the operator. The incidence of ecchymosis and hematoma formation can be decreased if pressure is placed on the injection site immediately after injection. The use of physical modalities including local heat as well as gentle range of motion exercises should be introduced several days after the patient undergoes this injection technique for shoulder pain. Vigorous exercises should be avoided because they will exacerbate the patient's symptomatology. Simple analgesics and nonsteroidal anti-inflammatory agents may be used concurrently with this injection technique.

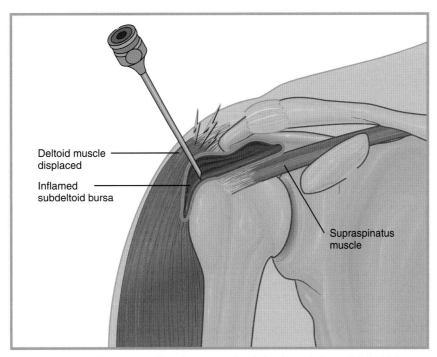

Deltoid muscle
displaced

Inflamed
subdeltoid bursa

Supraspinatus
muscle

Figure 20–2. Proper needle placement for injection of the subdeltoid bursa. (From Waldman SD: Atlas of Pain Management Injection Techniques. Philadelphia, WB Saunders, 2000, p 61.)

21

Bicipital Tendinitis

ICD-9 CODE 726.12

THE CLINICAL SYNDROME

The tendons of the long and short heads of the biceps either alone or together are particularly prone to the development of tendinitis, which is known as bicipital tendinitis. The etiology of this syndrome is usually at least in part due to impingement on the tendons of the biceps at the coracoacromial arch. The onset of bicipital tendinitis is usually acute, occurring after overuse or misuse of the shoulder joint. Inciting factors may include activities such as trying to start a recalcitrant lawn mower, practicing an overhead tennis serve, or overaggressive follow through when driving golf balls. The biceps muscle and tendons are susceptible to trauma and to wear and tear from overuse and misuse as mentioned. If the damage becomes severe enough, the tendon of the long head of the biceps can rupture, leaving the patient with a telltale "Popeye" biceps (named after the cartoon character with the unique biceps). This deformity can be accentuated by having the patient perform Luningston's maneuver, which is having the patient place his or her hands behind the head and flex the biceps muscle.

SIGNS AND SYMPTOMS

The pain of bicipital tendinitis is constant and severe and is localized in the anterior shoulder over the bicipital groove (Fig. 21–1). A catching sensation may also accompany the pain. Significant sleep disturbance is often reported. The patient may attempt to splint the inflamed tendons by internal rotation of the humerus, which moves the biceps tendon from beneath the coracoacromial arch. Patients with bicipital tendinitis will exhibit a positive Yergason's sign, which is production of pain on active supination of the forearm against resistance with the elbow flexed at a right angle (Fig. 21–2). Bursitis often accompanies bicipital tendinitis.

In addition to this pain, patients suffering from bicipital tendinitis will often experience a gradual decrease in functional ability with decreasing shoulder range of motion, making simple everyday tasks such as hair combing, fastening a brassiere, and reaching overhead quite difficult. With continued disuse, muscle wasting may occur and a frozen shoulder may develop.

TESTING

Plain radiographs are indicated for all patients who present with shoulder pain. Based on the patient's clinical presentation, additional testing, including complete blood count, sedimentation rate, and antinuclear antibody testing, may be indicated. Magnetic resonance imaging of the shoulder is indicated if rotator cuff tear is suspected. The following injection technique will serve as both a diagnostic and therapeutic maneuver.

DIFFERENTIAL DIAGNOSIS

Bicipital tendinitis is usually a straightforward clinical diagnosis. However, coexisting bursitis or tendinitis of the should from overuse or misuse may confuse the diagnosis. Occasional partial rotator cuff tear can be mistaken for bicipital tendinitis. If the clinical situation dictates, consideration should be given to primary or secondary tumors involving the shoulder, superior sulcus of the lung, or proximal humerus. The pain of acute herpes zoster, which occurs before the eruption of vesicular rash, can also mimic bicipital tendinitis.

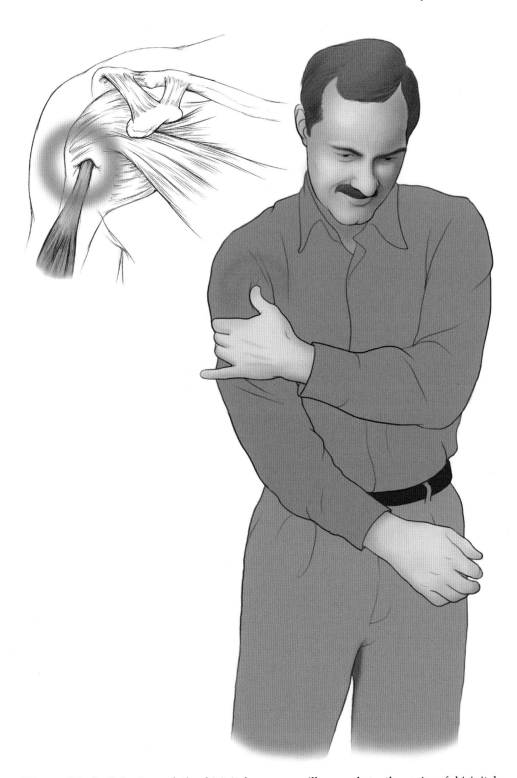

Figure 21–1. Palpation of the bicipital groove will exacerbate the pain of bicipital tendinitis.

TREATMENT

Initial treatment of the pain and functional disability associated with bicipital tendinitis should include a combination of the nonsteroidal anti-inflammatory drugs or cyclooxygenase-2 inhibitors and physical therapy. The local application of heat and cold may also be beneficial. For patients who do not respond to these treatment modalities, the following injection technique with local anesthetic and steroid may be a reasonable next step.

Injection for bicipital tendinitis is carried out by placing the patient in the supine position. The arm is then externally rotated approximately 45 degrees. The coracoid process is identified anteriorly. Just lateral to the coracoid process is the lesser tuberosity. The lesser tuberosity will be more easily palpated as the arm is passively rotated. The point overlying the tuberosity is marked with a sterile marker.

Proper preparation with antiseptic solution of the skin overlying the anterior shoulder is carried out. A sterile syringe containing 1.0 mL of 0.25% preservative-free bupivacaine and 40 mg methylprednisolone is attached to a 1½-inch 25-gauge needle using strict aseptic technique. With strict aseptic technique, the previously marked point is palpated and the insertion of the bicipital tendon is reidentified with the gloved finger. The needle is then carefully advanced at this point through the skin and subcutaneous tissues and underlying tendon until it impinges on bone. The needle is then withdrawn 1 to 2 mm out of the periosteum of the humerus, and the contents of the syringe are gently injected. There should be slight resistance to injection. If no resistance is encountered, the needle tip is either in the joint space itself or the tendon is ruptured. If there is significant resistance to injection, the needle tip is probably in the substance of a ligament or tendon and should be advanced or withdrawn slightly until the injection proceeds without significant resistance. The needle is then removed, and a sterile pressure dressing and ice pack are placed at the injection site.

SIDE EFFECTS AND COMPLICATIONS

The major complication of this injection technique is infection. This complication should be exceedingly rare if strict aseptic technique is followed. Trauma to the bicipital tendon from the injection itself remains an ever-present possibility. Tendons that are highly inflamed or previously damaged are subject to rupture if they are directly injected. This complication can be greatly decreased if the clinician uses gentle technique and stops injecting immediately if significant resistance to injection is encountered. Approximately 25% of patients will complain of a transient increase in pain after intra-articular injection of the shoulder joint and should be warned of such.

CLINICAL PEARLS

The musculotendinous unit of the shoulder joint is susceptible to the development of tendinitis for several reasons. First, the joint is subjected to a wide range of motions that are often repetitive in nature. Second, the space in which the musculotendinous unit functions is restricted by the coracoacromial arch, making impingement a likely possibility with extreme movements of the joint. Third, the blood supply to the musculotendinous unit is poor, making the healing of microtrauma more difficult. All of these factors can contribute to tendinitis of one or more of the tendons of the shoulder joint. Calcium deposition around the tendon may occur if the inflammation continues, making subsequent treatment more difficult. Tendinitis of the biceps tendon frequently coexists with bursitis of the associated bursae of the shoulder joint, creating additional pain and functional disability.

This injection technique is extremely effective in the treatment of pain secondary to the aforementioned causes of shoulder pain. Coexistent bursitis and arthritis may also contribute to shoulder pain and may require additional treatment with a more localized injection of local anesthetic and methylprednisolone acetate steroid. This technique is a safe procedure if careful attention is paid to the clinically relevant anatomy in the areas to be injected. Care must be taken to use sterile technique to avoid infection, as well as the use of universal precautions to avoid risk to the operator. The incidence of ecchymosis and hematoma formation can be decreased if pressure is placed on the injection site immediately after injection. The use of physical modalities including local heat as well as gentle range of motion exercises should be introduced several days after the patient undergoes this injection technique for shoulder pain. Vigorous exercises should be avoided because they will exacerbate the patient's symptomatology. Simple analgesics and the nonsteroidal anti-inflammatory drugs or a cyclooxygenase-2 inhibitor may be used concurrently with this injection technique.

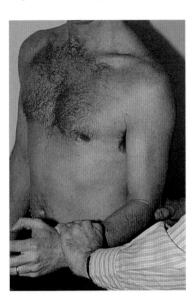

Figure 21–2. Yergason's test for bicipital tendinitis. (From Klippel JH, Dieppe PA: Rheumatology, 2nd ed. London, Mosby, 1998.)

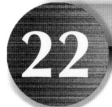

Rotator Cuff Tear

ICD-9 CODE
ROTATOR CUFF TEAR
TRAUMATIC 840.4

ROTATOR CUFF TEAR
DEGENERATIVE 726.10

THE CLINICAL SYNDROME

Rotator cuff tears represent a common cause of shoulder pain and dysfunction encountered in clinical practice. A rotator cuff tear will frequently occur after seemingly minor trauma to the musculotendinous unit of the shoulder. However, in most cases, the pathology responsible for the tear is usually a long time in the making and the most often is the result of ongoing tendinitis. The rotator cuff is made up of the subscapularis, supraspinatus infraspinatus, and teres minor muscles and associated tendons. The function of the rotator cuff is to rotate the arm to help provide shoulder joint stability along the other muscles, tendons, and ligaments of the shoulder.

The supraspinatus and infraspinatus muscle tendons are particularly susceptible to the development of tendinitis for several reasons. First, the joint is subjected to a wide variety of motions that are often repetitive in nature. Second, the space in which the musculotendinous unit functions is restricted by the coracoacromial arch, making impingement a likely possibility with extreme movements of the joint. Third, the blood supply to the musculotendinous unit is poor, making healing of microtrauma more difficult. All of these factors can contribute to tendinitis of one or more of the tendons of the shoulder joint.

Calcium deposition around the tendon may occur if the inflammation continues, making subsequent treatment more difficult.

Bursitis often accompanies rotator cuff tears and may require specific treatment. In addition to the pain, patients suffering from rotator cuff tear will often experience a gradual decrease in functional ability with decreasing shoulder range of motion, making simple everyday tasks such as hair combing, fastening a brassiere, or reaching overhead quite difficult. With continued disuse, muscle wasting may occur and a frozen shoulder may develop.

SIGNS AND SYMPTOMS

The patient presenting with rotator cuff tear will frequently complain that he or she cannot lift the arm above the level of the shoulder without using the other arm to lift it (Fig. 22-1). On physical examination, the patient will have weakness on external rotation if the infraspinatus is involved and weakness in abduction above the level of the shoulder if the supraspinatus is involved. Tenderness to palpation in the subacromial region is often present. Patients with partial rotator cuff tears will exhibit loss of the ability to smoothly reach overhead. Patients with complete tears will exhibit anterior migration of the humeral head as well as a complete inability to reach above the level of the shoulder. A positive drop arm test, which is the inability to hold the arm abducted at the level of the shoulder after the supported arm is released, will often be seen with complete tears of the rotator cuff. Moseley's test for rotator cuff tear, which is performed by having the patient actively abduct the arm to 80 degrees and then adding gentle resistance, which will force the arm to drop if complete rotator cuff tear is present, will also be positive.

Passive range of motion of the shoulder is normal, but active range of motion is limited.

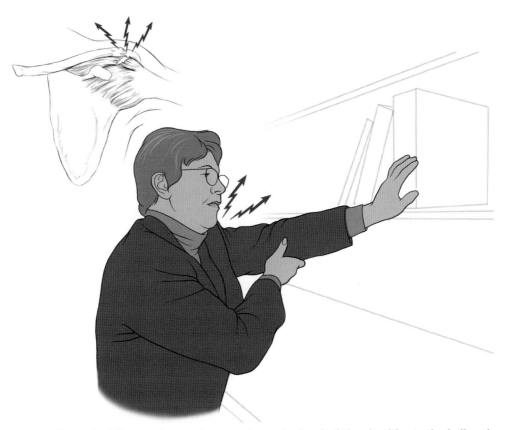

Figure 22–1. Inability to elevate the arm above the level of the shoulder is the hallmark of rotator cuff disturbance.

The pain of rotator cuff tear is constant and severe and is made worse with abduction and external rotation of the shoulder. Significant sleep disturbance is often reported. The patient may attempt to splint the inflamed subscapularis tendon by limiting medial rotation of the humerus.

TESTING

Plain radiographs are indicated in all patients who present with shoulder pain. Based on the patient's clinical presentation, additional testing, including complete blood count, sedimentation rate, and antinuclear antibody testing, may be indicated. Magnetic resonance imaging of the shoulder is indicated if rotator cuff tear is suspected.

DIFFERENTIAL DIAGNOSIS

Because rotator cuff tears may occur after seemingly minor trauma, the diagnosis will often be delayed. The tear may be either partial or complete, further confusing the diagnosis, although a careful physical examination can help distinguish the two. Tendinitis of the musculotendinous unit of the shoulder frequently coexists with bursitis of the associated bursae of the shoulder joint, creating additional pain and functional disability. This ongoing pain and functional disability can cause the patient to splint the shoulder group with resultant abnormal movement of the shoulder, which puts additional stress on the rotator cuff. This can lead to further trauma to the rotator cuff. It should be remembered that with rotator cuff tears, passive range of motion is normal but active range of motion is limited, in contradistinction to frozen shoulder, where both passive and active range of motion is limited. Rotator cuff tear rarely occurs before the age of 40 except in cases of severe acute trauma to the shoulder.

TREATMENT

Initial treatment of the pain and functional disability associated with rotator cuff tear should include a combination of the nonsteroidal anti-inflammatory drugs or cyclooxygenase-2 inhibitors and physical therapy. The local application of heat and cold may also be beneficial. For patients who do not respond to these treatment modalities, the following injection technique may be a reasonable next step before surgical intervention.

Injection for rotator cuff tear is carried out by placing the patient in the supine position and preparing with antiseptic solution the skin overlying the superior shoulder, acromion, and distal clavicle. A sterile syringe containing 4.0 mL of 0.25% preservative-free bupivacaine and 40 mg methylprednisolone is attached to a 1½-inch 25-gauge needle using strict aseptic technique. With strict aseptic technique, the lateral edge of the acromion is identified, and at the midpoint of the lateral edge, the injection site is identified. At this point, the needle is carefully advanced in a slightly cephalad trajectory through the skin, subcutaneous tissues, and deltoid muscle beneath the acromion process. If bone is encountered, the needle is withdrawn into the subcutaneous tissues and redirected slightly more inferiorly. After the needle is in place, the contents of the syringe are gently injected. There should be minimal resistance to injection unless calcification of the subacromial bursal sac is present. Calcification of the bursal sac will be identified as a resistance to needle advancement with an associated gritty feel. Significant calcific bursitis may ultimately require surgical excision to effect complete relief of symptoms. The needle is then removed, and a sterile pressure dressing and ice pack are placed at the injection site.

SIDE EFFECTS AND COMPLICATIONS

The major side effect or complication when treating patients with suspected rotator cuff tears is failure to correctly identify partial rotator cuff tears and treat them before they become complete. This problem usually occurs because a magnetic resonance image of the shoulder was not obtained and the diagnosis of shoulder pain and dysfunction was made on clinical grounds.

The major complication of the injection technique just discussed is infection. This complication should be exceedingly rare if strict aseptic technique is followed. The possibility of trauma to the rotator cuff from the injection itself remains an ever-present possibility. Tendons that are highly inflamed or previously damaged are subject to rupture if they are directly injected. This could convert a partial rotator cuff tear into a complete tear. This complication can be greatly decreased if the clinician uses gentle technique and stops injecting immediately if significant resistance to injection is encountered. Approximately 25% of patients will complain of a transient increase in pain after the injection technique and should be warned of such.

CLINICAL PEARLS

This injection technique is extremely effective in the treatment of pain secondary to the rotator cuff tears. This technique is not a substitute for surgery but can be used to palliate the pain of partial tears or in patients with complete tears in whom surgery is not contemplated. Coexistent bursitis and arthritis may also contribute to shoulder pain and may require additional treatment with a more localized injection of local anesthetic and methylprednisolone acetate steroid. This technique is a safe procedure if careful attention is paid to the clinically relevant anatomy in the areas to be injected. Care must be taken to use sterile technique to avoid infection, as well as universal precautions to avoid risk to the operator. The incidence of ecchymosis and hematoma formation can be decreased if pressure is placed on the injection site immediately after injection. The use of physical modalities including local heat as well as gentle range of motion exercises should be introduced several days after the patient undergoes this injection technique for shoulder pain. Vigorous exercises should be avoided because they will exacerbate the patient's symptomatology and may lead to complete tendon rupture. Simple analgesics and nonsteroidal anti-inflammatory drugs may be used concurrently with this injection technique. It should be noted that partial tears may be amenable to arthroscopic or minimal incision surgery and the clinician should not wait until the tear is complete before obtaining orthopedic consultation.

V Elbow Pain Syndromes

23 *Arthritis Pain—Elbow*

THE CLINICAL SYNDROME

Elbow pain secondary to degenerative arthritis is a common problem encountered in clinical practice. Osteoarthritis of the joint is the most common form of arthritis that results in elbow joint pain. Frequently, tendinitis and bursitis will coexist with arthritis pain of the elbow, making correct diagnosis more difficult. The olecranon bursa lies in the posterior aspect of the elbow joint and may become inflamed as a result of direct trauma or overuse of the joint. Bursae susceptible to the development of bursitis also exist between the insertion of the biceps and the head of the radius as well as in the antecubital and cubital area.

In addition to the aforementioned pain, patients suffering from arthritis of the elbow joint will often experience a gradual decrease in functional ability with decreasing elbow range of motion, making simple everyday tasks such as using a computer keyboard, holding a coffee cup, or turning a door knob overhead quite difficult (Fig. 23–1). With continued disuse, muscle wasting may occur and an adhesive capsulitis with subsequent ankylosis may develop.

SIGNS AND SYMPTOMS

The majority of patients presenting with elbow pain secondary to osteoarthritis and post-traumatic arthritis pain will present with the complaint of pain that is localized around the elbow and forearm. Activity makes the pain worse, with rest and heat providing some relief. The pain is constant and characterized as aching in nature. The pain may interfere with sleep. Some patients will complain of a grating or popping sensation with use of the joint, and crepitus may be present on physical examination.

TESTING

Plain radiographs are indicated for all patients who present with elbow pain. Based on the patient's clinical presentation, additional testing, including complete blood count, sedimentation rate, and antinuclear antibody testing, may be indicated. Magnetic resonance imaging of the elbow is indicated if joint instability is suspected.

DIFFERENTIAL DIAGNOSIS

Rheumatoid arthritis, post-traumatic arthritis, and psoriatic arthritis are also common causes of elbow pain secondary to arthritis. Less common causes of arthritis-induced elbow pain include the collagen vascular diseases, infection, and Lyme disease. Acute infectious arthritis will usually be accompanied by significant systemic symptoms, including fever and malaise, and should be easily recognized by the astute clinician and treated appropriately with culture and antibiotics rather than with injection therapy. The collagen vascular diseases will generally present as a polyarthropathy rather than as a monoarthropathy limited to the elbow joint, although elbow pain secondary to collagen vascular disease responds exceedingly well to the intra-articular injection technique described here.

TREATMENT

Initial treatment of the pain and functional disability associated with arthritis pain of the elbow should include a combination of the nonsteroidal anti-inflammatory drugs or cyclooxygenase-2 inhibitors and physical therapy. The local application of heat and cold may also be beneficial. For patients who do not respond to these treatment modalities, an intra-articular injection of local anesthetic and steroid may be a reasonable next step.

Intra-articular injection of the elbow is carried out with the patient in a supine position with the arm fully adducted at the patient's side and the elbow flexed with the dorsum of the hand resting on a folded towel. A total of 5 mL of local anesthetic and 40 mg methylprednisolone is drawn up in a 12-mL sterile syringe.

After sterile preparation of skin overlying the posterolateral aspect of the joint, the head of the radius is identified. Just superior to the head of the radius is an indentation, which represents the space between the radial head and humerus. Using strict aseptic technique, a 1-inch 25-gauge needle is inserted just above the superior aspect of the head of the radius through the skin, subcutaneous tissues, and joint capsule into the joint (Fig. 23–2). If bone is encountered, the needle is withdrawn into the subcutaneous tissues and redirected superiorly. After entering the joint space, the contents of the syringe are gently injected. There should be little resistance to injection. If resistance is encountered, the needle is probably in a ligament or tendon and should be advanced slightly into the joint space until the injection proceeds without significant resistance. The needle is then removed, and a sterile pressure dressing and ice pack are placed at the injection site.

SIDE EFFECTS AND COMPLICATIONS

The major complication of intra-articular injection of the elbow is infection. This complication should be exceedingly rare if strict aseptic technique is followed. The ulnar nerve is especially susceptible to damage at the elbow, and care must be taken to avoid this structure when performing intra-articular injection of the elbow. Approximately 25% of patients will complain of a transient increase in pain after intra-articular injection of the elbow joint and should be warned of such.

CLINICAL PEARLS

Pain and functional disability of the elbow are often the result of degenerative arthritis of the joint. Coexistent bursitis and tendinitis may also contribute to elbow pain and may confuse the diagnosis. The aforementioned injection technique is a safe procedure if careful attention is paid to the clinically relevant anatomy in the areas to be injected. Care must be taken to use sterile technique to avoid infection, as well as the use of universal precautions to avoid risk to the operator. The use of physical modalities including local heat as well as gentle range of motion exercises should be introduced several days after the patient undergoes this injection technique for elbow pain. Vigorous exercises should be avoided because they will exacerbate the patient's symptomatology. Simple analgesics and the nonsteroidal anti-inflammatory drugs or cyclooxygenase-2 inhibitors may be used concurrently with this injection technique.

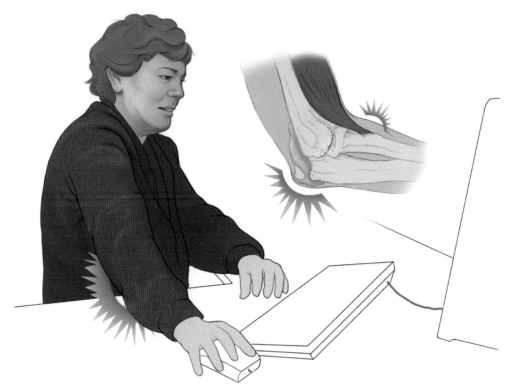

Figure 23–1. Arthritis of the elbow can cause pain and functional disability during common everyday tasks.

Figure 23–2. Proper needle placement for intra-articular injection of the elbow. (From Waldman SD: Atlas of Pain Management Injection Techniques. Philadelphia, WB Saunders, 2000, p 79.)

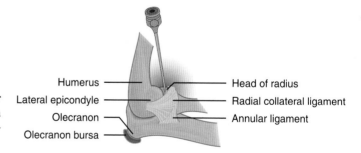

Humerus — Head of radius

Lateral epicondyle — Radial collateral ligament

Olecranon — Annular ligament

Olecranon bursa

24
Tennis Elbow

ICD-9 CODE 726.32

THE CLINICAL SYNDROME

Tennis elbow (also known as lateral epicondylitis) is caused by repetitive microtrauma to the extensor tendons of the forearm. The pathophysiology of tennis elbow is initially caused by microtearing at the origin of extensor carpi radialis and extensor carpi ulnaris. Secondary inflammation may occur that can become chronic as the result of continued overuse or misuse of the extensors of the forearm. Coexistent bursitis, arthritis, and gout may also perpetuate the pain and disability of tennis elbow.

Tennis elbow occurs in patients engaged in repetitive activities that include hand grasping, such as shaking hands by politicians, or high torque wrist turning, such as scooping ice cream at an ice cream parlor (Fig. 24–1). Tennis players develop tennis elbow via two separate mechanisms: (1) increased pressure grip strain as a result of playing with too heavy a racquet and (2) making backhand shots with a leading shoulder and elbow rather than keeping the shoulder and elbow parallel to the net. Other racquet sport players are also susceptible to the development of tennis elbow.

SIGNS AND SYMPTOMS

The pain of tennis elbow is localized to the region of the lateral epicondyle. It is constant and is made worse with active contraction of the wrist. Patients will note the inability to hold a coffee cup or hammer. Sleep disturbance is common. On physical examination, there will be tenderness along the extensor tendons at or just below the lateral epicondyle. Many patients with tennis elbow will exhibit a bandlike thickening within the affected extensor tendons. El-

bow range of motion will be normal. Grip strength on the affected side will be diminished. Patients with tennis elbow will demonstrate a positive tennis elbow test. The test is performed by stabilizing the patient's forearm and then having the patient clench his or her fist and actively extend the wrist. The examiner then attempts to force the wrist into flexion (Fig. 24–2). Sudden severe pain is highly suggestive of tennis elbow.

TESTING

Electromyography will help distinguish cervical radiculopathy and radial tunnel syndrome from tennis elbow. Plain radiographs are indicated in all patients who present with tennis elbow to rule out joint mice and other occult bony pathology. Based on the patient's clinical presentation, additional testing, including complete blood count, uric acid, sedimentation rate, and antinuclear antibody testing, may be indicated. Magnetic resonance imaging of the elbow is indicated if joint instability is suspected. The injection technique described below will serve as both a diagnostic and therapeutic maneuver.

DIFFERENTIAL DIAGNOSIS

Radial tunnel syndrome and, occasionally, C6-7 radiculopathy can mimic tennis elbow. Radial tunnel syndrome is an entrapment neuropathy that is the result of entrapment of the radial nerve below the elbow. Radial tunnel syndrome can be distinguished from tennis elbow in that with radial tunnel syndrome, the maximal tenderness to palpation is distal to the lateral epicondyle over the radial nerve, whereas with tennis elbow, the maximal tenderness to palpation is over the lateral epicondyle.

The most common nidus of pain from tennis elbow is the bony origin of the extensor tendon of extensor carpi radialis brevis at the anterior facet of the lateral epicondyle. Less commonly, tennis elbow pain can

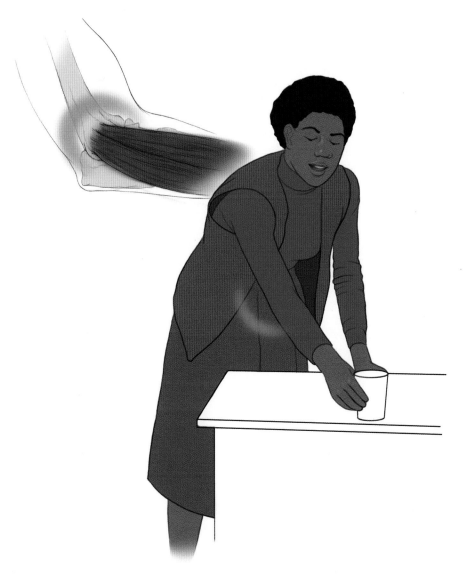

Figure 24–1. The pain of tennis elbow is localized to the lateral epicondyle.

originate from the origin of the extensor carpi radialis longus at the supracondylar crest or, rarely more distally, at the point where the extensor carpi radialis brevis overlies the radial head. As mentioned, bursitis may accompany tennis elbow. The olecranon bursa lies in the posterior aspect of the elbow joint and may also become inflamed as a result of direct trauma or overuse of the joint. Other bursae susceptible to the development of bursitis exist between the insertion of the biceps and the head of the radius as well as in the antecubital and cubital area.

TREATMENT

Initial treatment of the pain and functional disability associated with tennis elbow should include a combination of the nonsteroidal anti-inflammatory drugs or cyclooxygenase-2 inhibitors and physical therapy. The local application of heat and cold may also be beneficial. Any repetitive activity that may exacerbate the patient's symptomatology should be avoided. For patients who do not respond to these treatment modalities, the injection technique described here may be a reasonable next step.

Injection technique for tennis elbow is performed by placing the patient in a supine position with the arm fully adducted at the patient's side and the elbow flexed with the dorsum of the hand resting on a folded towel to relax the affected tendons. A total of 1 mL local anesthetic and 40 mg methylprednisolone is drawn up in a 5-mL sterile syringe.

After sterile preparation of skin overlying the posterolateral aspect of the joint, the lateral epicondyle is identified. Using strict aseptic technique, a 1-inch 25-gauge needle is inserted perpendicular to the lateral epicondyle through the skin and into the subcutaneous tissue overlying the affected tendon (Fig. 24–3). If bone is encountered, the needle is withdrawn back into the subcutaneous tissue. The contents of the syringe are then gently injected. There should be little resistance to injection. If resistance is encountered, the needle is probably in the tendon and should be withdrawn until the injection proceeds without significant resistance. The needle is then removed, and a sterile pressure dressing and ice pack are placed at the injection site.

SIDE EFFECTS AND COMPLICATIONS

The major complication associated with tennis elbow is the rupture of the affected inflamed tendons either from repetitive trauma or from injection directly into the tendon.

Inflamed and previously damaged tendons may rupture if directly injected, and needle position should be confirmed outside the tendon before injection to avoid this complication. Another complication of this injection technique is infection. This complication should be exceedingly rare if strict aseptic technique is followed. The ulnar nerve is especially susceptible to damage at the elbow, and care must be taken to avoid this nerve when injecting into the elbow. Approximately 25% of patients will complain of a transient increase in pain after this injection technique and should be warned of such.

CLINICAL PEARLS

This injection technique is extremely effective in the treatment of pain secondary to the tennis elbow. Coexistent bursitis and tendinitis may also contribute to elbow pain and may require additional treatment with more localized injection of local anesthetic and methylprednisolone acetate steroid. This technique is a safe procedure if careful attention is paid to the clinically relevant anatomy in the areas to be injected. The use of physical modalities including local heat as well as gentle range of motion exercises should be introduced several days after the patient undergoes this injection technique for tennis elbow pain. A Velcro band placed around the extensor tendons may also help relieve the symptoms of tennis elbow. Vigorous exercises should be avoided because they will exacerbate the patient's symptomatology. Simple analgesics and nonsteroidal anti-inflammatory drugs may be used concurrently with this injection technique. As mentioned, cervical radiculopathy and radial tunnel syndrome may mimic tennis elbow and must be ruled out to effectively treat the underlying pathology.

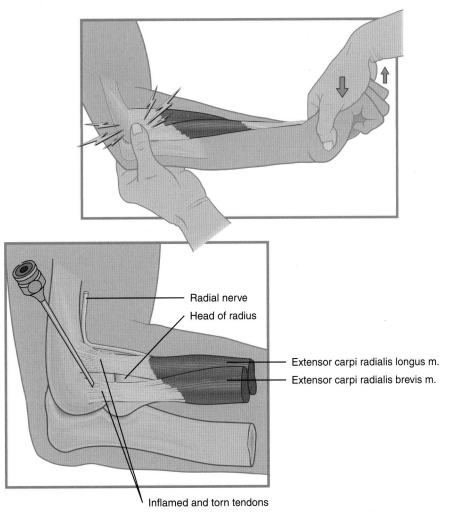

Radial nerve
Head of radius
Extensor carpi radialis longus m.
Extensor carpi radialis brevis m.
Inflamed and torn tendons

Figures 24–2 and 24–3. Palpation over the lateral epicondyle while the patient actively extends the wrist will elicit pain in patients with tennis elbow. Proper needle placement for injection of tennis elbows. (From Waldman SD: Atlas of Pain Management Injection Techniques. Philadelphia, WB Saunders, 2000, p 83.)

25

Golfer's Elbow

ICD-9 CODE 726.32

THE CLINICAL SYNDROME

Golfer's elbow (also known as medial epicondylitis) is caused by repetitive microtrauma to the flexor tendons of the forearm in a manner analogous to tennis elbow. The pathophysiology of golfer's elbow is initially caused by microtearing at the origin of the pronator teres, the flexor carpi radialis and flexor carpi ulnaris, and the palmaris longis. Secondary inflammation may occur, which can become chronic as the result of continued overuse or misuse of the flexors of the forearm. The most common nidus of pain from golfer's elbow is the bony origin of the flexor tendon of flexor carpi radialis and the humeral heads of the flexor carpi ulnarius and pronator teres at the medial epicondyle of the humerus. Less commonly, golfer's elbow pain can originate from the ulnar head of the flexor carpi ulnaris at the medial aspect of the olecranon process. Coexistent bursitis, arthritis, and gout may also perpetuate the pain and disability of golfer's elbow.

Golfer's elbow occurs in patients engaged in repetitive flexion activities that include throwing baseballs or footballs, carrying heavy suitcases, and driving golf balls. These activities have in common repetitive flexion of the wrist and strain on the flexor tendons due to excessive weight or sudden arrested motion. Interestingly, many of the activities that can cause tennis elbow can also cause golfer's elbow.

SIGNS AND SYMPTOMS

The pain of golfer's elbow is localized to the region of the medial epicondyle (Fig. 25–1). It is constant and is made worse with active contraction of the wrist. Patients will note the inability to hold a coffee cup or hammer. Sleep disturbance is common. On physical examination, there will be tenderness along the flexor tendons at or just below the medial epicondyle. Many patients with golfer's elbow will exhibit a bandlike thickening within the affected flexor tendons. Elbow range of motion will be normal. Grip strength on the affected side will be diminished. Patients with golfer's elbow will demonstrate a positive golfer's elbow test. The test is performed by stabilizing the patient's forearm and then having the patient actively flex the wrist. The examiner then attempts to force the wrist into extension. Sudden severe pain is highly suggestive of golfer's elbow.

TESTING

Plain radiographs are indicated in all patients who present with golfer's elbow to rule out joint mice and other occult bony pathology. Based on the patient's clinical presentation, additional testing, including complete blood count, uric acid, sedimentation rate, and antinuclear antibody testing, may be indicated. Magnetic resonance imaging of the elbow is indicated if joint instability is suspected. Electromyography is indicated to diagnosis entrapment neuropathy at the elbow and to help distinguish golfer's elbow from cervical radiculopathy. The injection technique described here will serve as both a diagnostic and therapeutic maneuver.

DIFFERENTIAL DIAGNOSIS

Occasionally, C6-7 radiculopathy can mimic golfer's elbow. The patient suffering from cervical radiculopathy will usually have neck pain and proximal upper extremity pain in addition to symptoms below the elbow. Electromyography will help distinguish radiculopathy from golfer's elbow. Bursitis, arthritis, and gout may also mimic golfer's elbow and may confuse the diagnosis. The olecranon bursa lies in the poste-

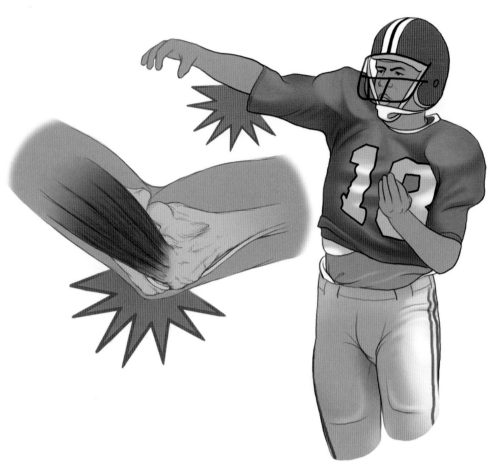

Figure 25–1. The pain of golfer's elbow occurs at the medial epicondyle.

rior aspect of the elbow joint and may also become inflamed as a result of direct trauma or overuse of the joint. Other bursae susceptible to the development of bursitis exist between the insertion of the biceps and the head of the radius as well as in the antecubital and cubital area.

TREATMENT

Initial treatment of the pain and functional disability associated with golfer's elbow should include a combination of the nonsteroidal anti-inflammatory drugs or cyclooxygenase-2 inhibitors and physical therapy. The local application of heat and cold may also be beneficial. Avoidance of any repetitive activity that may exacerbate the patient's symptomatology should be avoided. For patients who do not respond to these treatment modalities, the following injection technique may be a reasonable next step.

Injection for golfer's elbow is carried out by placing the patient in a supine position with the arm fully adducted at the patient's side and the elbow fully extended with the dorsum of the hand resting on a folded towel to relax the affected tendons. A total of 1 mL local anesthetic and 40 mg methylprednisolone is drawn up in a 5-mL sterile syringe.

After sterile preparation of skin overlying the medial aspect of the joint, the medial epicondyle is identified. Using strict aseptic technique, a 1-inch 25-gauge needle is inserted perpendicular to the medial epicondyle through the skin and into the subcutaneous tissue overlying the affected tendon. If bone is encountered, the needle is withdrawn into the subcutaneous tissue. The contents of the syringe are then gently injected. There should be little resistance to injection. If resistance is encountered, the needle is probably in the tendon and should be withdrawn until the injection proceeds without significant resistance. The needle is then removed, and a sterile pressure dressing and ice pack are placed at the injection site.

SIDE EFFECTS AND COMPLICATIONS

The major complications associated with this injection technique are related to trauma to the inflamed and previously damaged tendons. Such tendons may rupture if directly injected, and needle position should be confirmed outside the tendon before injection to avoid this complication. Another complication of this injection technique is infection. This complication should be exceedingly rare if strict aseptic technique is followed. The ulnar nerve is especially susceptible to damage at the elbow, and care must be taken to avoid this nerve when injecting the elbow. Approximately 25% of patients will complain of a transient increase in pain after intra-articular injection of the elbow joint and should be warned of such.

CLINICAL PEARLS

This injection technique is extremely effective in the treatment of pain secondary to the golfer's elbow. Coexistent bursitis and tendinitis may also contribute to elbow pain and may require additional treatment with more localized injection of local anesthetic and methylprednisolone acetate steroid. This technique is a safe procedure if careful attention is paid to the clinically relevant anatomy in the areas to be injected. The use of physical modalities including local heat as well as gentle range of motion exercises should be introduced several days after the patient undergoes this injection technique for elbow pain. A Velcro band placed around the flexor tendons may also help relieve the symptoms of golfer's elbow. Vigorous exercises should be avoided because they will exacerbate the patient's symptomatology. Simple analgesics and nonsteroidal anti-inflammatory drugs may be used concurrently with this injection technique. As mentioned, cervical radiculopathy may mimic golfer's elbow and must be ruled out to effectively treat the underlying pathology.

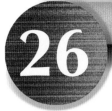

26

Ulnar Nerve Entrapment at the Elbow

ICD-9 CODE 354.2

THE CLINICAL SYNDROME

Ulnar nerve entrapment at the elbow is one of the most common entrapment neuropathies encountered in clinical practice. The causes include compression of the ulnar nerve by an aponeurotic band that runs from the medial epicondyle of the humerus to the medial border of the olecranon, direct trauma to the ulnar nerve at the elbow, and repetitive elbow motion. Ulnar nerve entrapment at the elbow is also called tardy ulnar palsy, cubital tunnel syndrome, and ulnar nerve neuritis. This entrapment neuropathy presents as pain and associated paresthesias in the lateral forearm that radiates to the wrist and ring and little finger (Fig. 26–1). Some patients suffering from ulnar nerve entrapment at the elbow may also notice pain referred to the medial aspect of the scapula on the affected side. Untreated, ulnar nerve entrapment at the elbow can result in a progressive motor deficit, and ultimately, flexion contracture of the affected fingers can result. The onset of symptoms usually occurs after repetitive elbow motions or from repeated pressure on the elbow, such as using the elbows to arise from bed. Direct trauma to the ulnar nerve as it enters the cubital tunnel may also result in a similar clinical presentation. Patients with vulnerable nerve syndrome, such as diabetics and alcoholics, are at greater risk for the development of ulnar nerve entrapment at the elbow.

SIGNS AND SYMPTOMS

Physical findings include tenderness over the ulnar nerve at the elbow. A positive Tinel's sign over the ulnar nerve as it passes beneath the aponeuroses is usually present. Weakness of the intrinsic muscles of the forearm and hand that are innervated by the ulnar nerve may be identified with careful manual muscle testing, although early in the course of the evolution of cubital tunnel syndrome, the only physical finding other than tenderness over the nerve may be the loss of sensation on the ulnar side of the little finger. Muscle wasting of the intrinsic muscles of the hand can best be identified by viewing the hand from above with the palm down (see Fig. 26–1). Tinel's sign at the elbow is often present when the ulnar nerve is stimulated.

TESTING

Electromyography and nerve conduction velocity testing are extremely sensitive tests, and the skilled electromyographer can diagnose ulnar nerve entrapment at the elbow with a high degree of accuracy as well as help sort out other neuropathic causes of pain that may mimic ulnar nerve entrapment at the elbow, including radiculopathy and plexopathy (see later). Plain radiographs are indicated in all patients who present with ulnar nerve entrapment at the elbow to rule out occult bony pathology. If surgery is contemplated, a magnetic resonance image of the affected elbow may help further delineate the pathologic process responsible for the nerve entrapment (e.g., bone spur or aponeurotic band thickening). If Pancoast's tumor or other tumors of the brachial plexus are suspected, chest radiographs with apical lordotic views may be helpful. Screening laboratory testing consisting of complete blood count, erythrocyte sedimentation rate, antinuclear antibody testing, and automated blood chemistry testing should be performed if the diagnosis of ulnar nerve entrapment at the elbow is in question to help rule out other causes of the patient's pain. The injection technique described here will serve as both a diagnostic and therapeutic maneuver.

DIFFERENTIAL DIAGNOSIS

Ulnar nerve entrapment at the elbow is often misdiagnosed as golfer's elbow, and this fact accounts for the many patients whose "golfer's elbow" fails to respond to conservative measures. Cubital tunnel syndrome can be distinguished from golfer's elbow in that in cubital tunnel syndrome, the maximal tenderness to palpation is over the ulnar nerve 1 inch below the medial epicondyle, whereas with golfer's elbow, the maximal tenderness to palpation is directly over the medial epicondyle. Cubital tunnel syndrome should also be differentiated from cervical radiculopathy involving the C7 or C8 roots and golfer's elbow. Furthermore, it should be remembered that cervical radiculopathy and ulnar nerve entrapment may coexist as the "double crush" syndrome. The double crush syndrome is seen most commonly with median nerve entrapment at the wrist or carpal tunnel syndrome.

TREATMENT

A short course of conservative therapy consisting of simple analgesics, nonsteroidal anti-inflammatory drugs, or cyclooxygenase-2 inhibitors, and splinting to avoid elbow flexion, is indicated in patients who present with ulnar nerve entrapment at the elbow. If the patient does not experience a marked improvement in symptoms within 1 week, careful injection of the ulnar nerve at the elbow using the following technique is a reasonable next step.

Ulnar nerve injection at the elbow is carried out by placing the patient in a supine position with the arm fully adducted at the patient's side and the elbow slightly flexed with the dorsum of the hand resting on a folded towel. A total of 5 to 7 mL local anesthetic is drawn up in a 12-mL sterile syringe. A total of 80 mg methylprednisolone acetate steroid is added to the local anesthetic with the first block, and 40 mg depot steroid is added with subsequent blocks.

The clinician then identifies the olecranon process and the medial epicondyle of the humerus. The ulnar nerve sulcus between these two bony landmarks is then identified. After preparation of the skin with antiseptic solution, a ⅝-inch 25-gauge needle is inserted just proximal to the sulcus and is slowly advanced in a slightly cephalad trajectory. As the needle advances approximately ½ inch, a strong paresthesia in the distribution of the ulnar nerve will be elicited. The patient should be warned that a paresthesia will occur and to say "There!!!!" as soon as the paresthesia is felt. After paresthesia is elicited and its distribution is identified, gentle aspiration is carried out to identify blood. If the aspiration test is negative and no persistent paresthesia into the distribution of the ulnar nerve remains, 5 to 7 mL of solution is slowly injected, with the patient being monitored closely for signs of local anesthetic toxicity. If no paresthesia can be elicited, a similar amount of solution is slowly injected in a fanlike manner just proximal to the notch, with care being taken to avoid intravascular injection.

If the patient does not respond to these treatments or if the patient is experiencing progressive neurologic deficit, strong consideration of surgical decompression of the ulnar nerve is indicated. As mentioned, magnetic resonance imaging of the affected elbow should help clarify the pathology responsible for compression of the ulnar nerve.

COMPLICATIONS AND PITFALLS

Failure to promptly identify and treat ulnar nerve entrapment at the elbow can result in permanent neurologic deficit. To avoid harm to the patient, it is also important to rule out other causes of pain and numbness that may mimic the symptoms of ulnar nerve entrapment at the elbow, such as Pancoast's tumor.

Ulnar nerve block at the elbow is a relatively safe block, with the major complications being inadvertent intravascular injection into the ulnar artery and persistent paresthesia secondary to needle trauma to the nerve. Because the nerve passes through the ulnar nerve sulcus and it is enclosed by a dense fibrous band, care should be taken to slowly inject just proximal to the sulcus to avoid additional compromise of the nerve.

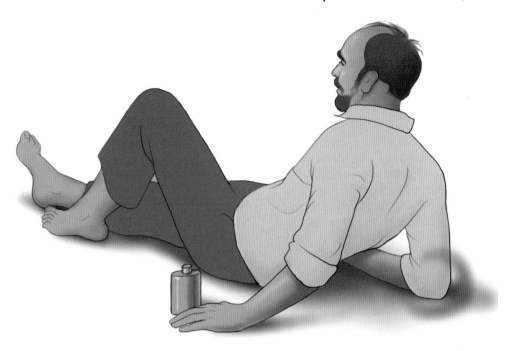

Figure 26–1. The ulnar nerve is susceptible to compression at the elbow.

CLINICAL PEARLS

Ulnar nerve entrapment at the elbow is often misdiagnosed as golfer's elbow, and this fact accounts for the many patients whose "golfer's elbow" fails to respond to conservative measures. Ulnar nerve entrapment at the elbow can be distinguished from golfer's elbow in that in cubital tunnel syndrome, the maximal tenderness to palpation is over the ulnar nerve 1 inch below the medial epicondyle, whereas with golfer's elbow, the maximal tenderness to palpation is directly over the medial epicondyle. If cubital tunnel syndrome is suspected, injection of the ulnar nerve at the elbow with local anesthetic and steroid will provide almost instantaneous relief.

Ulnar nerve block at the elbow is a simple and safe technique in the evaluation and treatment of ulnar nerve entrapment at the elbow. A careful neurologic examination to identify preexisting neurologic deficits that may later be attributed to the nerve block should be performed on all patients before beginning ulnar nerve block at the elbow, because there seems to be a propensity for the development of persistent paresthesia when the nerve is blocked at this level. The incidence of persistent paresthesia can be decreased by blocking the nerve proximal to the ulnar nerve sulcus and injecting slowly.

Cubital tunnel syndrome should also be differentiated from cervical radiculopathy involving the C8 spinal root, which may mimic ulnar nerve compression. Furthermore, it should be remembered that cervical radiculopathy and ulnar nerve entrapment may coexist in the double crush syndrome. The double crush syndrome is seen most commonly with median nerve entrapment at the wrist or carpal tunnel syndrome. Pancoast's tumor invading the medial cord of the brachial plexus may also mimic an isolated ulnar nerve entrapment and should be ruled out by apical lordotic chest radiography.

27

Olecranon Bursitis

ICD-9 726.33

THE CLINICAL SYNDROME

Olecranon bursitis may develop gradually due to repetitive irritation of the olecranon bursa or acutely due to trauma or infection. The olecranon bursa lies in the posterior aspect of the elbow between the olecranon process of the ulna and the overlying skin. It may exist as a single bursal sac or, in some patients, as a multisegmented series of sacs that may be loculated in nature. With overuse or misuse, these bursae may become inflamed, enlarged, and, on rare occasions, infected. The swelling associated with olecranon bursitis may at times be quite impressive, and the patient may complain about difficulty in wearing a long-sleeved shirt.

The olecranon bursa is vulnerable to injury from both acute trauma and repeated microtrauma. Acute injuries frequently take the form of direct trauma to the elbow in patients who play sports such as hockey or fall directly onto the olecranon process. Repeated pressure from leaning on the elbow to arise or from working long hours at a drafting table may result in inflammation and swelling of the olecranon bursa. Gout or bacterial infection may rarely precipitate acute olecranon bursitis. If the inflammation of the olecranon bursa becomes chronic, calcification of the bursa may occur with resultant residual nodules called gravel.

SIGNS AND SYMPTOMS

The patient suffering from olecranon bursitis will frequently complain of pain and swelling with any movement of the elbow but especially with extension. The pain is localized to the olecranon area, with referred pain often noted above the elbow joint. Often, the patient will be more concerned about the swelling around the bursa than with the pain. Physical examination will reveal point tenderness over the olecranon and swelling of the bursa that at times can be quite extensive (Figs. 27–1 and 27–2). Passive extension and resisted flexion shoulder will reproduce the pain as will any pressure over the bursa. Fever and chills will usually accompany infection of the bursa. If infection is suspected, aspiration, Gram stain, and culture of the bursal fluid followed by treatment with appropriate antibiotics are indicated on an emergency basis.

TESTING

The diagnosis of olecranon bursitis is usually made on clinical grounds alone. Plain radiographs of the posterior elbow are indicated if there is a history of elbow trauma or if arthritis of the elbow is suspected. Plain radiographs may also reveal calcification of the bursa and associated structures consistent with chronic inflammation. Magnetic resonance imaging is indicated if joint instability is suspected. Complete blood count, automated chemistry profile including uric acid, sedimentation rate, and antinuclear antibody testing are indicated if collagen vascular disease is suspected. If infection is considered, aspiration, Gram stain, and culture of bursal fluid are indicated on an emergency basis.

DIFFERENTIAL DIAGNOSIS

Olecranon bursitis is usually a straightforward clinical diagnosis. Occasionally, rheumatoid nodules or gouty arthritis of the elbow may confuse the clinician. Also, synovial cysts of the elbow may mimic olecranon bursitis. It should be remembered that coexistent tendinitis (e.g., tennis elbow and golfer's elbow) may require additional treatment.

TREATMENT

A short course of conservative therapy consisting of simple analgesics, nonsteroidal anti-inflammatory drugs or cyclooxygenase-2 inhibitors, and an elbow protector to prevent further trauma is a reasonable first step in the treatment of patients suffering from olecranon bursitis. If the patient does not experience rapid improvement, the following injection technique is a reasonable next step.

The patient is placed in a supine position with the arm fully adducted at the patient's side and the elbow flexed with the palm of the hand resting on the patients abdomen. A total of 2 mL local anesthetic and 40 mg methylprednisolone is drawn up in a 5-mL sterile syringe.

After sterile preparation of skin overlying the posterior aspect of the joint, the olecranon process and overlying bursa are identified. Using strict aseptic technique, a 1-inch 25-gauge needle is inserted through the skin and subcutaneous tissues directly into the bursa in the midline. If bone is encountered, the needle is withdrawn back into the bursa. After entering the bursa, the contents of the syringe are gently injected. There should be little resistance to injection. The needle is then removed, and a sterile pressure dressing and ice pack are placed at the injection site.

COMPLICATIONS AND PITFALLS

Failure to adequately treat olecranon bursitis may result in the development of chronic pain and loss of range of motion of the affected elbow. The major complication of the described injection of the olecranon bursa is infection. This complication should be exceedingly rare if strict aseptic technique is followed. As mentioned, the ulnar nerve is especially susceptible to damage at the elbow. Approximately 25% of patients will complain of a transient increase in pain after injection of the olecranon bursa and should be warned of such.

CLINICAL PEARLS

This injection technique is extremely effective in the treatment of pain and swelling secondary to the olecranon bursitis. Coexistent tendinitis and epicondylitis may also contribute to elbow pain and may require additional treatment with more localized injection of local anesthetic and methylprednisolone acetate steroid. This technique is a safe procedure if careful attention is paid to the clinically relevant anatomy in the areas to be injected, in particular, avoiding the ulnar nerve by keeping the needle trajectory in the midline. Care must be taken to use sterile technique to avoid infection, as well as the use of universal precautions to avoid risk to the operator. The incidence of ecchymosis and hematoma formation can be decreased if pressure is placed on the injection site immediately after injection. The use of physical modalities including local heat as well as gentle range of motion exercises should be introduced several days after the patient undergoes this injection technique for elbow pain. Vigorous exercises should be avoided because they will exacerbate the patient's symptomatology. Simple analgesics and nonsteroidal anti-inflammatory drugs may be used concurrently with this injection technique.

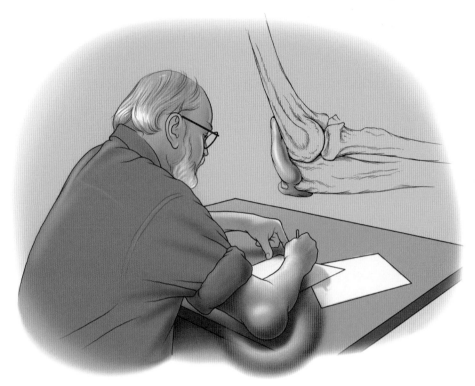

Figure 27–1. Olecranon bursitis is often caused by repeated pressure on the elbow.

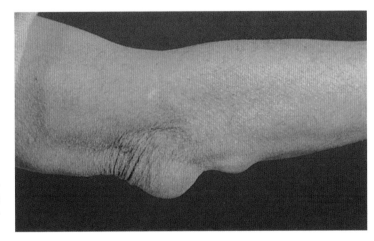

Figure 27–2. A case of olecranon bursitis in a patient with rheumatoid arthritis; a rheumatoid nodule is also shown. (From Klippel JH, Dieppe PA: Rheumatology, 2nd ed. London, Mosby, 1998.)

VI Wrist Pain Syndromes

28 Arthritis Pain at the Wrist

ICD-9 CODE 715.93

THE CLINICAL SYNDROME

Arthritis pain at the wrist is a commonly encountered complaint that can cause significant pain and suffering. The wrist joint is susceptible to the development of arthritis from a variety of conditions that have in common the ability to damage the joint cartilage. Patients with arthritis of the wrist will present with pain, swelling, and decreasing function of the wrist. Decreased grip strength is also a common finding. Osteoarthritis of the joint is the most common form of arthritis that results in wrist joint pain. However, rheumatoid arthritis, post-traumatic arthritis, and psoriatic arthritis are also common causes of wrist pain secondary to arthritis. These types of arthritis can result in significant alteration in the biomechanics of the wrist because they affect not only the joint but also the tendons and other connective tissues that make up the functional unit.

SIGNS AND SYMPTOMS

The majority of patients presenting with wrist pain secondary to osteoarthritis and post-traumatic arthritis pain will present with the complaint of pain that is localized around the wrist and hand. Activity makes the pain worse, with rest and heat providing some relief. The pain is constant and characterized as aching in nature. The pain may interfere with sleep. Some patients will complain of a grating or popping sensation with use of the joint, and crepitus may be present on physical examination. If the pain and dysfunction are secondary to rheumatoid arthritis, involvement of the metacarpophalangeal joints with characteristic deformity is often present.

In addition to this pain, patients suffering from arthritis of the wrist joint will often experience a gradual decrease in functional ability with decreasing wrist range of motion, making simple everyday tasks such as using a computer keyboard, holding a coffee cup, or turning a door knob quite difficult (Fig. 28–1). With continued disuse, muscle wasting may occur, and an adhesive capsulitis with subsequent ankylosis may develop.

TESTING

Plain radiographs are indicated in all patients who present with wrist pain. Based on the patient's clinical presentation, additional testing, including complete blood count, sedimentation rate, and antinuclear antibody testing, may be indicated. Magnetic resonance imaging of the wrist is indicated if joint instability is suspected. If infection is suspected, Gram stain and culture of the synovial fluid on an emergency basis and treatment with appropriate antibiotics are indicated.

DIFFERENTIAL DIAGNOSIS

Osteoarthritis of the joint is the most common form of arthritis that results in wrist joint pain. However, rheumatoid arthritis and post-traumatic arthritis are also common causes of wrist pain secondary to arthritis. Less common causes of arthritis-induced wrist pain include the collagen vascular diseases, infection, villonodular synovitis, and Lyme disease. Acute infectious arthritis will usually be accompanied by significant systemic symptoms, including fever and malaise, and should be easily recognized by the astute clinician and treated appropriately with antibiotics. The collagen vascular diseases will generally present as a polyarthropathy rather than as a monoarthropathy limited to the wrist joint, although wrist pain secondary to collagen vascular disease responds exceedingly well to the intra-articular injection technique described here.

TREATMENT

Initial treatment of the pain and functional disability associated with osteoarthritis of the wrist should include a combination of the nonsteroidal anti-inflammatory drugs or cyclooxygenase-2 inhibitors and physical therapy. The local application of heat and cold may also be beneficial. Splinting the wrist in neural position may also help provide symptomatic relief and protect the joint from additional trauma. For patients who do not respond to these treatment modalities, an intra-articular injection of local anesthetic and steroid may be a reasonable next step.

Intra-articular injection of the wrist is performed by placing the patient in a supine position with the arm fully adducted at the patient's side and the elbow slightly flexed with the palm of the hand resting on a folded towel. A total of 1.5 mL local anesthetic and 40 mg methylprednisolone is drawn up in a 5-mL sterile syringe.

After sterile preparation of skin overlying the dorsal joint, the midcarpus proximal to the indentation of the capitate bone is identified. Just proximal to the capitate bone is an indentation, which allows easy access to the wrist joint. Using strict aseptic technique, a 1-inch 25-gauge needle is inserted in the center of the midcarpal indentation through the skin, subcutaneous tissues, and joint capsule into the joint. If bone is encountered, the needle is withdrawn into the subcutaneous tissues and redirected superiorly. After entering the joint space, the contents of the syringe are gently injected. There should be little resistance to injection. If resistance is encountered, the needle is probably in a ligament or tendon and should be advanced slightly into the joint space until the injection proceeds without significant resistance. The needle is then removed, and a sterile pressure dressing and ice pack are placed at the injection site.

COMPLICATIONS AND PITFALLS

Joint protection is especially important in patients suffering from inflammatory arthritis of the wrist because repetitive trauma will result in further damage to the joint, tendons, and connective tissues. The major complication of intra-articular injection of the wrist is infection. This complication should be exceedingly rare if strict aseptic technique is followed. As mentioned, the ulnar nerve is especially susceptible to damage at the wrist. Approximately 25% of patients will complain of a transient increase in pain after intra-articular injection of the wrist joint and should be warned of such.

CLINICAL PEARLS

The use of physical modalities including local heat as well as gentle range of motion exercises should be introduced several days after the patient begins treatment for the pain and dysfunction of arthritis of wrist. Vigorous exercises should be avoided because they will exacerbate the patient's symptomatology. Simple analgesics and nonsteroidal anti-inflammatory drugs may be used concurrently with this injection technique. This injection technique is extremely effective in the treatment of pain secondary to the aforementioned causes of arthritis of the wrist joint. Coexistent bursitis and tendinitis may also contribute to wrist pain and may require additional treatment with more localized injection of local anesthetic and methylprednisolone acetate. This technique is a safe procedure if careful attention is paid to the clinically relevant anatomy in the areas to be injected.

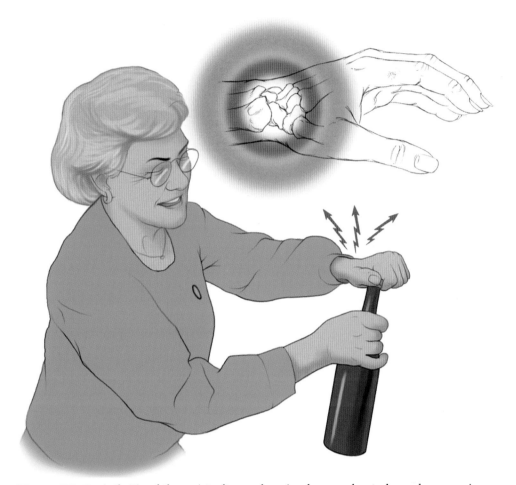

Figure 28–1. Arthritis of the wrist often makes simple everyday tasks such as opening a bottle painful.

29 *Carpal Tunnel Syndrome*

ICD-9 CODE 354.0

THE CLINICAL SYNDROME

Carpal tunnel syndrome is the most common entrapment neuropathy encountered in clinical practice. It is caused by compression of the median nerve as it passes through the carpal canal at the wrist. The most common causes of compression of the median nerve at this anatomic location include flexor tenosynovitis, rheumatoid arthritis, pregnancy, amyloidosis, and other space-occupying lesions that compromise the median nerve as it passes through this closed space. This entrapment neuropathy presents as pain, numbness, paresthesias, and associated weakness in the hand and wrist that radiates to the thumb, index finger, middle finger, and radial half of the ring finger (Fig. 29–1). These symptoms may also radiate proximal to the entrapment into the forearm. Untreated, progressive motor deficit and, ultimately, flexion contracture of the affected fingers can result. The onset of symptoms usually occurs after repetitive wrist motions or due to repeated pressure on the wrist such as resting the wrists on the edge of a computer keyboard. Direct trauma to the median nerve as it enters the carpal tunnel may result in a similar clinical presentation.

SIGNS AND SYMPTOMS

Physical findings include tenderness over the median nerve at the wrist. A positive Tinel's sign over the median nerve as it passes beneath the flexor retinaculum is usually present. A positive Phalen's test is highly suggestive of carpal tunnel syndrome. Phalen's test is performed by having the patient place the wrists in complete unforced flexion for at least 30 seconds (Fig. 29–2). If the median nerve is entrapped at the wrist, this maneuver will reproduce the symptoms of carpal tunnel syndromes. Weakness of thumb opposition and wasting of the thenar eminence are often seen in advanced carpal tunnel syndrome, although because of the complex motion of the thumb, subtle motor deficits may easily be missed. Early in the course of the evolution of carpal tunnel syndrome, the only physical finding other than tenderness over the median nerve may be the loss of sensation on the above-mentioned fingers.

TESTING

Electromyography will help distinguish cervical radiculopathy and diabetic polyneuropathy from carpal tunnel syndrome. Plain radiographs are indicated in all patients who present with carpal tunnel syndrome to rule out occult bony pathology. Based on the patient's clinical presentation, additional testing, including complete blood count, uric acid, sedimentation rate, and antinuclear antibody testing, may be indicated. Magnetic resonance imaging of the wrist is indicated if joint instability or a space-occupying lesion is suspected. The injection technique described here will serve as both a diagnostic and therapeutic maneuver.

DIFFERENTIAL DIAGNOSIS

Carpal tunnel syndrome is often misdiagnosed as arthritis of the carpometacarpal joint of the thumb, cervical radiculopathy, or diabetic polyneuropathy. Patients with arthritis of the carpometacarpal joint of the thumb will have a positive Watson's test and radiographic evidence of arthritis. Most patients suffering from a cervical radiculopathy will have reflex, motor, and sensory changes associated with neck pain, whereas patients with carpal tunnel syndrome will have no reflex changes and motor and sensory changes will be limited to the distal median nerve.

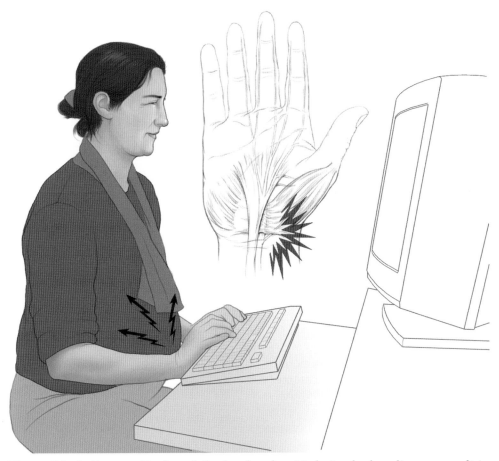

Figure 29–1. Poor positioning of the hand and wrist during keyboarding can result in carpal tunnel syndrome.

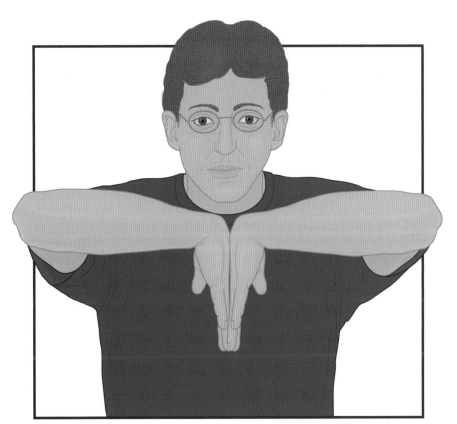

Figure 29–2. A positive Phalen's test is highly indicative of carpal tunnel syndrome. (From Waldman SD: Atlas of Pain Management Injection Techniques. Philadelphia, WB Saunders, 2000, p 145.)

Diabetic polyneuropathy will generally present as symmetrical sensory deficit involving the entire hand rather than limited just to the distribution of the median nerve. It should be remembered that cervical radiculopathy and median nerve entrapment may coexist as the "double crush" syndrome. Furthermore, because carpal tunnel syndrome is commonly seen in patients with diabetes, it is not surprising that diabetic polyneuropathy is usually present in diabetic patients with carpal tunnel syndrome.

TREATMENT

Mild cases of carpal tunnel syndrome will usually respond to conservative therapy, and surgery should be reserved for more severe cases. Initial treatment of carpal tunnel syndrome should consist of simple analgesics, nonsteroidal anti-inflammatory drugs, or cyclooxygenase inhibitors and splinting of the wrist. At a minimum, the splint should be worn at night, but 24 hours a day is ideal. Avoidance of repetitive activities thought to be responsible for the evolution of carpal tunnel syndrome (e.g., keyboarding, hammering) will also help ameliorate the patient's symptoms. If the patient fails to respond to these conservative measures, a next reasonable step is injection of the carpal tunnel with local anesthetic and steroid.

Carpal tunnel injection is performed by placing the patient in a supine position with the arm fully abducted at the patient's side and the elbow slightly flexed with the dorsum of the hand resting on a folded towel. A total of 3 mL local anesthetic and 40 mg methylprednisolone is drawn up in a 5-mL sterile syringe. The clinician then has the patient make a fist and at the same time flex his or her wrist to aid in identification of the palmaris longus tendon. After preparation of the skin with antiseptic solution, a ⅝-inch 25-gauge needle is inserted just medial to the tendon and just proximal to the crease of the wrist at a 30-degree angle (Fig. 29–3). The needle is slowly advanced until the tip is just beyond the tendon. A paresthesia in the distribution of the median nerve is often elicited, and the patient should be warned of such. The patient should be warned that should a paresthesia occur, he or she is to say "There!!!!" as soon as the paresthesia is felt. If a paresthesia is elicited, the needle is withdrawn slightly away from the median nerve. Gentle aspiration is then carried out to identify blood. If the aspiration test is negative and no persistent paresthesia into the distribution of the median nerve remains, 3 mL of solution is slowly injected, with the patient being monitored closely for signs of local anesthetic toxicity. If no paresthesia is elicited and the needle tips hits bone, the needle is

withdrawn out of the periosteum and after careful aspiration, 3 mL of solution is slowly injected.

For patients in whom these treatment modalities fail, surgical release of the median nerve at the carpal tunnel is indicated. Endoscopic techniques are showing promise and appear to result in less postoperative pain and dysfunction.

COMPLICATIONS AND PITFALLS

Failure to adequately treat carpal tunnel syndrome can result in permanent pain, numbness, and functional disability. This problem can be exacerbated if coexistent reflex sympathetic dystrophy is not aggressively treated with sympathetic neural blockade. Injection of the carpal tunnel is a relatively safe technique, with the major complications being inadvertent intravascular injection and persistent paresthesia secondary to needle trauma to the nerve. This technique can be safely performed in the presence of anticoagulation by using a 25- or 27-gauge needle, albeit at an increased risk of hematoma, if the clinical situation dictates a favorable risk-to-benefit ratio. These complications can be decreased if manual pressure is applied to the area of the block immediately after injection. The application of cold packs for 20-minute periods after the block will also decrease the amount of postprocedure pain and bleeding the patient may experience.

CLINICAL PEARLS

Carpal tunnel syndrome should always be differentiated from cervical radiculopathy involving the cervical nerve roots, which may at times mimic median nerve compression. Furthermore, it should be remembered that cervical radiculopathy and median nerve entrapment may coexist in the double crush syndrome. The double crush syndrome is seen most commonly with median nerve entrapment at the wrist or carpal tunnel syndrome.

Carpal tunnel injection is a simple and safe technique in the evaluation and treatment of these painful conditions. Careful neurologic examination to identify preexisting neurologic deficits that may later be attributed to the nerve block should be performed on all patients before beginning median nerve block at the wrist, especially in those patients with clinical symptoms of diabetes or clinically significant carpal tunnel syndrome.

Care should be taken to place the needle just beyond the flexor retinaculum and to inject slowly to allow the solution to flow easily into the carpal tunnel without further compromising the median nerve.

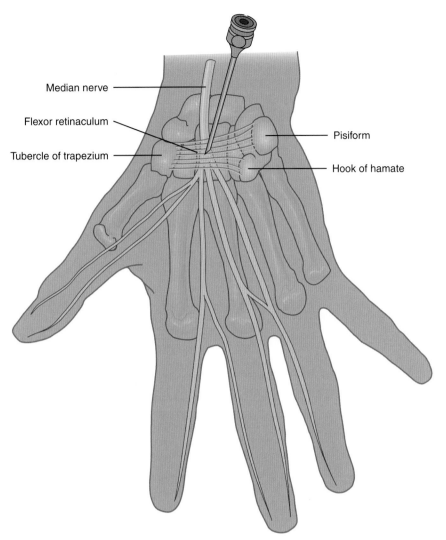

Figure 29–3. Proper needle placement for injection of the carpal tunnel. (From Waldman SD: Atlas of Pain Management Injection Techniques. Philadelphia, WB Saunders, 2000, p 145.)

30

de Quervain's Tenosynovitis

ICD-9 CODE 727.05

THE CLINICAL SYNDROME

de Quervain's tenosynovitis is caused by an inflammation and swelling of the tendons of the abductor pollicis longus and extensor pollicis brevis at the level of the radial styloid process. This inflammation and swelling is usually the result of trauma to the tendon from repetitive twisting motions. If the inflammation and swelling becomes chronic, a thickening of the tendon sheath occurs with a resulting constriction of the sheath. A triggering phenomenon may result with the tendon catching within the sheath, causing the thumb to lock, or "trigger." Arthritis and gout of the first metacarpal joint may also coexist with de Quervain's tenosynovitis and exacerbate its pain and disability.

de Quervain's tenosynovitis occurs in patients engaged in repetitive activities that include hand grasping, such as shaking hands by politicians, or high torque wrist turning, such as scooping ice cream at an ice cream parlor. de Quervain's tenosynovitis may also develop without obvious antecedent trauma in the parturient.

The pain of de Quervain's tenosynovitis is localized to the region of the radial styloid. It is constant and is made worse with active pinching activities of the thumb or ulnar deviation of the wrist. Patients will note the inability to hold a coffee cup or turn a screwdriver. Sleep disturbance is common.

SIGNS AND SYMPTOMS

On physical examination, there will be tenderness and swelling over the tendons and tendon sheaths along the distal radius with point tenderness over the radial styloid (Fig. 30-1). Many patients with de Quervain's tenosynovitis will exhibit a creaking sensation with flexion and extension of the thumb. Range of motion of the thumb may be decreased due to the pain, and a trigger thumb phenomenon may be noted. Patients with de Quervain's tenosynovitis demonstrate a positive Finkelstein test (Fig. 30-2). The Finkelstein test is performed by stabilizing the patient's forearm and then having the patient fully flex his or her thumb into the palm and then actively forcing the wrist toward the ulna. Sudden severe pain is highly suggestive of de Quervain's tenosynovitis.

TESTING

There is no specific test to diagnose de Quervain's tenosynovitis. The diagnosis is generally made on clinical grounds. Electromyography will help distinguish de Quervain's tenosynovitis from neuropathic processes such as cervical radiculopathy and cheiralgia paresthetica. Plain radiographs are indicated in all patients who present with de Quervain's tenosynovitis to rule out occult bony pathology. Based on the patient's clinical presentation, additional testing, including complete blood count, uric acid, sedimentation rate, and antinuclear antibody testing, may be indicated. Magnetic resonance imaging of the wrist is indicated if joint instability is suspected. The injection technique described here will serve as both a diagnostic and therapeutic maneuver.

DIFFERENTIAL DIAGNOSIS

Entrapment of the lateral antebrachial cutaneous nerve, arthritis of the first metacarpal joint, gout, cheiralgia paresthetica, and occasionally C6-7 radiculopathy can mimic de Quervain's tenosynovitis. Cheiralgia paresthetica is an entrapment neuropathy that is the result of entrapment of the superficial branch of the radial nerve at the wrist. All of these

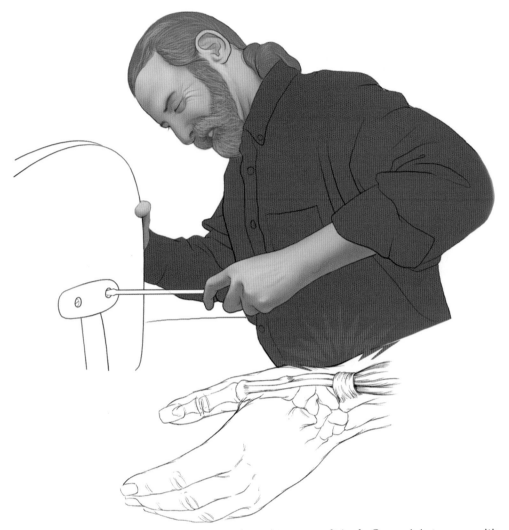

Figure 30–1. Repetitive microtrauma to the wrist can result in de Quervain's tenosynovitis.

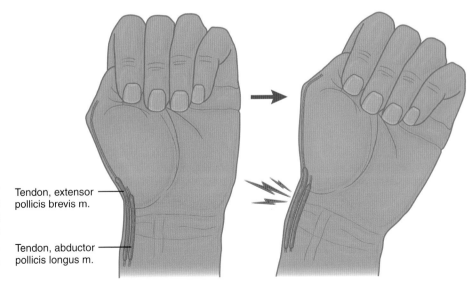

Figure 30–2. A positive Finkelstein's test is indicative of de Quervain's tenosynovitis. (From Waldman SD: Atlas of Pain Management Injection Techniques. WB Saunders, Philadelphia, 2000, p 123.)

Tendon, extensor pollicis brevis m.

Tendon, abductor pollicis longus m.

painful conditions can coexist with de Quervain's tenosynovitis.

TREATMENT

Initial treatment of the pain and functional disability associated with de Quervain's tenosynovitis should include a combination of the nonsteroidal anti-inflammatory drugs or cyclooxygenase-2 inhibitors and physical therapy. The local application of heat and cold may also be beneficial. Any repetitive activity that may exacerbate the patient's symptomatology should be avoided. Nighttime splinting of the affected thumb may also help avoid the "trigger finger" phenomenon that can occur on awakening in many patients suffering from this condition. For patients who do not respond to these treatment modalities, the following injection technique may be a reasonable next step.

Injection of de Quervain's tenosynovitis is carried out by placing the patient in a supine position, with the arm fully adducted at the patient's side and the ulnar surface of the wrist and hand resting on a folded towel to relax the affected tendons. A total of 2 mL local anesthetic and 40 mg methylprednisolone is drawn up in a 5-mL sterile syringe.

After sterile preparation of skin overlying the affected tendons, the radial styloid is identified. Using strict aseptic technique, a 1-inch 25-gauge needle is inserted at a 45-degree angle toward the radial styloid through the skin and into the subcutaneous tissue overlying the affected tendon. If bone is encountered, the needle is withdrawn into the subcutaneous tissue. The contents of the syringe are then gently injected. There should be little resistance to injection. If resistance is encountered, the needle is probably in the tendon and should be withdrawn until the injection proceeds without significant resistance. The needle is then removed, and a sterile pressure dressing and ice pack are placed at the injection site.

COMPLICATIONS AND PITFALLS

The major complications associated with this injection technique are related to trauma to the inflamed and previously damaged tendons. Such tendons may rupture if directly injected, and needle position should be confirmed outside the tendon before injection to avoid this complication. Another complication of this injection technique is infection. This complication should be exceedingly rare if strict aseptic technique is followed. The radial artery and superficial branch of the radial nerve are susceptible to damage if the needle is placed too medially, and care must be taken to avoid these structures when performing this injection technique. Approximately 25% of patients will complain of a transient increase in pain after this injection technique and should be warned of such.

CLINICAL PEARLS

The use of physical modalities including local heat as well as gentle range of motion exercises should be introduced several days after the patient undergoes this injection technique for elbow pain. A hand splint to immobilize the thumb may also help relieve the symptoms of de Quervain's tenosynovitis. Vigorous exercises should be avoided because they will exacerbate the patient's symptomatology. Simple analgesics and nonsteroidal anti-inflammatory drugs may be used concurrently with this injection technique. This injection technique is extremely effective in the treatment of pain secondary to the de Quervain's tenosynovitis. Coexistent arthritis and gout may also contribute to the pain and may require additional treatment with more localized injection of local anesthetic and methylprednisolone acetate. This technique is a safe procedure if careful attention is paid to the clinically relevant anatomy in the areas to be injected. Care must be taken to use sterile technique to avoid infection as well as universal precautions to avoid risk to the operator. The incidence of ecchymosis and hematoma formation can be decreased if pressure is placed on the injection site immediately after injection. As mentioned, arthritis of the first metacarpal joint, gout, cheiralgia paresthetica, and cervical radiculopathy may mimic de Quervain's tenosynovitis and must be ruled out to effectively treat the underlying pathology.

31
Arthritis Pain at the Carpometacarpal Joints

ICD-9 CODE 715.94

THE CLINICAL SYNDROME

Pain and dysfunction from arthritis of the carpometacarpal joints is a common complaint encountered in clinical practice. The carpometacarpal joints are susceptible to the development of arthritis from a variety of conditions that have in common the ability to damage the joint cartilage. Osteoarthritis of the joint is the most common form of arthritis that results in carpometacarpal joint pain. It occurs more commonly in females, and although the carpometacarpal joint of the thumb is most commonly affected, arthritis may also develop in the other carpometacarpal joints, especially after trauma. Rheumatoid arthritis, post-traumatic arthritis, and psoriatic arthritis are also common causes of carpometacarpal pain secondary to arthritis. Less common causes of arthritis-induced carpometacarpal pain include the collagen vascular diseases, infection, and Lyme disease. Acute infectious arthritis will usually be accompanied by significant systemic symptoms including fever and malaise and should be easily recognized by the astute clinician and treated appropriately with culture and antibiotics, rather than injection therapy. The collagen vascular diseases will generally present as a polyarthropathy rather than as a monoarthropathy limited to the carpometacarpal joint, although carpometacarpal pain secondary to collagen vascular disease responds exceedingly well to the intra-articular injection technique described here.

The carpometacarpal joints of the fingers are synovial plane joints that serve as the articulation between the carpals and the metacarpals and allow articulation of the bases of the metacarpal bones with one another. Movement of the joints is limited to a slight gliding motion, with the carpometacarpal joint of the little finger possessing the greatest range of motion. The primary function of the joint is to optimize the grip function of the hand. In most patients, there is a common joint space.

SIGNS AND SYMPTOMS

The majority of patients presenting with carpometacarpal pain secondary to osteoarthritis and post-traumatic arthritis pain will present with the complaint of pain that is localized to dorsum of the wrist. Activity associated especially with flexion, extension, and ulnar deviation of the carpometacarpal joints will exacerbate the pain, with rest and heat providing some relief (Fig. 31–1). The pain is constant and characterized as aching in nature. The pain may interfere with sleep. Some patients complain of a grating or popping sensation with use of the joint, and crepitus may be present on physical examination.

In addition the aforementioned pain, patients suffering from arthritis of the carpometacarpal joint will often experience a gradual decrease in functional ability with decreasing pinch and grip strength, making everyday tasks such as using a pencil or opening a jar quite difficult. With continued disuse, muscle wasting may occur, and an adhesive capsulitis with subsequent ankylosis may develop.

TESTING

Plain radiographs are indicated in all patients who present with carpometacarpal pain. Based on the patient's clinical presentation, additional testing, including complete blood count, sedimentation rate, and antinuclear antibody testing, may be indicated. Magnetic resonance imaging of the carpometacarpal joint is indicated if joint instability is suspected. If infection is suspected, Gram stain and culture of the synovial fluid on an emergency basis and treatment with appropriate antibiotics are indicated. If there is a history of trauma, radionucleotide bone scanning may be useful, because fractures of the navicular bone are often missed on plain radiographs of the wrist.

DIFFERENTIAL DIAGNOSIS

Arthritis pain of the carpometacarpal joints is usually diagnosed on clinical grounds with plain radiographs confirming the clinical findings. Occasionally, arthritis pain of the carpometacarpal joints may be confused with de Quervain's syndrome or other forms of tendinitis involving the wrist and fingers. These painful conditions as well as gout may coexist and make the diagnosis more difficult. If trauma is present, occult fractures of the metacarpals should always be considered.

TREATMENT

Initial treatment of the pain and functional disability associated with osteoarthritis of the carpometacarpal joints should include a combination of the nonsteroidal anti-inflammatory drugs or cyclooxygenase-2 inhibitors and physical therapy. The local application of heat and cold may also be beneficial. Splinting the wrist in neural position may also help provide symptomatic relief and protect the joint from additional trauma. For patients who do not respond to these treatment modalities, an intra-articular injection of local anesthetic and steroid may be a reasonable next step.

Intra-articular injection of the wrist is performed by placing the patient in a supine position, with the arm fully adducted at the patient's side and the hand in neutral position with the palmar aspect resting on a folded towel. A total of 1.5 mL local anesthetic and 40 mg methylprednisolone is drawn up in a 5-mL sterile syringe.

After sterile preparation of skin overlying the affected carpometacarpal joint, the space between the carpal and metacarpal is identified. The joint can be more easily identified by gliding the joint back and forth. Using strict aseptic technique, a 1-inch 25-gauge needle is inserted into the center of the joint through the skin, subcutaneous tissues, and joint capsule into the joint (Fig. 31–2). If bone is encountered, the needle is withdrawn into the subcutaneous tissues and redirected medially. After entering the joint space, the contents of the syringe are gently injected. There should be little resistance to injection. If resistance is encountered, the needle is probably in a tendon and should be advanced slightly into the joint space until the injection proceeds without significant resistance. The needle is then removed, and a sterile pressure dressing and ice pack are placed at the injection site.

COMPLICATIONS AND PITFALLS

Joint protection is especially important in patients suffering from inflammatory arthritis of the carpometacarpal joints because repetitive trauma will result in further damage to the joint, tendons, and connective tissues. The major complication associated with this intra-articular injection technique is infection. This complication should be exceedingly rare if strict aseptic technique is followed. Approximately 25% of patients will complain of a transient increase in pain after intra-articular injection of the carpometacarpal joints and should be warned of such.

CLINICAL PEARLS

The use of physical modalities including local heat as well as gentle range of motion exercises should be introduced several days after the patient begins treatment for the pain and dysfunction of arthritis of carpometacarpal joints. Vigorous exercises should be avoided because they will exacerbate the patient's symptomatology. Simple analgesics and nonsteroidal anti-inflammatory drugs may be used concurrently with this injection technique. This injection technique is extremely effective in the treatment of pain secondary to the aforementioned causes of arthritis of the wrist joint. Coexistent bursitis and tendinitis may also contribute to the patient's pain and may require additional treatment with more localized injection of local anesthetic and methylprednisolone acetate. This technique is a safe procedure if careful attention is paid to the clinically relevant anatomy in the areas to be injected.

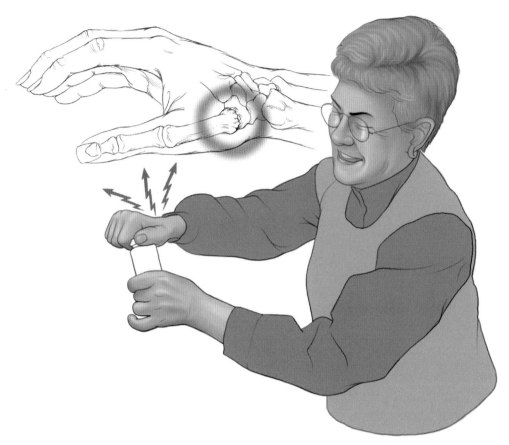

Figure 31–1. Arthritis of the carpometacarpal joints may cause pain and decreased grip strength.

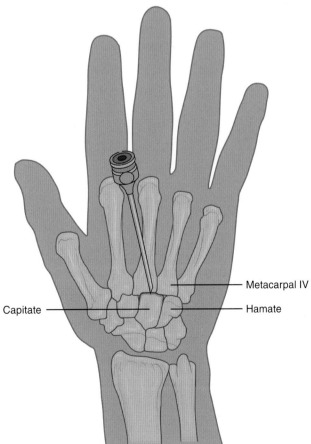

Figure 31–2. Proper needle placement for injection of the carpometacarpal joints. (From Waldman SD: Atlas of Pain Management Injection Techniques. WB Saunders, Philadelphia, 2000, p 129.)

VII Hand Pain Syndromes

32

Trigger Thumb

ICD-9 CODE 727.03

THE CLINICAL SYNDROME

Trigger thumb is caused by an inflammation and swelling of the tendon of the flexor pollicis longus due to compression by the head of the first metacarpal bone. Sesamoid bones in this region may also cause compression and trauma to the tendon. The inflammation and swelling of the tendon is usually the result of trauma to the tendon from repetitive motion or pressure overlying the tendon as it passes over these bony prominences. If the inflammation and swelling becomes chronic, a thickening of the tendon sheath occurs with a resulting constriction of the sheath. Frequently, a nodule develops on the tendon due to chronic pressure and irritation. These nodules can often be palpated when the patient flexes and extends the thumb. Such nodules may catch in the tendon sheath and produce a triggering phenomenon that causes the thumb to catch or lock (Fig. 32–1).

Arthritis and gout of the first metacarpal joint may also coexist with trigger thumb and exacerbate the pain and disability of trigger thumb. Trigger thumb occurs in patients engaged in repetitive activities that include hand grasping, such as shaking hands by politicians, or activities that require repetitive pinching movements of the thumb. Video games and frequent card playing have also been implicated in the evolution of trigger thumb.

SIGNS AND SYMPTOMS

The pain of trigger thumb is localized to the palmar aspect of the base of the thumb in contradistinction to the pain of de Quervain's tenosynovitis, in which the pain is most pronounced more proximally over the radial styloid. The pain of trigger thumb is constant and is made worse with active pinching activities of the thumb. Patients will note the inability to hold a coffee cup or a pen. Sleep disturbance is common, and patients often will awaken to find that the thumb has become locked in a flexed position during sleep. On physical examination, there will be tenderness and swelling over the tendon with maximal point tenderness over the base of the thumb. Many patients with trigger thumb exhibit a creaking sensation with flexion and extension of the thumb. Range of motion of the thumb may be decreased due to the pain, and a trigger thumb phenomenon may be noted. Patients with trigger thumb often demonstrate a nodule on the tendon of the flexor pollicis longus.

TESTING

Plain radiographs are indicated in all patients who present with trigger thumb to rule out occult bony pathology. Based on the patient's clinical presentation, additional testing, including complete blood count, uric acid, sedimentation rate, and antinuclear antibody testing, may be indicated. Magnetic resonance imaging of the hand is indicated if first metacarpal joint instability is suspected. The injection technique described here will serve as both a diagnostic and therapeutic maneuver.

DIFFERENTIAL DIAGNOSIS

The diagnosis of trigger thumb is usually made on clinical grounds. Coexistent arthritis of the metocarpocarpal joint of the thumb and gout of the first metacarpal joint may accompany trigger thumb and exacerbate the patient's pain symptomatology. The nidus of pain from trigger thumb is the tendon flexor pollicis longus at the level of the base of the first metacarpal. Occasionally, this may be confused with de Quervain's tenosynovitis.

TREATMENT

Initial treatment of the pain and functional disability associated with trigger thumb should include a combination of the nonsteroidal anti-inflammatory drugs or cyclooxygenase-2 inhibitors and physical therapy. The use of physical modalities including local heat as well as gentle range of motion exercises should be introduced several days after the patient undergoes the following injection technique. A quilter's glove to protect the thumb may also help relieve the symptoms of trigger thumb. Vigorous exercises should be avoided because they will exacerbate the patient's symptomatology.

Injection of trigger thumb is carried out by placing the patient in a supine position, with the arm fully adducted at the patient's side and the dorsal surface of the hand resting on a folded towel. A total of 2 mL local anesthetic and 40 mg methylprednisolone is drawn up in a 5-mL sterile syringe.

After sterile preparation of the skin overlying the affected tendon, the metacarpophalangeal joint of the thumb is identified. Using strict aseptic technique, at a point just proximal to the joint, a 1-inch 25-gauge needle is inserted at a 45-degree angle parallel to the affected tendon through the skin and into the subcutaneous tissue overlying the affected tendon. If bone is encountered, the needle is withdrawn into the subcutaneous tissue. The contents of the syringe are then gently injected. The tendon sheath will distend as the injection proceeds. There should be little resistance to injection. If resistance is encountered, the needle is probably in the tendon and should be withdrawn until the injection proceeds without significant resistance. The needle is then removed, and a sterile pressure dressing and ice pack are placed at the injection site.

COMPLICATIONS AND PITFALLS

Failure to adequately treat trigger thumb early in the course of the disease can result in permanent pain and functional disability due to continued trauma to the tendon and tendon sheath. The major complications associated with this injection technique are related to trauma to the inflamed and previously damaged tendon. Such tendons may rupture if directly injected, and needle position should be confirmed outside the tendon before injection to avoid this complication. Another complication of this injection technique is infection. This complication should be exceedingly rare if strict aseptic technique is followed. The radial artery and superficial branch of the radial nerve are susceptible to damage if the needle is placed too medially, and care must be taken to avoid these structures when performing this injection technique. Approximately 25% of patients will complain of a transient increase in pain after this injection technique and should be warned of such.

CLINICAL PEARLS

This injection technique is extremely effective in the treatment of pain secondary to the trigger thumb. Coexistent arthritis and gout may also contribute to the pain and may require additional treatment with more localized injection of local anesthetic and methylprednisolone acetate. This technique is a safe procedure if careful attention is paid to the clinically relevant anatomy in the areas to be injected. The radial artery and the superficial branch of the radial nerve are in proximity to the injection site for trigger thumb and may be traumatized if the needle is placed too medially. de Quervain's tenosynovitis may be confused with trigger thumb but can be distinguished by the location of pain and the motions that cause the triggering phenomenon.

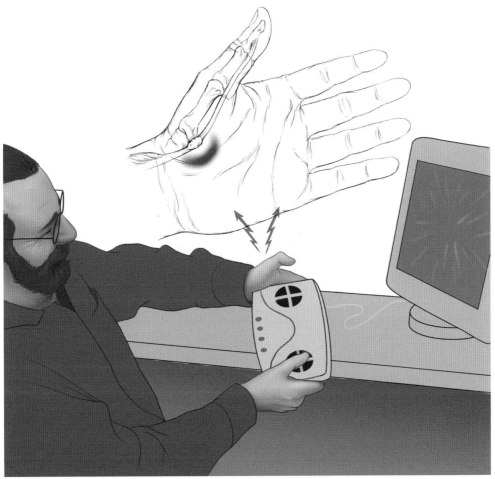

Figure 32–1. Trigger thumb is caused by microtrauma from repetitive pinching movement of the thumb.

33
Trigger Finger

ICD-9 CODE 727.03

THE CLINICAL SYNDROME

Trigger finger is caused by an inflammation and swelling of the tendons of the flexor digitorum superficialis due to compression by the heads of the metacarpal bones. Sesamoid bones in this region may also cause compression and trauma to the tendons. The inflammation and swelling of the tendon is usually the result of trauma to the tendon from repetitive motion or pressure overlying the tendon as it passes over these bony prominences. If the inflammation and swelling becomes chronic, a thickening of the tendon sheath occurs with a resulting constriction of the sheath. Frequently, a nodule develops on the tendon due to chronic pressure and irritation. These nodules can often be palpated when the patient flexes and extends the fingers. Such nodules may catch in the tendon sheath as the nodule passes under a restraining tendon pulley and produce a triggering phenomenon that causes the finger to catch or lock as the nodule catches on the pulley (Fig. 33–1).

Coexistent arthritis and gout of the metacarpal and interphalangeal joints may also be present with trigger finger and exacerbate the pain and disability of trigger finger. Trigger finger occurs in patients engaged in repetitive activities that include hand clenching such as gripping a steering wheel or holding a horse's reins too tightly.

SIGNS AND SYMPTOMS

The pain of trigger finger is localized to the distal palm with tender tendon nodules often being pal-pated. The pain of trigger finger is constant and is made worse with active gripping activities of the hand. Patients will note significant stiffness when flexing the fingers. Sleep disturbance is common, and often the patient will awaken to find the finger has become locked in a flexed position during sleep. On physical examination, there will be tenderness and swelling over the tendon with maximal point tenderness over the heads of the metacarpals. Many patients with trigger finger will exhibit a creaking sensation with flexion and extension of the fingers. Range of motion of the fingers may be decreased due to the pain, and a trigger finger phenomenon may be noted. Patients with trigger finger will often demonstrate nodules on the tendons of the flexor digitorum superficialis.

TESTING

Plain radiographs are indicated in all patients who present with trigger finger to rule out occult bony pathology. Based on the patient's clinical presentation, additional testing including complete blood count, uric acid, sedimentation rate, and antinuclear antibody testing may be indicated. Magnetic resonance imaging of the hand is indicated if joint instability is suspected. The injection technique described here will serve as both a diagnostic and therapeutic maneuver.

DIFFERENTIAL DIAGNOSIS

The diagnosis of trigger finger is usually made on clinical grounds. Coexistent arthritis or gout of the metacarpocarpal joints may accompany trigger finger and exacerbate the patient's pain symptomatology. Occult fractures may occasionally confuse the clinical presentation.

134

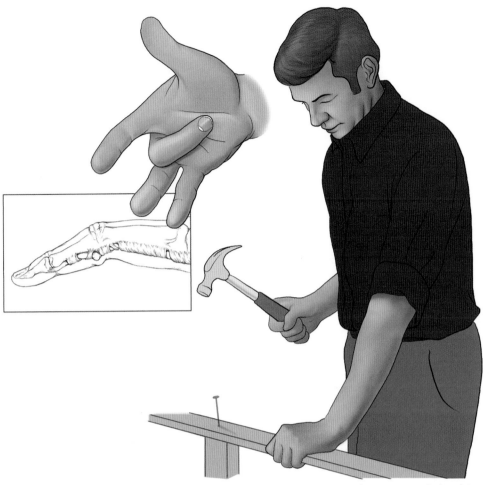

Figure 33–1. Trigger finger is caused by repetitive microtrauma from repeated clenching of the hand.

TREATMENT

Initial treatment of the pain and functional disability associated with trigger finger should include a combination of the nonsteroidal anti-inflammatory drugs or cyclooxygenase-2 inhibitors and physical therapy. The use of physical modalities including local heat as well as gentle range of motion exercises should be introduced several days after the patient undergoes the following injection technique. A nighttime splint to protect the fingers may also help relieve the symptoms of trigger thumb. Vigorous exercises should be avoided because they will exacerbate the patient's symptomatology.

Injection of trigger finger is carried out by placing the patient in a supine position, with the arm fully adducted at the patient's side and the dorsal surface of the hand resting on a folded towel. A total of 2 mL local anesthetic and 40 mg methylprednisolone is drawn up in a 5-mL sterile syringe.

After sterile preparation of the skin overlying the affected tendon, the head of the metacarpal beneath the tendon is identified. Using strict aseptic technique, at a point just proximal to the joint, a 1-inch 25-gauge needle is inserted at a 45-degree angle parallel to the affected tendon through the skin and into the subcutaneous tissue overlying the affected tendon. If bone is encountered, the needle is withdrawn into the subcutaneous tissue. The contents of the syringe are then gently injected. The tendon sheath will distend as the injection proceeds. There should be little resistance to injection. If resistance is encountered, the needle is probably in the tendon and should be withdrawn until the injection proceeds without significant resistance. The needle is then removed, and a sterile pressure dressing and ice pack are placed at the injection site.

COMPLICATIONS AND PITFALLS

Failure to adequately treat trigger finger early in the course of the disease can result in permanent pain and functional disability due to continued trauma to the tendon and tendon sheath. The major complications associated with this injection technique are related to trauma to the inflamed and previously damaged tendon. Such tendons may rupture if directly injected, and needle position should be confirmed outside the tendon before injection to avoid this complication. Another complication of this injection technique is infection. This complication should be exceedingly rare if strict aseptic technique is followed. The radial artery and superficial branch of the radial nerve are susceptible to damage if the needle is placed too medially, and care must be taken to avoid these structures when this injection technique is performed. Approximately 25% of patients will complain of a transient increase in pain after this injection technique and should be warned of such.

CLINICAL PEARLS

The use of physical modalities including local heat as well as gentle range of motion exercises should be introduced several days after the patient undergoes this injection technique. A hand splint to protect the fingers may also help relieve the symptoms of trigger finger. Vigorous exercises should be avoided because they will exacerbate the patient's symptomatology. Simple analgesics and nonsteroidal anti-inflammatory drugs may be used concurrently with this injection technique.

This injection technique is extremely effective in the treatment of pain secondary to the trigger finger. Co-existent arthritis and gout may also contribute to the pain and may require additional treatment with more localized injection of local anesthetic and methylprednisolone acetate. This technique is a safe procedure if careful attention is paid to the clinically relevant anatomy in the areas to be injected. Care must be taken to use sterile technique to avoid infection, as well as universal precautions to avoid risk to the operator. The incidence of ecchymosis and hematoma formation can be decreased if pressure is placed on the injection site immediately after injection. Surgical treatment should be considered for patients who fail to respond to these treatment modalities.

34

Ganglion Cysts of the Hand and Wrist

ICD-9 CODE 727.41

THE CLINICAL SYNDROME

The dorsum of the wrist is especially susceptible to the development of ganglion cysts. Ganglion cysts usually appear on the dorsum of the wrist in the area overlying the extensor tendons or joint space, with a predilection for the joint space of the lunate or from the tendon sheath of the extensor carpi radialis. These cysts are thought to form as the result of herniation of synovial-containing tissues from joint capsules or tendon sheaths. This tissue may then become irritated and begin producing increased amounts of synovial fluid, which can pool in cyst-like cavities overlying the tendons and joint space. A one-way valve phenomenon may cause these cyst-like cavities to expand because the fluid cannot freely flow back into the synovial cavity.

SIGNS AND SYMPTOMS

Activity, especially extreme flexion and extension, makes the pain worse, with rest and heat providing some relief. The pain is constant and characterized as aching in nature. It is often the unsightly nature of the ganglion cyst rather than the pain that causes the patient to seek medical attention (Fig. 34–1). The ganglion will be smooth to palpation and will transilluminate with a penlight, in contradistinction to solid tumors, which will not transilluminate. Palpation of the ganglion may increase the pain.

TESTING

Plain radiographs of the wrist are indicated in all patients who present with ganglion cysts to rule out bony abnormalities, including tumors. Based on the patient's clinical presentation, additional testing, including complete blood count, sedimentation rate, and antinuclear antibody testing, may be indicated. Magnetic resonance imaging of the wrist is indicated if the etiology of the wrist mass is suspect.

DIFFERENTIAL DIAGNOSIS

Ganglion cysts of the wrist and hand generally present in a clinically distinct manner, making diagnosis easy. The clinician should be aware that coexistent bursitis and tendinitis may confuse the clinical picture if the ganglion cyst is small. Noncystic masses should always undergo magnetic resonance imaging to help rule out primary or metastatic tumors.

TREATMENT

Initial treatment of the pain and functional disability associated with ganglion cyst of the hand and wrist should include a combination of the nonsteroidal anti-inflammatory drugs or cyclooxygenase-2 inhibitors and physical therapy. The use of physical modalities including local heat as well as gentle range of motion exercises should be introduced several days after the patient undergoes the following injection technique. A nighttime splint to protect the fingers may also help relieve the morning symptoms of ganglion cyst. Vigorous exercises should be avoided because they will exacerbate the patient's symptomatology.

If the patient does not respond to these conservative modalities, a trial of injection therapy with local anesthetic and steroid is a reasonable next step. To inject a ganglion cyst, the patient is placed in a supine position with the arm fully adducted at the patient's side and the elbow slightly flexed with the palm of the hand resting on a folded towel. A total of

1.5 mL local anesthetic and 40 mg methylprednisolone is drawn up in a 5-mL sterile syringe.

After sterile preparation of skin overlying the ganglion, a 1-inch 22-gauge needle is inserted in the center of the ganglion, and the contents of the cyst are aspirated. If bone is encountered, the needle is withdrawn into the ganglion cyst, and aspiration is carried out.

After aspiration of the ganglion cyst, the contents of the syringe are gently injected. There should be little resistance to injection. The needle is then removed, and a sterile pressure dressing and ice pack are placed at the injection site. If the ganglion reappears, surgical treatment may ultimately be required.

COMPLICATIONS AND PITFALLS

The major complication of injection of a ganglion is infection. This complication should be exceedingly rare if strict aseptic technique is followed. Care must be taken to avoid injection directly into tendons, which may already be inflamed from irritation due to the ganglion rubbing against the tendon.

CLINICAL PEARLS

Although an initial trial of conservative therapy is indicated, ganglion cysts of the wrist and hand will often require surgical treatment. If conservative therapy fails, the aforementioned injection technique is extremely effective in the treatment of pain secondary to ganglion cysts. Coexistent bursitis and tendinitis may also contribute to wrist pain and may require additional treatment with more localized injection of local anesthetic and methylprednisolone acetate. This technique is a safe procedure if careful attention is paid to the clinically relevant anatomy in the areas to be injected. Care must be taken to use sterile technique to avoid infection, as well as universal precautions to avoid risk to the operator. The incidence of ecchymosis and hematoma formation can be decreased if pressure is placed on the injection site immediately after injection. The use of physical modalities including local heat as well as gentle range of motion exercises should be introduced several days after the patient undergoes this injection technique. Vigorous exercises should be avoided because they will exacerbate the patient's symptomatology. Simple analgesics and nonsteroidal anti-inflammatory drugs may be used concurrently with this injection technique.

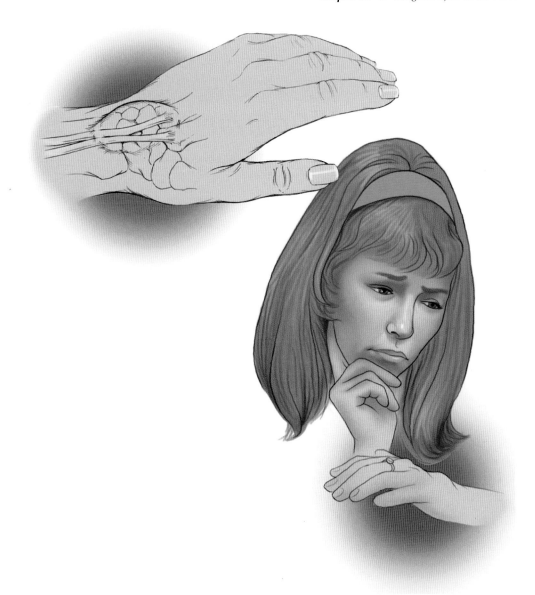

Figure 34–1. The appearance of a ganglion cyst will often cause the patient to seek medical attention out of fear of cancer.

35

Dupuytren's Contracture

ICD-9 CODE 728.6

THE CLINICAL SYNDROME

Dupuytren's contracture is a common complaint encountered in clinical practice. Although it is initially painful, patients suffering from Dupuytren's contracture generally seek medical help due to the functional disability rather than the pain. Dupuytren's contracture is caused by a progressive fibrosis of the palmar fascia. Initially, the patient may notice fibrotic nodules along the course of the flexor tendons of the hand that are tender to palpation. These nodules arise from the palmar fascia and initially do not involve the flexor tendons. As the disease advances, these fibrous nodules coalesce and form fibrous bands that gradually thicken and contract around the flexor tendons, which has the effect of drawing the affected fingers into flexion. While all fingers can develop Dupuytren's contracture, the ring and little finger are most commonly affected (Fig. 35–1). If untreated, the fingers will develop permanent flexion contractures. The pain of Dupuytren's contracture seems to burn itself out as the disease progresses.

Dupuytren's contracture is thought to have a genetic basis and occurs most frequently in males of northern Scandinavian descent. The disease may also be associated with trauma to the palm, diabetes, alcoholism, and chronic barbiturate use. The disease rarely occurs before the fourth decade. The plantar fascia may also be concurrently affected.

SIGNS AND SYMPTOMS

In the early stages of the disease, hard fibrotic nodules along the path of the flexor tendons may be palpated. These nodules are often misdiagnosed as calluses or warts. At this early stage, pain is invariably present. As the disease progresses, the clinician will note taut fibrous bands that may cross the metacarpophalangeal joint and ultimately the proximal interphalangeal joint. These bands are not painful to palpation, and while they limit finger extension, finger flexion remains relatively normal. It is at this point that patients will often seek medical advice as they begin having difficulty putting on gloves and reaching into their pocket to retrieve keys. In the final stages of the disease, the flexion contracture develops with its attendant negative impact on function. Coexistent arthritis, gout of the metacarpal and interphalangeal joints, and trigger finger may also be present with Dupuytren's contracture and exacerbate the pain and disability of Dupuytren's contracture.

TESTING

Plain radiographs are indicated for all patients who present with Dupuytren's contracture to rule out underlying occult bony pathology. Based on the patient's clinical presentation, additional testing, including complete blood count, uric acid, sedimentation rate, and antinuclear antibody testing, may be indicated. Magnetic resonance imaging of the hand is indicated if joint instability or tumor is suspected. Electromyography is indicated if coexistent ulnar or carpal tunnel is suspected. The injection technique described here will provide transient improvement in the pain and disability of this disease, but surgical treatment may ultimately be required to restore function.

DIFFERENTIAL DIAGNOSIS

Dupuytren's contracture is the result of the thickening of the palmar fascia and its effect on the flexor tendons and represents a clinically distinct entity that is rarely misdiagnosed once the syndrome is well es-

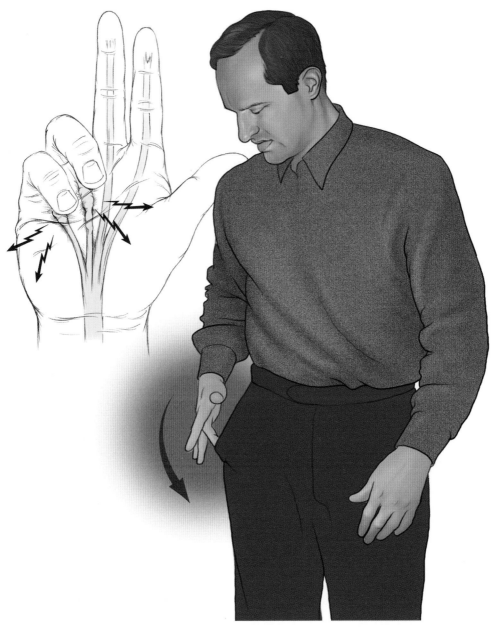

Figure 35-1. Dupuytren's contracture usually affects the fourth and fifth digits in males over 40 years of age.

tablished. Coexistent flexor tendinitis or occasionally trigger finger may be confused with Dupuytren's contracture early in the course of the disease.

TREATMENT

Initial treatment of the pain and functional disability associated with Dupuytren's contracture should include a combination of the nonsteroidal anti-inflammatory drugs or cyclooxygenase-2 inhibitors and physical therapy. The use of physical modalities including local heat as well as gentle range of motion exercises should be introduced several days after the patient undergoes the following injection technique. A nighttime splint to protect the fingers may also help relieve the symptoms of trigger thumb. Vigorous exercises should be avoided because they will exacerbate the patient's symptomatology.

Injection of Dupuytren's contracture is carried out by placing the patient in a supine position with the arm fully adducted at the patient's side with the dorsal surface of the hand resting on a folded towel. A total of 2 mL local anesthetic and 40 mg methylprednisolone is drawn up in a 5-mL sterile syringe.

Sterile preparation of the skin overlying the fibrous band or nodule is carried out at a point just lateral to the fibrosis, and a 1-inch 25-gauge needle is inserted at a 45-degree angle parallel to the fibrosis through the skin and into the subcutaneous tissue overlying the fibrotic area. If bone is encountered, the needle is withdrawn into the subcutaneous tissue and again advanced in proximity of the fibrosis. The contents of the syringe are then gently injected. There may be some resistance to injection due to fibrosis of the surrounding tissue. If significant resistance is encountered, the needle is probably in the tendon or fibrotic nodule and should be withdrawn until the injection proceeds without significant resistance. The needle is then removed, and a sterile pressure dressing and ice pack are placed at the injection site. As mentioned, while these treatment modalities will help provide symptomatic relief, Dupuytren's contracture will usually require surgical treatment.

COMPLICATIONS AND PITFALLS

The major complications associated with this injection technique are related to trauma to an inflamed or previously damaged tendon. Such tendons may rupture if directly injected, and needle position should be confirmed outside the tendon before injection to avoid this complication. Another complication of this injection technique is infection. This complication should be exceedingly rare if strict aseptic technique is followed. Approximately 25% of patients will complain of a transient increase in pain after this injection technique and should be warned of such.

CLINICAL PEARLS

The aforementioned treatment modalities are useful in providing symptomatic relief of the pain and disability of Dupuytren's contracture. However, most patients will ultimately require surgical treatment of this syndrome. This injection technique is extremely effective in the palliation of pain and dysfunction secondary to the Dupuytren's contracture. Coexistent arthritis and gout may also contribute to the pain and may require additional treatment with more localized injection of local anesthetic and methylprednisolone acetate. This technique is a safe procedure if careful attention is paid to the clinically relevant anatomy in the areas to be injected. Care must be taken to use sterile technique to avoid infection, as well as universal precautions to avoid risk to the operator. The incidence of ecchymosis and hematoma formation can be decreased if pressure is placed on the injection site immediately after injection. The use of physical modalities including local heat, massage, as well as gentle range of motion exercises should be introduced several days after the patient undergoes this injection technique. Vigorous exercises should be avoided because they will exacerbate the patient's symptomatology. Simple analgesics and nonsteroidal anti-inflammatory drugs may be used concurrently with this injection technique.

VIII Chest Wall Pain Syndromes

36

Costosternal Syndrome

ICD-9 CODE 733.6

THE CLINICAL SYNDROME

A significant number of patients who suffer from noncardiogenic chest pain suffer from costosternal joint pain. Most commonly, the costosternal joints become a source of pain due to inflammation as a result of overuse or misuse or due to trauma secondary to acceleration/deceleration injuries or blunt trauma to the chest wall. With severe trauma, the joints may sublux or dislocate. The costosternal joints are also susceptible to the development of arthritis, including osteoarthritis, rheumatoid arthritis, ankylosing spondylitis, Reiter's syndrome, and psoriatic arthritis. The joints are also subject to invasion by tumor either from primary malignancies, including thymoma, or from metastatic disease.

SIGNS AND SYMPTOMS

Physical examination of the patient suffering from costosternal syndrome will reveal that the patient will vigorously attempt to splint the joints by keeping the shoulders stiffly in neutral position (Fig. 36–1). Pain is reproduced with active protraction or retraction of the shoulder, deep inspiration, and full elevation of the arm. Shrugging of the shoulder may also reproduce the pain. Coughing may be difficult, and this may lead to inadequate pulmonary toilet in patients who have sustained trauma to the anterior chest wall. The costosternal joints and adjacent intercostal muscles may also be tender to palpation. The patient may also complain of a clicking sensation with movement of the joint.

TESTING

Plain radiographs are indicated for all patients who present with pain that is thought to be emanating from the costosternal joints to rule out occult bony pathology including tumor. If trauma is present, radionucleotide bone scanning may be useful to rule out occult fractures of the ribs, sternum, or both. Based on the patient's clinical presentation, additional testing, including complete blood count, prostate-specific antigen, sedimentation rate, and antinuclear antibody testing, may be indicated. Magnetic resonance imaging of the joints is indicated if joint instability or occult mass is suspected. The following injection technique will serve as both a diagnostic and therapeutic maneuver.

DIFFERENTIAL DIAGNOSIS

As mentioned, the pain of costosternal syndrome is often mistaken for pain of cardiac origin and can lead to visits to the emergency department and unnecessary cardiac work-ups. If trauma has occurred, costosternal syndrome may coexist with fractured ribs or fractures of the sternum itself, which can be missed on plain radiographs and may require radionucleotide bone scanning for proper identification. Tietze's syndrome, which is painful enlargement of the upper costochondral cartilage associated with viral infections, can be confused with costosternal syndrome.

Neuropathic pain involving the chest wall may also be confused or coexist with costosternal syndrome. Examples of such neuropathic pain include diabetic polyneuropathies and acute herpes zoster involving the thoracic nerves. The possibility of diseases of the structures of the mediastinum remain ever present and at times can be difficult to diagnose. Pathologic processes that inflame the pleura, such as pulmonary

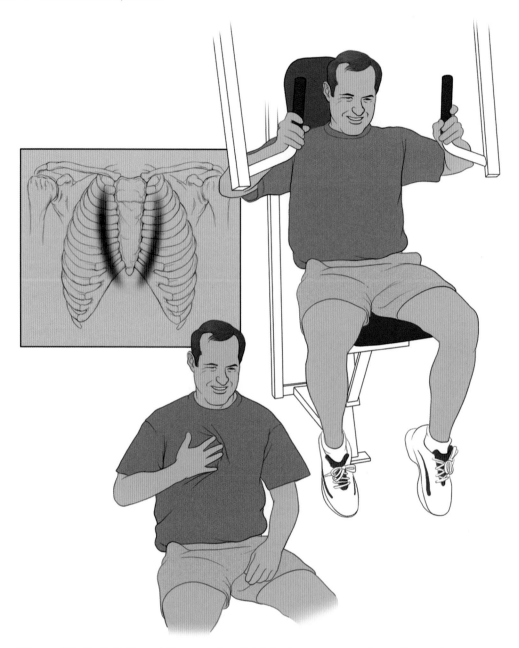

Figure 36–1. Irritation of the costosternal joints from overuse of exercise equipment can cause costosternal syndrome.

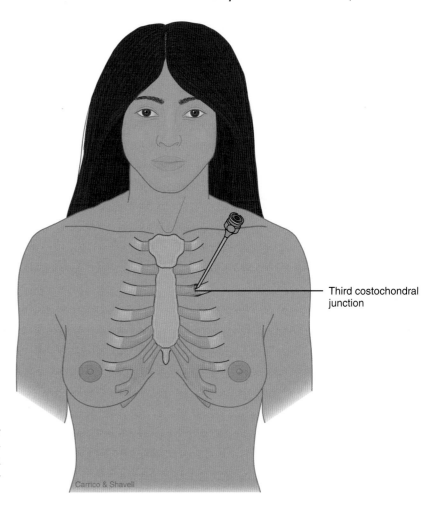

Third costochondral junction

Figure 36–2. Correct needle placement for injection technique for costosternal syndrome. (From Waldman SD: Atlas of Pain Management Injection Techniques. WB Saunders, Philadelphia, 2000, p 173.)

embolus, infection, and Bornholm's disease, may also confuse the diagnosis and complicate treatment.

TREATMENT

Initial treatment of the pain and functional disability associated with costosternal syndrome should include a combination of the nonsteroidal anti-inflammatory drugs or the cyclooxygenase-2 inhibitors. The local application of heat and cold may also be beneficial. The use of an elastic rib belt may also help provide symptomatic relief and help protect the costosternal joints from additional trauma. For patients who do not respond to these treatment modalities, the following injection technique with local anesthetic and steroid may be a reasonable next step.

Intra-articular injection of the costosternal joint is performed by placing the patient in the supine position; proper preparation with antiseptic solution of the skin overlying the affected costosternal joints is then carried out. A sterile syringe containing 1.0 mL of 0.25% preservative-free bupivacaine for each joint to be injected and 40 mg methylprednisolone acetate is attached to a 1½-inch 25-gauge needle using strict aseptic technique.

With strict aseptic technique, the costosternal joints are identified. The costosternal joints should be easily palpable as a slight bulging at the point where the rib attaches to the sternum. The needle is then carefully advanced through the skin and subcutaneous tissues medially with a slight cephalad trajectory into proximity with the joint (Fig. 36–2). If bone is encountered, the needle is withdrawn from the periosteum. After the needle is in proximity to the joint, 1 mL of solution is gently injected. There should be limited resistance to injection. If significant resistance is encountered, the needle should be withdrawn slightly until the injection proceeds with only limited resistance. This procedure is repeated for each affected joint. The needle is then removed, and a sterile pressure dressing and ice pack are placed at the injection site.

COMPLICATIONS AND PITFALLS

Because of the many pathologic processes that may mimic the pain of costosternal syndrome, the clinician must be careful to rule out underlying cardiac disease and diseases of the lung and structures of the mediastinum. Failure to do so could lead to disastrous results. The major complication of this injection technique is pneumothorax if the needle is placed too laterally or deeply and invades the pleural space. Infection, although rare, can occur if strict aseptic technique is not followed. The possibility of trauma to the contents of the mediastinum remains an ever-present possibility. This complication can be greatly decreased if the clinician pays close attention to accurate needle placement.

CLINICAL PEARLS

Patients suffering from pain emanating from the costosternal joint will often attribute their pain symptomatology to a heart attack. Reassurance is required, although it should be remembered that this musculoskeletal pain syndrome and coronary artery disease can coexist. Tietze's syndrome, which is painful enlargement of the upper costochondral cartilage associated with viral infections, can be confused with costosternal syndrome, although both respond to the aforementioned injection technique. The use of physical modalities including local heat as well as gentle range of motion exercises should be introduced several days after the patient undergoes this injection for costosternal joint pain. Vigorous exercises should be avoided because they will exacerbate the patient's symptomatology. Simple analgesics and nonsteroidal anti-inflammatory drugs may be used concurrently with this injection technique. Laboratory evaluation for collagen vascular disease is indicated in patients suffering from costosternal joint pain in whom other joints are involved.

37

Intercostal Neuralgia

ICD-9 CODE 354.8

THE CLINICAL SYNDROME

In contradistinction to most other causes of pain involving the chest wall that are musculoskeletal in nature, the pain of intercostal neuralgia is neuropathic. As with costosternal joint pain, Tietze's syndrome, and rib fractures, a significant number of patients who suffer from intercostal neuralgia first seek medical attention because they believe they are suffering a heart attack. If the subcostal nerve is involved, patients may believe they are suffering from gallbladder disease. The pain of intercostal neuralgia is due to damage or inflammation of the intercostal nerves. The pain is constant and burning in nature and may involve any of the intercostal nerves as well as the subcostal nerve of the twelfth rib. The pain usually begins at the posterior axillary line and radiates anteriorly into the distribution of the affected intercostal or subcostal nerves, or both (Fig. 37–1).

Deep inspiration or movement of the chest wall may slightly increase the pain of intercostal neuralgia, but to a much lesser extent compared with the pain associated with the musculoskeletal causes of chest wall pain, such as costosternal joint pain, Tietze's syndrome, and broken ribs.

SIGNS AND SYMPTOMS

Physical examination of the patient suffering from intercostal neuralgia will generally reveal minimal physical findings unless there is a history of previous thoracic or subcostal surgery or cutaneous findings of herpes zoster involving the thoracic dermatomes. In contradistinction to the aforementioned musculoskele-

tal causes of chest wall and subcostal pain, the patient suffering from intercostal neuralgia does not attempt to splint or protect the affected area. Careful sensory examination of the affected dermatomes may reveal decreased sensation or allodynia. With significant motor involvement of the subcostal nerve, the patient may complain that his or her abdomen bulges out.

TESTING

Plain radiographs are indicated for all patients who present with pain thought to be emanating from the intercostal nerve to rule out occult bony pathology including tumor. If trauma is present, radionucleotide bone scanning may be useful to rule out occult fractures of the ribs, sternum, or both. Based on the patient's clinical presentation, additional testing, including complete blood count, prostate-specific antigen, sedimentation rate, and antinuclear antibody testing, may be indicated. Computed tomography scanning of the thoracic contents is indicated if occult mass is suspected. The following injection technique will serve as both a diagnostic and therapeutic maneuver.

DIFFERENTIAL DIAGNOSIS

As mentioned, the pain of intercostal neuralgia is often mistaken for pain of cardiac or gallbladder origin and can lead to visits to the emergency department and unnecessary cardiac and gastrointestinal work-ups. If trauma has occurred, intercostal neuralgia may coexist with fractured ribs or fractures of the sternum itself, which can be missed on plain radiographs and may require radionucleotide bone scanning for proper identification. Tietze's syndrome, which is painful enlargement of the upper costochondral cartilage associated with viral infections, can be confused with intercostal neuralgia.

Neuropathic pain involving the chest wall may also be confused or coexist with costosternal syndrome. Examples of such neuropathic pain include diabetic polyneuropathies and acute herpes zoster involving the thoracic nerves. The possibility of diseases of the structures of the mediastinum remains ever present and at times these diseases can be difficult to diagnose. Pathologic processes that inflame the pleura, such as pulmonary embolus, infection, and Bornholm's disease, may also confuse the diagnosis and complicate treatment.

TREATMENT

Initial treatment of intercostal neuralgia should include a combination of simple analgesics and the nonsteroidal anti-inflammatory drugs or the cyclooxygenase-2 inhibitors. If these medications do not adequately control the patient's symptomatology, a tricyclic antidepressant or gabapentin should be added.

Traditionally, the *tricyclic antidepressants* have been a mainstay in the palliation of pain secondary to intercostal neuralgia. Controlled studies have demonstrated the efficacy of amitriptyline for this indication. Other tricyclic antidepressants, including nortriptyline and desipramine, have also shown to be clinically useful. Unfortunately, this class of drugs is associated with significant anticholinergic side effects, including dry mouth, constipation, sedation, and urinary retention. These drugs should be used with caution in those suffering from glaucoma, cardiac arrhythmia, and prostatism. To minimize side effects and encourage compliance, the primary care physician should start amitriptyline or nortriptyline at a 10-mg dose at bedtime. The dose can be then titrated upward to 25 mg at bedtime as side effects allow. Upward titration of dosage in 25-mg increments can be carried out each week as side effects allow. Even at lower doses, patients will generally report a rapid improvement in sleep disturbance and will begin to experience some pain relieve in 10 to 14 days. If the patient does not experience any improvement in pain as the dose is being titrated upward, the addition of gabapentin alone or in combination with nerve blocks with local anesthetic or steroid, or both, is recommended (see later). The *selective serotonin reuptake inhibitors* such as fluoxetine have also been used to treat the pain of diabetic neuropathy, and although they are better tolerated than the tricyclic antidepressants, they appear to be less efficacious.

If the antidepressant compounds are ineffective or contraindicated, *gabapentin* represents a reasonable alternative. Gabapentin should be started with a 300-mg dose at bedtime for 2 nights. The patient should be cautioned about potential side effects, including dizziness, sedation, confusion, and rash. The drug is then increased in 300-mg increments, given in equally divided doses over 2 days, as side effects allow until pain relief is obtained or a total dosage of 2400 mg daily is reached. At this point, if the patient has experienced partial relief of pain, blood values are measured, and the drug is carefully titrated upward using 100-mg tablets. Rarely will more than 3600 mg daily be required.

The local application of *heat and cold* may also be beneficial to provide symptomatic relief of the pain of intercostal neuralgia. The use of an elastic rib belt may also help provide symptomatic relief. For patients who do not respond to these treatment modalities, the following injection technique using local anesthetic and steroid may be a reasonable next step.

The patient is placed in the prone position with the patient's arms hanging loosely off the side of the cart. Alternatively, this block can be done with the patient in the sitting or lateral position. The rib to be blocked is identified by palpating its path at the posterior axillary line. The index and middle fingers are then placed on the rib bracketing the site of needle insertion. The skin is then prepped with antiseptic solution. A 1½-inch 22-gauge needle is attached to a 12-mL syringe and is advanced perpendicular to the skin, aiming for the middle of the rib between the index and middle fingers. The needle should impinge on bone after being advanced approximately ¾ inch. After bony contact is made, the needle is withdrawn into the subcutaneous tissues, and the skin and subcutaneous tissues are retracted with the palpating fingers inferiorly. This allows the needle to be walked off the inferior margin of the rib. As soon as bony contact is lost, the needle is slowly advanced approximately 2 mm deeper. This will place the needle in proximity to the costal groove, which contains the intercostal nerve as well as the intercostal artery and vein. After careful aspiration reveals no blood or air, 3 to 5 mL of 1.0% preservative-free lidocaine is injected. If there is an inflammatory component to the pain, the local anesthetic is combined with 80 mg methylprednisolone acetate and is injected in incremental doses. Subsequent daily nerve blocks are carried out in a similar manner, substituting 40 mg methylprednisolone for the initial 80-mg dose. Because of the overlapping innervation of the chest and upper abdominal wall, the intercostal nerves above and below the nerve suspected of subserving the painful condition will have to be blocked.

COMPLICATIONS AND PITFALLS

The major problem in the care of patients thought to suffer from intercostal neuralgia is the failure to

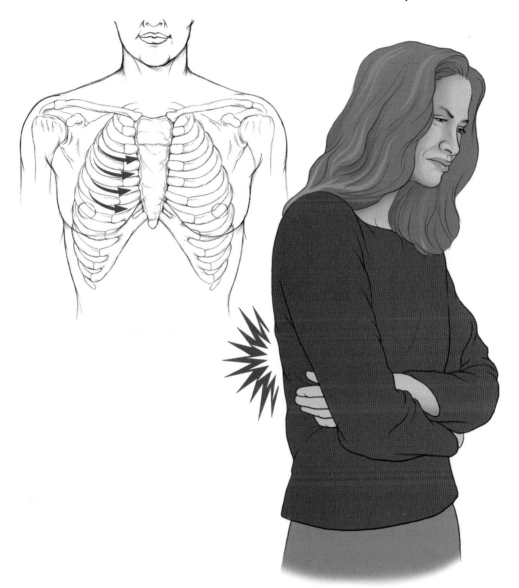

Figure 37–1. The pain of intercostal neuralgia is neuropathic rather than musculoskeletal in origin.

identify potentially serious pathology of the thorax or upper abdomen. Given the proximity of the pleural space, pneumothorax after intercostal nerve block is a distinct possibility. The incidence of the complication is less than 1%, but it occurs with greater frequency in patients with chronic obstructive pulmonary disease. Due to the proximity to the intercostal nerve and artery, the clinician should carefully calculate the total milligram dosage of local anesthetic administered, because vascular uptake via these vessels is high. Although uncommon, infection remains an ever-present possibility, especially in the immunocompromised patient with cancer. Early detection of infection is crucial to avoid potentially life-threatening sequelae.

CLINICAL PEARLS

Intercostal neuralgia is a commonly encountered cause of chest wall and thoracic pain. Correct diagnosis is necessary to properly treat this painful condition and to avoid overlooking serious intrathoracic or intra-abdominal pathology. The use of the pharmacologic agents mentioned, including gabapentin, will allow the clinician to adequately control the pain of intercostal neuralgia. Intercostal nerve block is a simple technique that can produce dramatic relief for patients suffering from intercostal neuralgia. As mentioned, the proximity of the intercostal nerve to the pleural space makes careful attention to technique mandatory.

38

Diabetic Truncal Neuropathy

ICD-9 CODE 250.6

THE CLINICAL SYNDROME

Diabetic neuropathy is the name used by clinicians to describe a heterogeneous group of diseases that affect the autonomic and peripheral nervous systems of patients suffering from diabetes mellitus. Diabetic neuropathy is now thought to be the most common form of peripheral neuropathy that afflicts humankind, with an estimated 220 million people suffering from this malady worldwide.

One of the most commonly encountered forms of diabetes neuropathy is diabetic truncal neuropathy. The pain and motor dysfunction of diabetic truncal neuropathy are often attributed to intrathoracic or intra-abdominal pathology leading to extensive work-ups for appendicitis, cholecystitis, renal calculi, and so on. The onset of symptoms will frequently coincide with periods of extreme hypoglycemia or hyperglycemia or with weight loss or weight gain. The patient who presents with diabetic truncal neuropathy will complain of severe dysesthetic pain with patchy sensory deficits in the distribution of the lower thoracic and/or upper thoracic dermatomes. The pain will often be worse at night and significant sleep disturbance may result, further worsening the patient's pain symptomatology. The symptoms of diabetic truncal neuropathy will often spontaneously resolve over a period of 6 to 12 months. However, due to the severity of symptoms associated with this condition, aggressive symptomatic relief with pharmacotherapy and neural blockade with local anesthetic and steroid is indicated.

SIGNS AND SYMPTOMS

Physical examination of the patient suffering from diabetic truncal neuropathy will generally reveal minimal physical findings unless there was a history of previous thoracic or subcostal surgery or cutaneous findings of herpes zoster involving the thoracic dermatomes. In contradistinction to the patient suffering from musculoskeletal causes of chest wall and subcostal pain, the patient suffering from diabetic truncal neuropathy does not attempt to splint or protect the affected area. Careful sensory examination of the affected dermatomes may reveal decreased sensation or allodynia. With significant motor involvement of the subcostal nerve, the patient may complain that his or her abdomen bulges out (Fig. 38–1).

TESTING

The presence of diabetes should raise a high index of suspicion that diabetic truncal neuropathy is present given the high incidence of this condition in patients suffering from diabetes mellitus. The targeted history and physical examination should allow the primary care physician to make the diagnosis of peripheral neuropathies in a large percentage of his or her patients suffering from diabetes.

If a diagnosis of diabetic truncal neuropathy is entertained on the basis of the targeted history and physical examination, screening laboratory testing, including a complete blood count, chemistry profile, sedimentation rate, thyroid function studies, antinuclear antibody testing, and urinalysis, should help rule out most peripheral neuropathies that may mimic diabetic truncal neuropathy and that are easily treatable. Electromyography and nerve conduction velocity testing are indicated in all patients suffering from peripheral neuropathy to help identify treatable entrapment neuropathies and further delineate the type of peripheral neuropathy that is present. Electromyography and nerve conduction velocity testing may also help quantify the severity of peripheral or entrapment neuropathy, or both. Additional laboratory testing is indicated as the clinical situation dictates (e.g., Lyme disease titers, heavy metal screens, and the like). Magnetic resonance imaging of the spi-

153

nal canal and cord should be performed if myelopathy is suspected. Nerve or skin biopsy is occasionally indicated if no etiology for the peripheral neuropathy can be ascertained. Lack of response to the therapies presented here should cause the primary care physician to reconsider the working diagnosis and to repeat testing as clinically indicated.

DIFFERENTIAL DIAGNOSIS

It should be remembered that diseases other than diabetic neuropathy may cause peripheral neuropathies in diabetic patients. These diseases may exist alone and may be clinically misdiagnosed as diabetic truncal neuropathy or may coexist with diabetic truncal neuropathy, making their identification and subsequent treatment more difficult.

Although uncommon in the United States, globally, Hansen's disease is a common cause of peripheral neuropathy that may mimic or coexist with diabetic truncal neuropathy. Other infectious etiologies of peripheral neuropathies include Lyme disease and human immunodeficiency virus infection. Substances that are toxic to nerves may also cause peripheral neuropathies that are indistinguishable from diabetic neuropathy on clinical grounds. Such substances include alcohol, heavy metals, chemotherapeutic agents, and hydrocarbons. Heritable disorders such as Charcot-Marie-Tooth disease and other familial diseases of the peripheral nervous system must also be considered, although treatment options are somewhat limited. Metabolic and endocrine causes of peripheral neuropathy that must be ruled out include vitamin deficiencies, pernicious anemia, hypothyroidism, uremia, and acute intermittent porphyria. Other causes of peripheral neuropathy that may confuse the clinical picture include Guillain-Barré syndrome, amyloidosis, entrapment neuropathies, carcinoid syndrome, paraneoplastic syndromes, and sarcoidosis. Because many of these causes of peripheral neuropathy are treatable, such as pernicious anemia, it is imperative that the clinician rule out these treatable diagnoses before attributing a patient's symptomatology solely to his or her diabetes.

Intercostal neuralgia and the musculoskeletal causes of chest wall and subcostal pain may also be confused with diabetic truncal neuropathy. As with these conditions, the patient's pain may be erroneously attributed to cardiac or upper abdominal pathology, leading to unnecessary testing and treatment.

TREATMENT

Control of Blood Sugar

Current thinking suggests that the better the glycemic control, the less severe is the symptomatology

of diabetic truncal neuropathy. Significant swings in blood sugars seem to predispose diabetic patients to the development of clinically significant diabetic truncal neuropathy. Some investigators believe that oral hypoglycemic agents, while controlling blood sugars, do not protect the patient from the development of diabetic truncal neuropathy as well as does insulin. In fact, some patients with diabetic truncal neuropathy who are on hypoglycemic agents will experience improvement in symptomatology when switched to insulin.

Pharmacologic Treatment

Antidepressant Agents

Traditionally, the tricyclic antidepressants have been a mainstay in the palliation of pain secondary to diabetic truncal neuropathy. Controlled studies have demonstrated the efficacy of amitriptyline for this indication. Other tricyclic antidepressants, including nortriptyline and desipramine, have also shown to be clinically useful. Unfortunately, this class of drugs is associated with significant anticholinergic side effects, including dry mouth, constipation, sedation, and urinary retention. These drugs should be used with caution in those suffering from glaucoma, cardiac arrhythmia, and prostatism. To minimize side effects and encourage compliance, the primary care physician should start amitriptyline or nortriptyline at a 10-mg dose at bedtime. The dose can be then titrated upward to 25 mg at bedtime as side effects allow. Upward titration of dosage in 25-mg increments can be carried out each week as side effects allow. Even at lower doses, patients will generally report a rapid improvement in sleep disturbance and will begin to experience some pain relief in 10 to 14 days. If the patient does not experience any improvement in pain as the dose is being titrated upward, the addition of gabapentin alone or in combination with nerve blocks with local anesthetic and steroid is recommended (see later). The selective serotonin reuptake inhibitors such as fluoxetine have also been used to treat the pain of diabetic truncal neuropathy, and although they are better tolerated that the tricyclic antidepressants, they appear to be less efficacious.

Anticonvulsant Agents

The anticonvulsants have long been used to treat neuropathic pain, including diabetic truncal neuropathy. Both phenytoin and carbamazepine have been used with varying degrees of success either alone or in combination with the antidepressant compounds. Unfortunately, the side effect profiles of these drugs have limited their clinical usefulness. The anticonvulsant *gabapentin* has been shown to be highly effica-

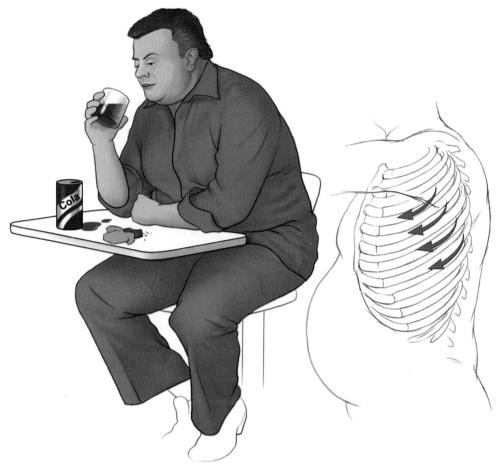

Figure 38–1. The pain of diabetic truncal neuropathy is neuropathic in nature and is often made worse by poorly controlled blood sugar.

cious in the treatment of a variety of neuropathic painful conditions, including postherpetic neuralgia and diabetic truncal neuropathy. Used properly, gabapentin is extremely well tolerated compared with other drugs, including the antidepressant compounds and anticonvulsants mentioned here that previously were used routinely to treat diabetic truncal neuropathy. In fact, in most pain centers, gabapentin has become the adjuvant analgesic of choice in the treatment of diabetic truncal neuropathy. Gabapentin has a large therapeutic window, but the primary care physician is cautioned to start this medication at the lower end of the dosage spectrum and to titrate upward slowly to avoid central nervous system side effects, including sedation and fatigue. The following recommended dosage schedule will minimize side effects and encourage compliance. A single bedtime dose of 300 mg for 2 nights can be followed with a 300-mg twice daily dose for an additional 2 days. If the patient is tolerating this twice-daily dosing, the dosage may be increased to 300 mg three times daily. It has been our experience that most patients will begin to experience pain relief at this dosage range. Additional titration upward can be carried out in 300-mg increments as side effects allow. Daily doses above 3600 mg in divided doses are not currently recommended. Tablets of 600 and 800 mg have been made available to simplify maintenance dosing after titration has been completed. Clinical trials are under way with a gabapentin analogue that may provide additional therapeutic options for patients suffering from diabetic truncal neuropathy.

Antiarrhythmic Agents

Mexilitene is an antiarrhythmic compound that has been shown to be possibly effective in the management of diabetic truncal neuropathy. Some pain specialists believe that mexilitene is especially useful in those patients with diabetic truncal neuropathy whose pain manifests primarily as sharp lancinating or burning pain. Unfortunately, this drug is poorly tolerated by most patients and should be reserved for those patients in whom there was lack of response to first-line pharmacologic treatments such as gabapentin or nortriptyline alone or in combination with neural blockade.

Topical Agents

Some clinicians have reported success in the treatment of diabetic truncal neuropathy with topical application of capsaicin. An extract of chili peppers, capsaicin is thought to relieve neuropathic pain by depleting substance P. The side effects of capsaicin include significant burning and erythema and limit the use of this substance by many patients.

Topical lidocaine administered via transdermal patch or in a gel have also been shown to provide short-term relief of the pain of diabetic truncal neuropathy. This drug should be used with caution in patients who are on mexilitene because there is the potential for cumulative local anesthetic toxicity. Whether topical lidocaine will have a role in the long-term treatment of diabetic truncal neuropathy remains to be seen.

Analgesic Agents

In general, neuropathic pain such as diabetic truncal neuropathy responds poorly to analgesic compounds. The simple analgesics, including acetaminophen and aspirin, can be used in combination with the antidepressant and anticonvulsant compounds, but care must be taken not to exceed the recommended daily dose or renal or hepatic side effects may occur. The nonsteroidal anti-inflammatory drugs may also provide a modicum of pain relief when used with the antidepressants and anticonvulsant compounds, but given the nephrotoxicity of this class of drugs, they should be used with extreme caution in diabetic patients due to the high incidence of diabetic nephropathy, even early in the course of the disease. The role of the cyclooxygenase-2 inhibitors in the palliation of the pain has not been adequately studied.

The pain of diabetic truncal neuropathy responds poorly to treatment with opioid analgesics. Given the significant central nervous system and gastrointestinal side effects coupled with the problems of tolerance, dependence, and addiction, the narcotic analgesics should rarely if ever be used as a primary treatment for the pain of diabetic truncal neuropathy. If a narcotic analgesic is being considered in the setting, consideration should be given to the analgesic tramadol, which binds weakly to the opioid receptors and may provide some symptomatic relief. Tramadol should be used with care in combination with the antidepressant compounds to avoid the increased risk of seizures.

Neural Blockade

The use of neural blockade with local anesthetic either alone or in combination with steroid has been shown to be useful in the management of both the acute and chronic pain associated with diabetic truncal neuropathy. For truncal neuropathic pain, thoracic epidural or intercostal nerve block with local anesthetic or steroid, or both, may be beneficial. Occasionally, neuroaugmentation via spinal cord stimulation may provide significant relief of the pain of diabetic truncal neuropathy in those patients whom more conservative measures have not helped. Neurodestructive procedures are rarely if ever indicated to treat the pain of diabetic truncal neuropathy because they will often worsen the patient's pain and cause functional disability.

COMPLICATIONS AND PITFALLS

The major problem in the care of patients thought to suffer from diabetic truncal neuropathy is the failure to identify potentially serious pathology of the thorax or upper abdomen. Given the proximity of the pleural space, pneumothorax after intercostal nerve block is a distinct possibility. The incidence of the complication is less than 1%, but it occurs with greater frequency in patients with chronic obstructive pulmonary disease. Due to the proximity to the intercostal nerve and artery, the clinician should carefully calculate the total milligram dosage of local anesthetic administered, because vascular uptake via these vessels is high. Although uncommon, infection remains an ever-present possibility, especially in the immunocompromised patient with cancer. Early detection of infection is crucial to avoid potentially life-threatening sequelae.

CLINICAL PEARLS

Diabetic truncal neuropathy is a commonly encountered cause of thoracic pain and subcostal pain. Correct diagnosis is necessary to properly treat this painful condition and to avoid overlooking serious intrathoracic or intra-abdominal pathology. The use of the pharmacologic agents mentioned, including gabapentin, will allow the clinician to adequately control the pain of diabetic truncal neuropathy. Intercostal or epidural nerve blocks are simple techniques that can produce dramatic relief for patients suffering from intercostal neuralgia. As mentioned, the proximity of the intercostal nerve to the pleural space makes careful attention to technique mandatory when performing intercostal nerve block.

39

Tietze's Syndrome

ICD-9 CODE 733.6

THE CLINICAL SYNDROME

Tietze's syndrome is a common cause of chest wall pain encountered in clinical practice. Distinct from costosternal syndrome, Tietze's syndrome was first described in 1921 and is characterized by acute painful swelling of the costal cartilages. The second and third costal cartilages are most commonly involved, and in contradistinction to costosternal syndrome, which usually occurs no earlier than the fourth decade, Tietze's syndrome is a disease of the second and third decades. The onset is acute and is often associated with a concurrent viral respiratory tract infection. It has been postulated that microtrauma to the costosternal joints from serve coughing or heavy labor may be the cause of Tietze's syndrome. Painful swelling of the second and third costochondral joints is the sine qua non of Tietze's syndrome (Fig. 39–1). Such swelling is absent in costosternal syndrome, which occurs much more frequently than Tietze's syndrome.

SIGNS AND SYMPTOMS

Physical examination will reveal that the patient suffering from Tietze's syndrome will vigorously attempt to splint the joints by keeping the shoulders stiffly in neutral position. Pain is reproduced with active protraction or retraction of the shoulder, deep inspiration, and full elevation of the arm. Shrugging of the shoulder may also reproduce the pain. Coughing may be difficult, and this may lead to inadequate pulmonary toilet in patients suffering from Tietze's syndrome. The costosternal joints, especially the second and third, will be swollen and exquisitely tender to palpation. The adjacent intercostal muscles may also be tender to palpation. The patient may also complain of a clicking sensation with movement of the joint.

TESTING

Plain radiographs are indicated for all patients who present with pain thought to be emanating from the costosternal joints to rule out occult bony pathology including tumor. If trauma is present, radionucleotide bone scanning should be considered to rule out occult fractures of the ribs, sternum, or both. Based on the patient's clinical presentation, additional testing, including complete blood count, prostate-specific antigen, sedimentation rate, and antinuclear antibody testing, may be indicated. Magnetic resonance imaging of the joints is indicated if joint instability or occult mass is suspected. The following injection technique will serve as both a diagnostic and therapeutic maneuver.

DIFFERENTIAL DIAGNOSIS

It should be remembered that there are a variety of other painful conditions that affect the costosternal joints that occur with a much greater frequency than does Tietze's syndrome. The costosternal joints are susceptible to the development of arthritis, including osteoarthritis, rheumatoid arthritis, ankylosing spondylitis, Reiter's syndrome, and psoriatic arthritis. The joints are often traumatized during acceleration/deceleration injuries and blunt trauma to the chest. With severe trauma, the joints may sublux or dislocate. Overuse or misuse can also result in acute inflammation of the costosternal joint, which can be quite debilitating for the patient. The joints are also subject to invasion by tumor either from primary malignancies, including thymoma, or from metastatic disease.

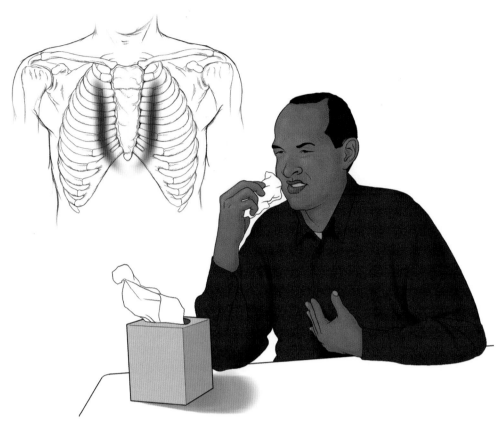

Figure 39–1. Swelling of the second and third costochondral joints is the sine qua non of Tietze's syndrome.

TREATMENT

Initial treatment of the pain and functional disability associated with Tietze's syndrome should include a combination of the nonsteroidal anti-inflammatory drugs or the cyclooxygenase-2 inhibitors. The local application of heat and cold may also be beneficial. The use of an elastic rib belt may also help provide symptomatic relief and help protect the costovertebral joints from additional trauma. For patients who do not respond to these treatment modalities, the following injection technique using local anesthetic and steroid may be a reasonable next step.

Injection for Tietze's syndrome is performed by placing the patient in the supine position, and proper preparation with antiseptic solution of the skin overlying the affected costosternal joints is carried out. A sterile syringe containing the 1.0 mL of 0.25% preservative-free bupivacaine for each joint to be injected and 40 mg methylprednisolone is attached to a 1½-inch 25-gauge needle using strict aseptic technique.

With strict aseptic technique, the costovertebral joints are identified. The costosternal joints should be easily palpable as a slight bulging at the point where the rib attaches to the sternum. The needle is then carefully advanced through the skin and subcutaneous tissues medially with a slight cephalad trajectory into proximity with the joint. If bone is encountered, the needle is withdrawn out of the periosteum. After the needle is in proximity to the joint, 1 mL of solution is gently injected. There should be limited resistance to injection. If significant resistance is encountered, the needle should be withdrawn slightly until the injection proceeds with only limited resistance. This procedure is repeated for each affected joint. The needle is then removed, and a sterile pressure dressing and ice pack are placed at the injection site.

COMPLICATIONS AND PITFALLS

Because of the many pathologic processes that may mimic the pain of Tietze's syndrome, the clinician must be careful to rule out underlying cardiac disease and diseases of the lung and structures of the mediastinum. Failure to do so could lead to disastrous results. The major complication of this injection technique is pneumothorax if the needle is placed too laterally or deeply and invades the pleural space. Infection, although rare, can occur if strict aseptic technique is not followed. The possibility of trauma to the contents of the mediastinum remains ever present. This complication can be greatly decreased if the clinician pays close attention to accurate needle placement.

CLINICAL PEARLS

Patients suffering from pain emanating from the costosternal joint will often attribute their pain to a heart attack. Reassurance is required, although it should be remembered that this musculoskeletal pain syndrome and coronary artery disease can coexist. Tietze's syndrome, which is painful enlargement of the upper costochondral cartilage associated with viral respiratory tract infections, can be confused with the more commonly occurring costosternal syndrome, although both respond to the aforementioned injection technique. Care must be taken to use sterile technique to avoid infection, as well as universal precautions to avoid risk to the operator. The incidence of ecchymosis and hematoma formation can be decreased if pressure is placed on the injection site immediately after injection. The use of physical modalities including local heat as well as gentle range of motion exercises should be introduced several days after the patient undergoes this injection technique for costosternal joint pain. Vigorous exercises should be avoided as they will exacerbate the patient's symptomatology. Simple analgesics and nonsteroidal anti-inflammatory drugs may be used concurrently with this injection technique. Laboratory evaluation for collagen vascular disease is indicated in patients suffering from costosternal joint pain in whom other joints are involved.

40 *Fractured Ribs*

ICD-9 CODE 807.0

THE CLINICAL SYNDROME

Fractured ribs are one of the most common causes of chest wall pain. They are most commonly associated with trauma to the chest wall. In osteoporotic patients or in patients with primary tumors or metastatic disease involving the ribs, they may occur with coughing (tussive fractures) or spontaneously.

The pain and functional disability associated with fractured ribs is determined in large part by the severity of injury (e.g., the number of ribs involved), the nature of the injury (e.g., partial or complete fractures, free-floating fragments), and the amount of damage to surrounding structures including the intercostal nerves and pleura. The severity of pain associated with fractured ribs may range from a dull, deep ache with partial osteoporotic fractures to severe sharp, stabbing pain that limits the patient's ability to maintain adequate pulmonary toilet.

SIGNS AND SYMPTOMS

Rib fractures are aggravated by deep inspiration, coughing, and any movement of the chest wall. Palpation of the affected ribs may elicit pain and reflex spasm of the musculature of the chest wall. Ecchymosis overlying the fractures may be present (Fig. 40–1). The clinician should be aware of the possibility of pneumothorax or hemopneumothorax. Damage to the intercostal nerves may produce severe pain and result in reflex splinting of the chest wall, further compromising the patient's pulmonary status. Failure to aggressively treat this pain and splinting may result in a negative cycle of hypoventilation, atelectasis, and ultimately pneumonia.

TESTING

Plain radiographs of the ribs and chest are indicated for all patients who present with pain from fractured ribs to rule out occult fractures and other bony pathology including tumor as well as pneumothorax and hemopneumothorax. If trauma is present, radionucleotide bone scanning may be useful to rule out occult fractures of the ribs, sternum, or both. If no trauma is present, bone density testing to rule out osteoporosis is appropriate as are serum protein electrophoresis and testing for hyperparathyroidism. Based on the patient's clinical presentation, additional testing, including complete blood count, prostate-specific antigen, sedimentation rate, and antinuclear antibody testing, may be indicated. Computed tomography scanning of the thoracic contents is indicated if occult mass or significant trauma to the thoracic contents is suspected. Electrocardiography to rule out cardiac contusion is indicated for all patients with traumatic sternal fractures or significant anterior chest wall trauma. The following injection technique should be used early to avoid pulmonary complications.

DIFFERENTIAL DIAGNOSIS

In the setting of trauma, the diagnosis of fractured ribs usually is easily made. It is in the setting of spontaneous rib fracture secondary to osteoporosis or metastatic disease that the diagnosis may be confusing. In this setting, the pain of occult rib fracture is often mistaken for pain of cardiac or gallbladder origin and can lead to visits to the emergency department and unnecessary cardiac and gastrointestinal work-ups. Tietze's syndrome, which is painful enlargement of the upper costochondral cartilage associated with viral infections, can be confused with fractured ribs, especially if the patient has been coughing.

TREATMENT

Initial treatment of rib fracture pain should include a combination of simple analgesics and the nonsteroidal anti-inflammatory drugs or the cyclooxygenase-2 inhibitors. If these medications do not adequately control the patient's symptomatology, short-acting potent opioid analgesics such as hydrocodone represent a reasonable next step. Because the opioid analgesics have the potential to suppress the cough reflex and respiration, the clinician must be careful to monitor the patient closely and to instruct the patient in adequate pulmonary toilet techniques.

The local application of heat and cold may also be beneficial to provide symptomatic relief of the pain of rib fracture. The use of an elastic rib belt may also help provide symptomatic relief. For patients who do not respond to these treatment modalities, the following injection technique using local anesthetic and steroid should be implemented to avoid pulmonary complications.

The patient is placed in the prone position with the patient's arms hanging loosely off the side of the cart. Alternatively, this block can be done with the patient in the sitting or lateral position. The rib to be blocked is identified by palpating its path at the posterior axillary line. The index and middle fingers are then placed on the rib, bracketing the site of needle insertion. The skin is then prepped with antiseptic solution. A 1½-inch 22-gauge needle is attached to a 12-mL syringe and is advanced perpendicular to the skin, aiming for the middle of the rib in between the index and middle fingers. The needle should impinge on bone after being advanced approximately ¾ inch. After bony contact is made, the needle is withdrawn into the subcutaneous tissues, and the skin and subcutaneous tissues are retracted with the palpating fingers inferiorly. This allows the needle to be walked off the inferior margin of the rib. As soon as bony contact is lost, the needle is slowly advanced approximately 2 mm deeper. This will place the needle in proximity to the costal groove, which contains the intercostal nerve as well as the intercostal artery and vein. After careful aspiration reveals no blood or air, 3 to 5 mL of 1.0% preservative-free lidocaine is injected. If there is an inflammatory component to the

pain, the local anesthetic is combined with 80 mg methylprednisolone and is injected in incremental doses. Subsequent daily nerve blocks are carried out in a similar manner, substituting 40 mg methylprednisolone for the initial 80-mg dose. Because of the overlapping innervation of the chest and upper abdominal wall, the intercostal nerves above and below the nerve suspected of subserving the painful condition will have to be blocked.

COMPLICATIONS AND PITFALLS

The major problem in the care of patients thought to suffer from rib fracture is the failure to identify potentially serious pathology of the thorax or upper abdomen, such as occult tumor, pneumothorax, or hemopneumothorax. Given the proximity of the pleural space, pneumothorax after intercostal nerve block is a distinct possibility. The incidence of the complication is less than 1%, but it occurs with greater frequency in patients with chronic obstructive pulmonary disease. Due to the proximity to the intercostal nerve and artery, the clinician should carefully calculate the total milligram dosage of local anesthetic administered, because vascular uptake via these vessels is high. Although uncommon, infection remains an ever-present possibility, especially in the immunocompromised patient with cancer. Early detection of infection is crucial to avoid potentially life-threatening sequelae.

CLINICAL PEARLS

Rib fracture is a commonly encountered cause of chest wall and thoracic pain. Correct diagnosis is necessary to properly treat this painful condition and to avoid overlooking serious intrathoracic or intra-abdominal pathology. The use of the aforementioned pharmacologic agents including opioid analgesics will allow the clinician to adequately control the pain of rib fracture. Intercostal nerve block is a simple technique that can produce dramatic relief for patients suffering from rib fracture. As mentioned, the proximity of the intercostal nerve to the pleural space makes careful attention to technique mandatory.

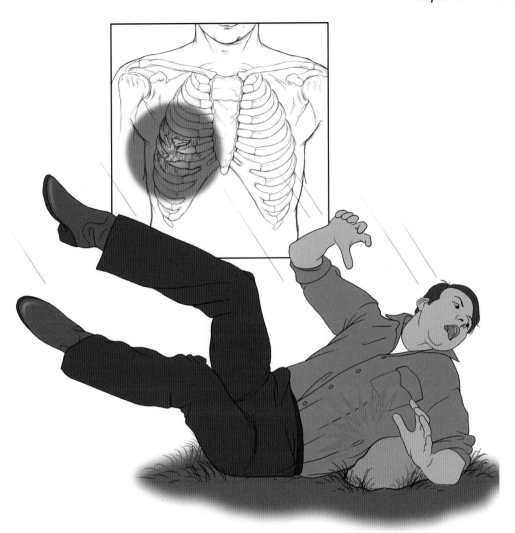

Figure 40-1. The pain of fractured ribs is amenable to intercostal nerve block with local anesthetic and steroid.

41

Post-Thoracotomy Pain

ICD-9 CODE 786.52

THE CLINICAL SYNDROME

Essentially all patients who undergo thoracotomy will suffer from acute postoperative pain. This acute pain syndrome will invariably respond to the rational use of systemic and spinal opioids as well as intercostal nerve block. Unfortunately, a small percentage of patients who undergo thoracotomy will suffer persistent pain beyond the usual course of postoperative pain. This pain syndrome is called post-thoracotomy pain syndrome and can be difficult to treat. The causes of post-thoracotomy pain are listed in Table 41–1 and include direct surgical trauma to the intercostal nerves, fractured ribs due to the rib spreader, compressive neuropathy of the intercostal nerves due to direct compression to the intercostal nerves, cutaneous neuroma formation, and stretch injuries to the intercostal nerves at the costovertebral junction. With the exception of fractured ribs, which produce characteristic local pain that is worse with deep inspiration, coughing, or movement of the affected ribs, the other causes of post-thoracotomy pain result in moderate to severe pain that is constant in nature and follows the distribution of the affected intercostal nerves. The

pain may be characterized at neuritic and may occasionally have a dysesthetic quality.

SIGNS AND SYMPTOMS

Physical examination of the patient suffering from post-thoracotomy syndrome will generally reveal tenderness along the healed thoracotomy incision. Occasionally, palpation of the scar will elicit paresthesias suggestive of neuroma formation. The patient suffering from post-thoracotomy syndrome may attempt to splint or protect the affected area (Fig. 41–1). Careful sensory examination of the affected dermatomes may reveal decreased sensation or allodynia. With significant motor involvement of the subcostal nerve, the patient may complain that his or her abdomen bulges out. Occasionally, patients suffering from post-thoracotomy syndrome will develop a reflex sympathetic dystrophy of the ipsilateral upper extremity. If the reflex sympathetic dystrophy is left untreated, a frozen shoulder may develop.

TESTING

Plain radiographs are indicated for all patients who present with pain that is thought to be emanating from the intercostal nerve to rule out occult bony pathology including tumor. Radionucleotide bone scanning may be useful to rule out occult fractures of the ribs, sternum, or both. Based on the patient's clinical presentation, additional testing, including complete blood count, prostate specific antigen, sedimentation rate, and antinuclear antibody testing, may be indicated. Computed tomography scanning of the thoracic contents is indicated if occult mass or pleural disease is suspected. The following injection technique will serve as both a diagnostic and therapeutic maneuver. Electromyography is useful in distinguishing injury of the distal intercostal nerve from stretch

Table 41–1. Causes of Post-thoracotomy Pain Syndrome

Direct surgical trauma to the intercostal nerves
Fractured ribs due to the rib spreader
Compressive neuropathy of the intercostal nerves due to direct compression of the intercostal nerves by retractors
Cutaneous neuroma formation
Stretch injuries to the intercostal nerves at the costovertebral junction

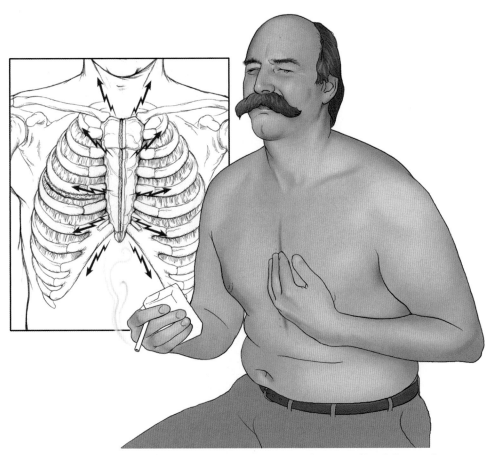

Figure 41–1. The patient with post-thoracotomy syndrome will exhibit tenderness to palpation of the scar.

injuries of the intercostal nerve at the costovertebral junction.

DIFFERENTIAL DIAGNOSIS

The pain of post-thoracotomy syndrome may be mistaken for pain of cardiac or gallbladder origin and can lead to visits to the emergency department and unnecessary cardiac and gastrointestinal work-ups. If trauma has occurred, post-thoracotomy syndrome may coexist with fractured ribs or fractures of the sternum itself, which can be missed on plain radiographs and may require radionucleotide bone scanning for proper identification. Tietze's syndrome, which is painful enlargement of the upper costochondral cartilage associated with viral infections, can be confused with post-thoracotomy syndrome.

Neuropathic pain involving the chest wall may also be confused or coexist with post-thoracotomy syndrome. Examples of such neuropathic pain include diabetic polyneuropathies and acute herpes zoster involving the thoracic nerves. The possibility of diseases of the structures of the mediastinum remains ever present and at times these diseases can be difficult to diagnose. Pathologic processes that inflame the pleura, such as pulmonary embolus, infection, and Bornholm's disease, may also confuse the diagnosis and complicate treatment.

TREATMENT

Initial treatment of post-thoracotomy syndrome should include a combination of simple analgesics and the nonsteroidal anti-inflammatory drugs or the cyclooxygenase-2 inhibitors. If these medications do not adequately control the patient's symptomatology, a tricyclic antidepressant or gabapentin should be added.

Traditionally, the *tricyclic antidepressants* have been a mainstay in the palliation of pain secondary to post-thoracotomy syndrome. Controlled studies have demonstrated the efficacy of amitriptyline for this indication. Other tricyclic antidepressants, including nortriptyline and desipramine, have also shown to be clinically useful. Unfortunately, this class of drugs is associated with significant anticholinergic side effects, including dry mouth, constipation, sedation, and urinary retention. These drugs should be used with caution in those suffering from glaucoma, cardiac arrhythmia, and prostatism. To minimize side effects and encourage compliance, the primary care physician should start amitriptyline or nortriptyline at a 10-mg dose at bedtime. The dose can be then titrated upward to 25 mg at bedtime as side effects allow. Upward titration of dosage in 25-mg increments can

be carried out each week as side effects allow. Even at lower doses, patients will generally report a rapid improvement in sleep disturbance and will begin to experience some pain relief in 10 to 14 days. If the patient does not experience any improvement in pain as the dose is being titrated upward, the addition of gabapentin alone or in combination with nerve blocks with local anesthetics or steroid, or both, is recommended (see later). The *selective serotonin reuptake inhibitors* such as fluoxetine have also been used to treat the pain of diabetic neuropathy, and although they are better tolerated than the tricyclic antidepressants, they appear to be less efficacious.

If the antidepressant compounds are ineffective or contraindicated, *gabapentin* represents a reasonable alternative. Gabapentin should be started at a 300-mg dose at bedtime for 2 nights. The patient should be cautioned about potential side effects, including dizziness, sedation, confusion, and rash. The drug is then increased in 300-mg increments, given in equally divided doses over 2 days, as side effects allow until pain relief is obtained or a total dosage of 2400 mg daily is reached. At this point, if the patient has experienced partial relief of pain, blood values are measured and the drug is carefully titrated upward using 100-mg tablets. Rarely will more than 3600 mg daily be required.

The local application of *heat and cold* may also be beneficial to provide symptomatic relief of the pain of post-thoracotomy syndrome. The use of an elastic rib belt may also help provide symptomatic relief. For patients who do not respond to these treatment modalities, the following injection technique using local anesthetic and steroid may be a reasonable next step.

The patient is placed in the prone position with the patient's arms hanging loosely off the side of the cart. Alternatively, this block can be done with the patient in the sitting or lateral position. The rib to be blocked is identified by palpating its path at the posterior axillary line. The index and middle fingers are then placed on the rib, bracketing the site of needle insertion. The skin is then prepped with antiseptic solution. A 1½-inch 22-gauge needle is attached to a 12-ml syringe and is advanced perpendicular to the skin, aiming for the middle of the rib between the index and middle fingers. The needle should impinge on bone after being advanced approximately ¾ inch. After bony contact is made, the needle is withdrawn into the subcutaneous tissues, and the skin and subcutaneous tissues are retracted with the palpating fingers inferiorly. This allows the needle to be walked off the inferior margin of the rib. As soon as bony contact is lost, the needle is slowly advanced approximately 2 mm deeper. This will place the needle in proximity to the costal groove, which contains the intercostal nerve as well as the intercostal artery and vein. After careful aspiration reveals no blood or air,

3 to 5 ml of 1.0% preservative-free lidocaine is injected. If there is an inflammatory component to the pain, the local anesthetic is combined with 80 mg methylprednisolone and is injected in incremental doses. Subsequent daily nerve blocks are carried out in a similar manner, substituting 40 mg methylprednisolone for the initial 80-mg dose. Because of the overlapping innervation of the chest and upper abdominal wall, the intercostal nerves above and below the nerve suspected of subserving the painful condition will have to be blocked.

It should be remembered that stretch injury of the intercostal nerve may result in post-thoracotomy pain syndrome. Electromyography may be useful to help identify this problem. If such an injury exists, it may respond to thoracic steroid epidural nerve block.

COMPLICATIONS AND PITFALLS

The major problem in the care of patients thought to suffer from post-thoracotomy syndrome is the failure to identify potentially serious pathology of the thorax or upper abdomen. Given the proximity of the pleural space, pneumothorax after intercostal nerve block is a distinct possibility. The incidence of the complication is less than 1%, but it occurs with greater frequency in patients with chronic obstructive pulmonary disease. Due to the proximity to the intercostal nerve and artery, the clinician should carefully calculate the total milligram dosage of local anesthetic administered, because vascular uptake via these vessels is high. Although uncommon, infection remains an ever-present possibility, especially in the immunocompromised patient with cancer. Early detection of infection is crucial to avoid potentially life-threatening sequelae.

CLINICAL PEARLS

Post-thoracotomy syndrome is a commonly encountered cause of chest wall and thoracic pain. Correct diagnosis is necessary to properly treat this painful condition and to avoid overlooking serious intrathoracic or intra-abdominal pathology. The use of the aforementioned pharmacologic agents, including gabapentin, will allow the clinician to adequately control the pain of post-thoracotomy syndrome. Intercostal nerve block is a simple technique that can produce dramatic relief for patients suffering from post-thoracotomy syndrome. As mentioned, the proximity of the intercostal nerve to the pleural space makes careful attention to technique mandatory.

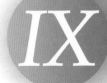

IX Thoracic Spine Pain Syndromes

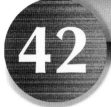

Acute Herpes Zoster of the Thoracic Dermatome

ICD-9 CODE 053.9

THE CLINICAL SYNDROME

Herpes zoster is an infectious disease that is caused by the varicella-zoster virus (VZV), which also is the causative agent of chickenpox (varicella). The thoracic nerve roots are the most common site for the development of acute herpes zoster. Primary infection in the nonimmune host manifests itself clinically as the childhood disease chickenpox. It is postulated that during the course of primary infection with VZV, the virus migrates to the dorsal root of the thoracic nerves. The virus then remains dormant in the ganglia, producing no clinically evident disease. In some individuals, the virus may reactivate and travel along the sensory pathways of the first division of the trigeminal nerve, producing the pain and skin lesions characteristic of shingles. The reason that reactivation occurs in only some individuals is not fully understood, but it is theorized that a decrease in cell-mediated immunity may play an important role in the evolution of this disease entity by allowing the virus to multiply in the ganglia and spread to the corresponding sensory nerves, producing clinical disease. Patients who are suffering from malignancies (particularly lymphoma), receiving immunosuppressive therapy (chemotherapy, steroids, radiation), or suffering from chronic diseases are generally debilitated and much more likely than the healthy population to develop acute herpes zoster. These patients all have in common a decreased cell-mediated immune response, which may be the reason for their propensity to develop shingles. This may also explain why the incidence of shingles increases dramatically in patients older than 60 years and is relatively uncommon in persons younger than 20 years.

SIGNS AND SYMPTOMS

As viral reactivation occurs, ganglionitis and peripheral neuritis cause pain, which is generally localized to the segmental distribution of the thoracic nerve roots. This pain may be accompanied by flulike symptoms and generally progresses from a dull, aching sensation to dysesthetic to neuritic pain in the distribution of the thoracic nerve roots. In most patients, the pain of acute herpes zoster precedes the eruption of rash by 3 to 7 days, often leading to erroneous diagnosis (see Differential Diagnosis). However, in most patients, the clinical diagnosis of shingles is readily made when the characteristic rash appears. Like chickenpox, the rash of herpes zoster appears in crops of macular lesions, which rapidly progress to papules and then to vesicles (Fig. 42–1). As the disease progresses, the vesicles coalesce and crusting occurs. The area affected by the disease can be extremely painful, and the pain tends to be exacerbated by any movement or contact (e.g., with clothing or sheets). As healing takes place, the crusts fall away, leaving pink scars in the distribution of the rash that gradually become hypopigmented and atrophic.

In most patients, the hyperesthesia and pain generally resolve as the skin lesions heal. In some, however, pain may persist beyond lesion healing. This most common and feared complication of acute herpes zoster is called postherpetic neuralgia, and the elderly are affected at a higher rate than the general population suffering from acute herpes zoster (see Fig. 1–2). The symptoms of postherpetic neuralgia can vary from a mild self-limited problem to a debilitating, constantly burning pain that is exacerbated by light touch, movement, anxiety, or temperature change or a combination. This unremitting pain may be so severe that it completely devastates the patient's life, and ultimately it can lead to suicide. It is the desire to avoid this disastrous sequel to a usually benign self-limited disease that dictates the clinician use all possible therapeutic efforts for the patient suffering from acute herpes zoster in the thoracic nerve roots.

TESTING

Although in most instances the diagnosis of acute herpes zoster involving the thoracic nerve roots is easily made on clinical grounds, occasionally, confirmatory testing is required. Such testing may be desirable in patients with other skin lesions that confuse the clinical picture, such as patients with HIV infection who are suffering from Kaposi's sarcoma. In such patients, the diagnosis of acute herpes zoster may be confirmed by obtaining a Tzanck smear from the base of a fresh vesicle, which will reveal multinucleated giant cells and eosinophilic inclusions. To differentiate acute herpes zoster from localized herpes simplex infection, the clinician can obtain fluid from a fresh vesicle and submit it for immunofluorescent testing.

DIFFERENTIAL DIAGNOSIS

Careful initial evaluation, including a thorough history and physical examination, is indicated in all patients suffering from acute herpes zoster involving the thoracic nerve roots to rule out occult malignancy or systemic disease that may be responsible for the patient's immunocompromised state and to allow early recognition of changes in clinical status that may presage the development of complications, including myelitis or dissemination of the disease. Other causes of pain in the distribution of the thoracic nerve roots include thoracic radiculopathy and peripheral neuropathy. Intrathoracic and intra-abdominal pathology may also mimic the pain of acute herpes zoster involving the thoracic dermatomes.

TREATMENT

The therapeutic challenge of the patient presenting with acute herpes zoster involving the thoracic nerve roots is twofold: (1) the immediate relief of acute pain and symptoms and (2) the prevention of complications, including postherpetic neuralgia. It is the consensus of most pain specialists that the earlier in the natural course of the disease that treatment is initiated, the less likely the patient will develop postherpetic neuralgia. Furthermore, because the older patient is at highest risk for developing postherpetic

neuralgia, early and aggressive treatment of this group of patients is mandatory.

Nerve Blocks

Sympathetic neural blockade with local anesthetic and steroid via thoracic epidural nerve block appears to be the treatment of choice to relieve the symptoms of acute herpes zoster involving the thoracic nerve roots as well as to prevent the occurrence of postherpetic neuralgia. Sympathetic nerve block is thought to achieve these goals by blocking the profound sympathetic stimulation that is a result of the viral inflammation of the nerve and dorsal root ganglion. If untreated, this sympathetic hyperactivity can cause ischemia secondary to decreased blood flow of the intraneural capillary bed. If this ischemia is allowed to persist, endoneural edema forms, increasing endoneural pressure and causing a further reduction in endoneural blood flow with irreversible nerve damage.

As vesicular crusting occurs, the addition of steroids to the local anesthetic may decrease neural scarring and further decrease the incidence of postherpetic neuralgia. These sympathetic blocks should be continued aggressively until the patient is pain free and should be reimplemented at the return of pain. Failure to use sympathetic neural blockade immediately and aggressively, especially in the elderly, may sentence the patient to a lifetime of suffering from postherpetic neuralgia. Occasionally, some patients suffering from acute herpes zoster involving the thoracic nerve roots may not experience pain relief from thoracic epidural nerve block but will respond to blockade of the thoracic sympathetic nerves.

Opioid Analgesics

Opioid analgesics may be useful in relieving the aching pain that is often present during the acute stages of herpes zoster as sympathetic nerve blocks are being implemented. They are less effective in the relief of the neuritic pain that is often present. Careful administration of potent, long-acting narcotic analgesics (e.g., oral morphine elixir or methadone) on a time contingent rather than an as-needed basis may represent a beneficial adjunct to the pain relief provided by sympathetic neural blockade. Because many patients suffering from acute herpes zoster are elderly or may have severe multisystem disease, close monitoring for the potential side effects of potent narcotic analgesics (e.g., confusion or dizziness, which may cause a patient to fall) is warranted. Daily dietary fiber supplementation and milk of magnesia should

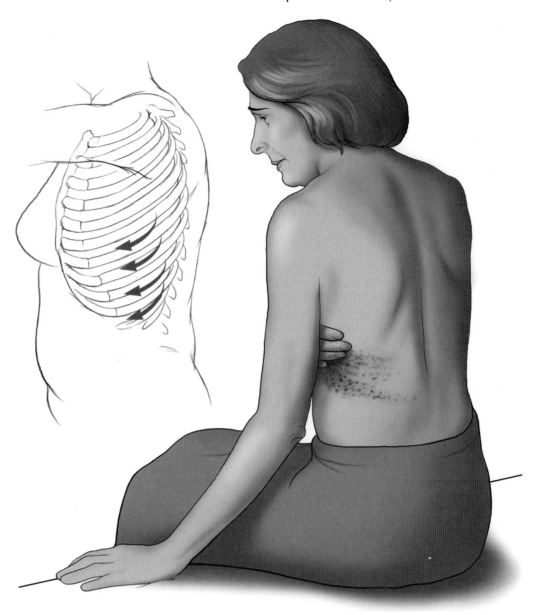

Figure 42–1. Acute herpes zoster occurs most commonly in the thoracic dermatomes.

be started along with opioid analgesics to prevent the side effect of constipation.

Adjuvant Analgesics

The anticonvulsant gabapentin represents a first-line treatment in the palliation of neuritic pain of acute herpes zoster involving the thoracic nerve roots. Studies also suggest that gabapentin may help prevent the development of postherpetic neuralgia. Treatment with gabapentin should begin early in the course of the disease, and this drug may be used concurrently with neural blockade, opioid analgesics, and other adjuvant analgesics, including the antidepressant compounds if care is taken to avoid central nervous system side effects. Gabapentin is started at a dose of 300 mg at bedtime and is titrated upward in 300-mg increments to a maximum dosage of 3600 mg daily given in divided doses as side effects allow. Carbamazepine should be considered in patients suffering from severe neuritic pain who have failed to respond to nerve blocks and gabapentin. If this drug is used, rigid monitoring for hematologic parameters, especially in patients receiving chemotherapy or radiation therapy, is indicated. Phenytoin may also be beneficial to treat neuritic pain but should not be used in patients with lymphoma because the drug may induce a pseudolymphoma-like state that is difficult to distinguish from the actual lymphoma itself.

Antidepressant Compounds

Antidepressants may also be useful adjuncts in the initial treatment of the patient suffering from acute herpes zoster. On an acute basis, these drugs will help alleviate the significant sleep disturbance that is commonly seen in this setting. In addition, the antidepressants may be valuable in helping ameliorate the neuritic component of the pain, which is treated less effectively with narcotic analgesics. After several weeks of treatment, the antidepressants may exert a mood-elevating effect that may be desirable in some patients. Care must be taken to observe closely for central nervous system side effects in this patient population. These drugs may cause urinary retention and constipation that may be mistakenly attributed to herpes zoster myelitis.

Antiviral Agents

A limited number of antiviral agents, including famciclovir and acyclovir, have been shown to shorten the course of acute herpes zoster and may help prevent the development of acute herpes zoster. They are probably useful in attenuating the disease in immunosuppressed patients. These antiviral agents can be used in conjunction with the aforementioned treatment modalities. Careful monitoring for side effects is mandatory with the use of these drugs.

Adjunctive Treatments

The application of ice packs to the lesions of acute herpes zoster may provide relief in some patients. The application of heat will increase pain in most patients, presumably because of increased conduction of small fibers, but is beneficial in an occasional patient and may be worth trying if the application of cold is ineffective. Transcutaneous electrical nerve stimulation and vibration may also be effective in a limited number of patients. The favorable risk-to-benefit ratio of all these modalities makes them reasonable alternatives for patients who cannot or will not undergo sympathetic neural blockade or tolerate pharmacologic interventions.

Topical application of aluminum sulfate as a tepid soak provides excellent drying of the crusting and weeping lesions of acute herpes zoster, and most patients find these soaks to be soothing. Zinc oxide ointment may also be used as a protective agent, especially during the healing phase, when temperature sensitivity is a problem. Disposable diapers can be used as an absorbent padding to protect healing lesions from contact with clothing and sheets.

COMPLICATIONS AND PITFALLS

In most patients, acute herpes zoster involving the thoracic nerve roots is a self-limited disease. In the elderly and the immunosuppressed, however, complications may occur. Cutaneous and visceral dissemination may range from a mild rash resembling chickenpox to an overwhelming, life-threatening infection in those already suffering from severe multisystem disease. Myelitis may cause bowel, bladder, and lower extremity paresis. Ocular complications from trigeminal nerve involvement may range from severe photophobia to keratitis with loss of sight.

CLINICAL PEARLS

Because the pain of herpes zoster usually precedes the eruption of skin lesions by 5 to 7 days, an erroneous diagnosis of other painful conditions (e.g., thoracic radiculopathy, cholecystitis) may be made. In this setting, the astute clinician will advise the patient to call immediately should rash appear as the diagnosis of acute herpes zoster is a possibility. Some pain specialists believe that in a small number of immuno-competent patients, when reactivation of virus occurs, a rapid immune response may attenuate the natural course of the disease and the characteristic rash of acute herpes zoster may not appear. This pain in the distribution of the thoracic nerve roots without associated rash is called zoster sine herpete and is by necessity a diagnosis of exclusion. Therefore, other causes of thoracic and subcostal pain must be ruled out before invoking this diagnosis.

43

Postherpetic Neuralgia

ICD-9 CODE 053.19

THE CLINICAL SYNDROME

One of the most difficult pain syndromes to treat, postherpetic neuralgia will occur in 10% of patients after a bout of acute herpes zoster. The reason that this painful condition occurs in some patients but not others is unknown, but it occurs more frequently in older patients and appears to occur more frequently after acute herpes zoster of the trigeminal nerve as opposed to acute herpes zoster involving the thoracic dermatomes. Conditions that cause vulnerable nerve syndrome, such as diabetes, may also predispose the patient to develop postherpetic neuralgia. It is the consensus among pain specialists that aggressive treatment of acute herpes zoster will help the patient avoid postherpetic neuralgia.

The pain of postherpetic neuralgia is characterized as a constant, dysesthetic pain that may be exacerbated by movement or stimulation of the affected cutaneous regions. There may be sharp, shooting neuritic pain superimposed on the constant dysesthetic symptoms. Some patients suffering from postherpetic neuralgia will also note a burning component reminiscent of reflex sympathetic dystrophy.

SIGNS AND SYMPTOMS

As the lesions of acute herpes zoster heal, the crusts fall away, leaving pink scars in the distribution of the rash that gradually become hypopigmented and atrophic (Fig. 43–1). These affected cutaneous areas are often allodynic, although hypesthesia and rarely anesthesia of the affected areas may occur. In most patients, these sensory abnormalities and pain generally resolve as the skin lesions heal. In some, however, pain may persist beyond lesion healing.

TESTING

In most instances, the diagnosis of postherpetic neuralgia roots is easily made on clinical grounds. Testing is generally used to identify other treatable coexisting diseases such as vertebral compression fractures or to rule out the underlying disease responsible for the patient's immunocompromised state. Such testing should include basic screening laboratory testing, rectal examination, mammography, and testing for collagen vascular diseases and human immunodeficiency infection. Skin biopsy may help confirm the presence of previous infection with herpes zoster if the history is in question.

DIFFERENTIAL DIAGNOSIS

Careful initial evaluation, including a thorough history and physical examination, is indicated for all patients suffering from postherpetic neuralgia to rule out occult malignancy or systemic disease that may be responsible for the patient's immunocompromised state and to allow early recognition of changes in clinical status that may presage the development of complications, including myelitis or dissemination of the disease. Other causes of pain in the distribution of the thoracic nerve roots include thoracic radiculopathy and peripheral neuropathy. Intrathoracic and intra-abdominal pathology may also mimic the pain of acute herpes zoster involving the thoracic dermatomes. For pain in the distribution of the first division of the trigeminal nerve, the clinician must rule out diseases of the eye, ear, nose, and throat as well as intracranial pathology.

TREATMENT

The primary goal of all clinicians caring for patients with acute herpes zoster is the rapid and aggressive

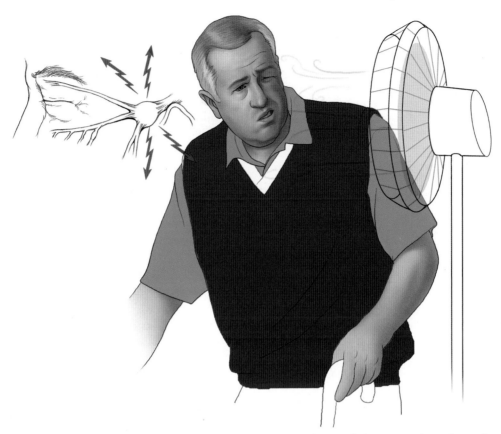

Figure 43–1. Allodynia and dysesthesia are characteristic of the pain of postherpetic neuralgia.

treatment of symptoms to help decrease the incidence of postherpetic neuralgia. It is the consensus of most pain specialists that the earlier in the natural course of the disease that treatment is initiated, the less likely the patient will develop postherpetic neuralgia. Furthermore, because the older patient is at highest risk for the development of postherpetic neuralgia, early and aggressive treatment of this group of patients is mandatory. Should despite everyone's best efforts postherpetic neuralgia occur, the following treatments are appropriate.

Adjuvant Analgesics

The anticonvulsant gabapentin represents a first-line treatment in the palliation of pain of postherpetic neuralgia. Treatment with gabapentin should begin early in the course of the disease, and this drug may be used concurrently with neural blockade, opioid analgesics, and other adjuvant analgesics, including the antidepressant compounds if care is taken to avoid central nervous system side effects. Gabapentin is started at a dose of 300 mg at bedtime and is titrated upward in 300-mg increments to a maximum dosage of 3600 mg daily given in divided doses as side effects allow.

Carbamazepine should be considered in patients suffering from severe neuritic pain in whom nerve blocks and gabapentin have failed to bring relief. If this drug is used, rigid monitoring for hematologic parameters, especially in patients receiving chemotherapy or radiation therapy, is indicated. Phenytoin may also be beneficial to treat neuritic pain but should not be used in patients with lymphoma because the drug may induce a pseudolymphoma-like state that is difficult to distinguish from the actual lymphoma itself.

Antidepressant Compounds

Antidepressants may also be useful adjuncts in the initial treatment of the patient suffering from postherpetic neuralgia. On an acute basis, these drugs will help alleviate the significant sleep disturbance that is commonly seen in this setting. In addition, the antidepressants may be valuable in helping ameliorate the neuritic component of the pain, which is treated less effectively with narcotic analgesics. After several weeks of treatment, the antidepressants may exert a mood-elevating effect that may be desirable in some patients. Care must be taken to observe closely for central nervous system side effects in this patient population. These drugs may cause urinary retention and constipation that may be mistakenly attributed to herpes zoster myelitis.

Nerve Blocks

Sympathetic neural blockade with local anesthetic and steroid via either epidural nerve block or blockade of the sympathetic nerves subserving the painful area appears to be a reasonable next step if the aforementioned pharmacologic modalities fail to control the pain of postherpetic neuralgia. The exact mechanism of pain relief from neural blockade when treating postherpetic neuralgia is unknown, but it may be related to modulation of pain transmission at the spinal cord level. In general, neurodestructive procedures have a very low success rate and should be used only after all other treatments have been optimized, if at all.

Opioid Analgesics

Opioid analgesics have a limited role in the management of postherpetic neuralgia and in the experience of this author frequently do more harm than good. Careful administration of potent, long-acting narcotic analgesics (e.g., oral morphine elixir or methadone) on a time-contingent rather than an as-needed basis may represent a beneficial adjunct to the pain relief provided by sympathetic neural blockade. Because many patients suffering from postherpetic neuralgia are elderly or may have severe multisystem disease, close monitoring for the potential side effects of potent narcotic analgesics (e.g., confusion or dizziness, which may cause a patient to fall) is warranted. Daily dietary fiber supplementation and milk of magnesia should be started along with opioid analgesics to prevent the side effect of constipation.

Adjunctive Treatments

The application of ice packs to the area affected with postherpetic neuralgia may provide relief in some patients. The application of heat will increase pain in most patients, presumably because of increased conduction of small fibers, but it is beneficial in an occasional patient and may be worth trying if the application of cold is ineffective. Transcutaneous electrical nerve stimulation and vibration may also be effective in a limited number of patients. The favorable risk-to-benefit ratio of all these modalities makes them reasonable alternatives for patients who cannot or will not undergo sympathetic neural blockade or tolerate pharmacologic interventions. The topical application of capsaicin may be beneficial in some patients suffering from postherpetic neuralgia. However, the burning associated with this drug when applied to the painful area will often limit the usefulness of this intervention.

COMPLICATIONS AND PITFALLS

Although there are no complications specifically associated with postherpetic neuralgia itself, the consequences of the unremitting pain are devastating. Failure to aggressively treat the pain of postherpetic neuralgia and the associated symptoms of sleep disturbance and depression can result in suicide.

CLINICAL PEARLS

Because the pain of postherpetic neuralgia is so devastating, the clinician must endeavor to rapidly and aggressively treat the pain of acute herpes zoster. If postherpetic neuralgia develops, aggressive treatment as outlined here with special attention to the insidious onset of severe depression should be undertaken. If serious depression occurs, hospitalization with suicide precautions is mandatory.

44

Thoracic Vertebral Compression Fracture

THE CLINICAL SYNDROME

Thoracic vertebral compression fracture is one of the most common causes of dorsal spine pain. Vertebral compression fracture is most often the result of osteoporosis of the dorsal spine. This is also associated with trauma to the dorsal spine due to acceleration/deceleration injuries. In osteoporotic patients or in patients with primary tumors or metastatic disease involving the thoracic vertebra, this may occur with coughing (tussive fractures) or spontaneously.

The pain and functional disability associated with fractured vertebra are determined in large part by the severity of injury (e.g., the number of vertebra involved) and the nature of the injury (e.g., whether the fracture allows impingement on the spinal nerves or the spinal cord itself). The severity of pain associated with thoracic vertebral compression fracture may range from a dull, deep ache with minimal compression of the vertebra without nerve impingement to severe sharp, stabbing pain that limits the patient's ability to ambulate and cough.

SIGNS AND SYMPTOMS

Compression fractures of the thoracic vertebra are aggravated by deep inspiration, coughing, and any movement of the dorsal spine (Fig. 44–1). Palpation of the affected vertebra may elicit pain and reflex spasm of the paraspinous musculature of the dorsal spine. If trauma has occurred, hematoma and ecchymosis overlying the fracture site may be present. If trauma has occurred, the clinician should be aware of the possibility of damage to the bony thorax and the intra-abdominal and intrathoracic contents. Damage to the spinal nerves may produce abdominal ileus and severe pain with resulting splinting of the paraspinous muscles of the dorsal spine, further compromising the patient's ability to walk and pulmonary status. Failure to aggressively treat this pain and splinting may result in a negative cycle of hypoventilation, atelectasis, and ultimately pneumonia.

TESTING

Plain radiographs of the vertebra are indicated for all patients who present with pain from thoracic vertebral compression fracture to rule out other occult fractures and other bony pathology including tumor. If trauma is present, radionucleotide bone scanning may be useful to rule out occult fractures of the vertebra, sternum, or both. If no trauma is present, bone density testing to rule out osteoporosis is appropriate, as are serum protein electrophoresis and testing for hyperparathyroidism. Based on the patient's clinical presentation, additional testing, including complete blood count, prostate specific antigen, sedimentation rate, and antinuclear antibody testing, may be indicated. Computed tomography scanning of the thoracic contents is indicated if occult mass or significant trauma to the thoracic contents is suspected. Electrocardiography to rule out cardiac contusion is indicated in all patients with traumatic sternal fractures or significant anterior dorsal spine trauma. The following injection technique should be used early on to avoid these pulmonary complications.

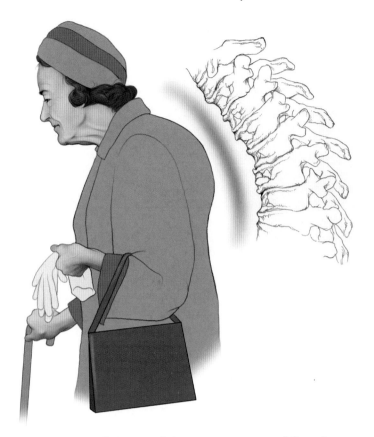

Figure 44–1. Osteoporosis is a common cause of thoracic vertebral fractures.

DIFFERENTIAL DIAGNOSIS

In the setting of trauma, the diagnosis of thoracic vertebral compression fracture usually is easily made. It is in the setting of spontaneous vertebral fracture secondary to osteoporosis or metastatic disease that the diagnosis may be confusing. In this setting, the pain of occult vertebral compression fracture is often mistaken for pain of cardiac or gallbladder origin and can lead to visits to the emergency department and unnecessary cardiac and gastrointestinal work-ups. Acute sprain of the thoracic paraspinous muscles can be confused with thoracic vertebral compression fracture, especially if the patient has been coughing. Because the pain of acute herpes zoster may precede the rash by 24 to 72 hours, the pain may be erroneously attributed to vertebral compression fracture.

TREATMENT

The initial treatment of pain secondary to compression fracture of the thoracic spine should include a combination of simple analgesics and the nonsteroidal anti-inflammatory drugs or the cyclooxygenase-2 inhibitors. If these medications do not adequately control the patient's symptomatology, short-acting potent opioid analgesics such as hydrocodone represent a reasonable next step. Because the opioid analgesics have the potential to suppress the cough reflex and respiration, the clinician must be careful to monitor the patient closely and to instruct the patient in adequate pulmonary toilet techniques.

The local application of heat and cold may also be beneficial to provide symptomatic relief of the pain of rib fracture. The use of an orthotic device (e.g., the Cash brace) may also help provide symptomatic relief. For patients who do not respond to these treatment modalities, thoracic epidural block with local anesthetic and steroid is a reasonable next step.

COMPLICATIONS AND PITFALLS

The major problem in the care of patients thought to suffer from compression fracture of the thoracic vertebra is the failure to identify potentially serious compression of the thoracic spinal cord or the fact that the fracture is due to metastatic disease. Failure to rapidly control pain and ambulate patients suffering from thoracic vertebral compression fractures due to senile osteoporosis puts the patient at risk for complications, including pneumonia and thrombophlebitis.

CLINICAL PEARLS

Compression fracture of the thoracic vertebra is a commonly encountered cause of dorsal spine pain. Correct diagnosis is necessary to properly treat this painful condition and to avoid overlooking serious intrathoracic or upper intra-abdominal pathology. The use of the aforementioned pharmacologic agents, including opioid analgesics, will allow the clinician to adequately control the pain of vertebral compression fracture. Thoracic steroid epidural block is a simple technique that can produce dramatic relief for patients suffering from vertebral compression fracture.

X Abdominal and Groin Pain Syndromes

Acute Pancreatitis

ICD-9 CODE 577.0

THE CLINICAL SYNDROME

Acute pancreatitis is one of the most common causes of abdominal pain. The incidence of acute pancreatitis is approximately 0.5% of the general population with a mortality rate of 1% to 1.5%. In the United States, acute pancreatitis is most commonly caused by alcohol, with gallstones being the most common cause in most European countries. There are many causes of acute pancreatitis, which are summarized in Table 45–1. In addition to alcohol and gallstones, other common causes of acute pancreatitis include viral infections, tumor, and medications.

Abdominal pain is a common feature in acute pancreatitis. It may range from mild to severe and is characterized by steady, boring epigastric pain that radiates to the flanks and chest. The pain is worse with the supine position, and the patient with acute pancreatitis will often prefer sitting with the dorsal spine flexed and the knees drawn up to the abdomen. Nausea, vomiting, and anorexia are also common features of acute pancreatitis.

Table 45–1. Common Causes of Acute Pancreatitis

Alcohol
Gallstones
Viral infections
Medications
Metabolic causes
Connective tissue diseases
Tumor obstruction of ampulla of Vater
Hereditary

SIGNS AND SYMPTOMS

The patient with acute pancreatitis will appear ill and anxious. Tachycardia and hypotension due to hypovolemia are common, as is low-grade fever. Saponification of subcutaneous fat is seen in approximately 15% of patients suffering from acute pancreatitis, as are pulmonary complications including pleural effusions and pleuritic pain that may compromise respiration. Diffuse abdominal tenderness with peritoneal signs are invariably present. A pancreatic mass or pseudocyst due to pancreatic edema may be palpable. If hemorrhage occurs, periumbilical ecchymosis (Cullen's sign) and flank ecchymosis (Turner's sign) may be present (Fig. 45–1). Both of these findings suggest severe necrotizing pancreatitis and indicate a poor prognosis. If hypocalcemia is present, Chvostek's or Trousseau's sign may be present.

TESTING

Elevation of the serum amylase levels is the sine qua non of acute pancreatitis. Levels tend to peak at 48 to 72 hours and then begin to drift toward normal. Serum lipase will remain elevated and may correlate better with the actual severity of the disease. Because elevated serum amylase levels may be caused by other diseases, such as parotitis, amylase isozymes may be necessary to confirm a pancreatic basis for this laboratory finding. Plain radiographs of the chest are indicated for all patients who present with pain from acute pancreatitis to identify pulmonary complications, including pleural effusion, that are the result of the acute pancreatitis. Given the extrapancreatic manifestations of acute pancreatitis (e.g., acute renal or hepatic failure), serial complete blood count, serum calcium, serum glucose, liver function tests, and electrolytes are indicated in all patients suffering from acute pancreatitis. Computed tomography scanning of the abdomen will help identify pancreatic pseudocyst and may help the clinician gauge the severity and progress of the disease. Gallbladder evaluation with radionucleotides is indicated if gallstones are being considered as a cause of acute pancreatitis. Arterial blood gases will help identify respiratory failure and metabolic acidosis.

DIFFERENTIAL DIAGNOSIS

The differential diagnosis should consider perforated peptic ulcer, acute cholecystitis, bowel obstruction, renal calculi, myocardial infarction, mesenteric infarction, diabetic ketoacidosis, and pneumonia. Rarely, the collagen vascular diseases, including systemic lupus erythematosus and polyarteritis nodosa, may mimic pancreatitis. Because the pain of acute herpes zoster may precede the rash by 24 to 72 hours, the pain may be erroneously attributed to acute pancreatitis.

TREATMENT

Most cases of acute pancreatitis are self-limited and will resolve within 5 to 7 days. Initial treatment of acute pancreatitis is aimed primarily at putting the pancreas at rest. This is accomplished by holding the patient NPO (nothing by mouth) to decrease serum gastrin secretion and, if ileus is present, by instituting nasogastric suction. Short-acting potent opioid analgesics such as hydrocodone represent a reasonable next step if conservative measures do not control the patient's pain. If ileus is present, parenteral narcotics such as meperidine are a good alternative. Because the opioid analgesics have the potential to suppress the cough reflex and respiration, the clinician must be careful to monitor the patient closely and to instruct the patient in adequate pulmonary toilet techniques. If the symptoms persist, computed tomography–guided celiac plexus block with local anesthetic and steroid is indicated and may help decrease the mortality and morbidity rates associated with the disease. As an alternative, continuous thoracic epidural block with local anesthetic, opioid, or both may provide adequate pain control and allow the patient to avoid the respiratory depression associated with systemic opioid analgesics.

Hypovolemia should be treated aggressively with crystalloid and colloid infusions. For prolonged cases of acute pancreatitis, parenteral nutrition is indicated to avoid malnutrition. Surgical drainage and removal of necrotic tissue may be required in severe necrotizing pancreatitis that fails to respond to these treatment modalities.

COMPLICATIONS AND PITFALLS

The major problem in the care of patients suffering from acute pancreatitis is a failure of the clinician to recognize the severity of the patient's condition and to identify and aggressively treat the extrapancreatic manifestations of acute pancreatitis. Hypovolemia, hypocalcemia, and renal and respiratory failure occur with sufficient frequency that the clinician must actively seek these potentially fatal complications and treat them aggressively.

CLINICAL PEARLS

Acute pancreatitis is a commonly encountered cause of abdominal pain. Correct diagnosis is necessary to properly treat this painful condition and to avoid overlooking serious extrapancreatic complications associated with this disease. The use of the aforementioned treatment modalities agents, including opioid analgesics, will allow the clinician to adequately control the pain of acute pancreatitis. Celiac plexus block and thoracic epidural block are straightforward techniques that can produce dramatic relief for patients suffering from acute pancreatitis.

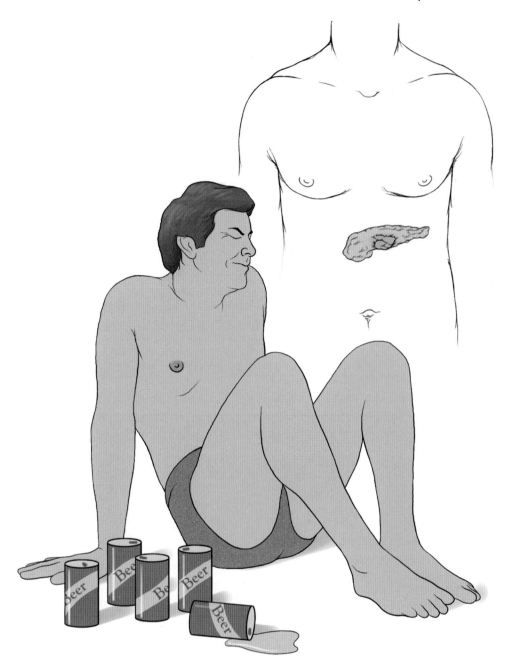

Figure 45-1. Excessive consumption of alcohol is only one of many causes of acute pancreatitis.

46

Chronic Pancreatitis

ICD-9 CODE 577.1

THE CLINICAL SYNDROME

Chronic pancreatitis is one result of acute pancreatitis. Chronic pancreatitis may present as recurrent episodes of acute inflammation of the pancreas superimposed on chronic pancreatic dysfunction or as a more constant problem. As the exocrine function of the pancreas deteriorates, malabsorption with steatorrhea and azorrhea develops. Abdominal pain is usually present, but it may be characterized by exacerbations and remissions. In the United States, chronic pancreatitis is most commonly caused by alcohol, followed by cystic fibrosis and pancreatic malignancies. Hereditary causes such as alpha-1 antitrypsin deficiency also are common causes of chronic pancreatitis. In the developing countries, the most common cause of chronic pancreatitis is severe protein calorie malnutrition.

Abdominal pain is a common feature in chronic pancreatitis. It mimics the pain of acute pancreatitis, may range from mild to severe, and is characterized by steady, boring epigastric pain that radiates to the flanks and chest. The pain is worse with alcohol and fatty meals. Nausea, vomiting, and anorexia are also common features of chronic pancreatitis, but as mentioned, the clinical symptoms frequently encountered in chronic pancreatitis are characterized by exacerbations and remissions.

SIGNS AND SYMPTOMS

The patient with chronic pancreatitis will present as does the patient with acute pancreatitis but may appear more chronically ill than acutely ill (Fig. 46–1). Tachycardia and hypotension due to hypovolemia are much less common in chronic pancreatitis and if present represent an extremely ominous prognostic indicator or suggest that another pathologic process, such as perforated peptic ulcer, is present. Diffuse abdominal tenderness with peritoneal signs may be present if acute inflammation occurs. A pancreatic mass or pseudocyst due to pancreatic edema may be palpable.

TESTING

Although elevation of serum amylase levels is the sine qua non of acute pancreatitis, amylase levels in chronic pancreatitis may be only mildly elevated or even within normal limits. Amylase levels tend to peak at 48 to 72 hours and then begin to drift toward normal. Serum lipase levels will also be attenuated in chronic pancreatitis compared with the findings seen in acute pancreatitis. Serum lipase may remain elevated longer than serum amylase in this setting and may correlate better with the actual severity of the disease. Because elevated serum amylase may be caused by other diseases, such as parotitis, amylase isozymes may be necessary to confirm a pancreatic basis for this laboratory finding. Plain radiographs of the chest are indicated for all patients who present with pain from chronic pancreatitis to identify pulmonary complications, including pleural effusion, that are the result of the chronic pancreatitis. Given the extrapancreatic manifestations of chronic pancreatitis (e.g., acute renal or hepatic failure), serial complete blood count, serum calcium, serum glucose, liver function tests, and electrolytes are indicated in all patients suffering from chronic pancreatitis. Computed tomography scanning of the abdomen will help identify pancreatic pseudocyst or pancreatic tumor that may have been previously overlooked and may help the clinician gauge the severity and progress of the disease. Gallbladder evaluation with radionucleotides is indicated if gallstones are being considered as a cause of chronic pancreatitis. Arterial blood gases will

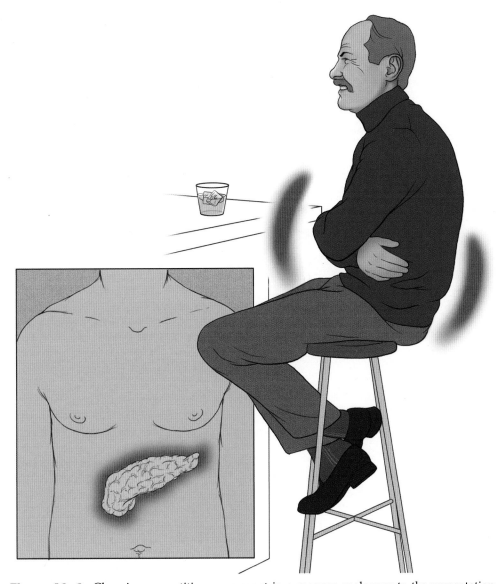

Figure 46–1. Chronic pancreatitis may present in a manner analogous to the presentation of acute pancreatitis, but can be more challenging to treat.

help identify respiratory failure and metabolic acidosis.

DIFFERENTIAL DIAGNOSIS

The differential diagnosis should consider perforated peptic ulcer, acute cholecystitis, bowel obstruction, renal calculi, myocardial infarction, mesenteric infarction, diabetic ketoacidosis, and pneumonia. Rarely, the collagen vascular diseases, including systemic lupus erythematosus and polyarteritis nodosa, may mimic chronic pancreatitis. Because the pain of acute herpes zoster may precede the rash by 24 to 72 hours, the pain may be erroneously attributed to chronic pancreatitis in patients who have had previous bouts of the disease. The clinician should always consider the possibility of pancreatic malignancy in patients who are thought to be suffering from chronic pancreatitis.

TREATMENT

The initial treatment of patients suffering from chronic pancreatitis should be focused on the treatment of the pain and malabsorption. As with acute pancreatitis, the treatment of chronic pancreatitis is aimed primarily at putting the pancreas at rest. This is accomplished by holding the patient NPO (nothing by mouth) to decrease serum gastrin secretion and, if ileus is present, instituting nasogastric suction. Short-acting potent opioid analgesics such as hydrocodone represent a reasonable next step if conservative measures do not control the patient's pain. If ileus is present, parenteral narcotics such as meperidine are a good alternative. Because the opioid analgesics have the potential to suppress the cough reflex and respiration, the clinician must be careful to monitor the patient closely and to instruct the patient in adequate pulmonary toilet techniques. As with all chronic diseases, the use of opioid analgesics must be monitored carefully as the potential for misuse and dependence is high.

If the symptoms persist, computed tomography–guided celiac plexus block with local anesthetic and steroid is indicated and may help decrease the mortality and morbidity rates associated with the disease

(Fig. 46–2). If the relief from this technique is short lived, neurolytic computed tomography–guided celiac plexus block with alcohol or phenol represents a reasonable next step. As an alternative, continuous thoracic epidural block with local anesthetic, opioid, or both may provide adequate pain control and allow the patient to avoid the respiratory depression associated with systemic opioid analgesics.

Hypovolemia should be treated aggressively with crystalloid and colloid infusions. For prolonged cases of chronic pancreatitis, parenteral nutrition is indicated to avoid malnutrition. Surgical drainage and removal of necrotic tissue may be required in patients with severe necrotizing pancreatitis that fails to respond to the above-mentioned treatment modalities.

COMPLICATIONS AND PITFALLS

The major problem in the care of patients suffering from chronic pancreatitis is a failure of the clinician to recognize the severity of the patient's condition and to identify and aggressively treat the extrapancreatic manifestations of chronic pancreatitis. Hypovolemia, hypocalcemia, and renal and respiratory failure occur with sufficient frequency that the clinician must actively seek this potentially fatal complications and treat them aggressively. If opioids are used, the clinician must constantly watch for overuse and dependence, especially if the underlying etiology of the chronic pancreatitis is alcohol abuse.

CLINICAL PEARLS

Chronic pancreatitis is a commonly encountered cause of abdominal pain. Correct diagnosis is necessary to properly treat this painful condition and to avoid overlooking serious extrapancreatic complications associated with this disease. The use of the above-mentioned treatment modalities agents, including the judicious use of opioid analgesics to treat the pain of acute exacerbations, will allow the clinician to adequately control the pain of chronic pancreatitis. Celiac plexus block and thoracic epidural block are straightforward techniques that can produce dramatic relief for patients suffering from chronic pancreatitis.

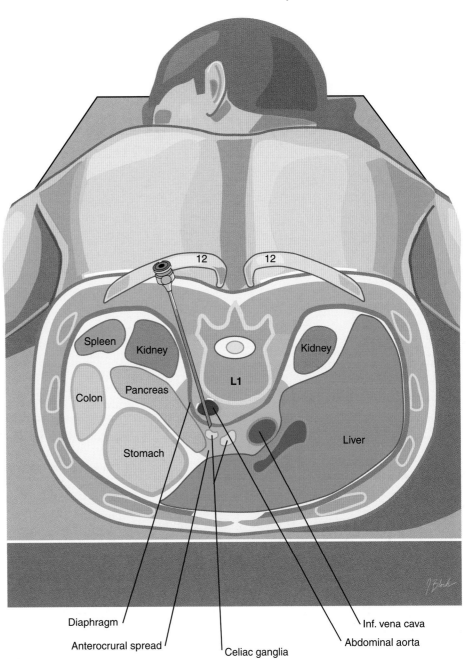

Figure 46–2. Proper needle placement for transaortic celiac plexus block. (From Waldman SD: Atlas of Interventional Pain Management. Philadelphia, WB Saunders, 1998, p 272.)

Ilioinguinal Neuralgia

THE CLINICAL SYNDROME

Ilioinguinal neuralgia is one of the most common causes of lower abdominal and pelvic pain encountered in clinical practice. Ilioinguinal neuralgia is caused by compression of the ilioinguinal nerve as it passes through the transverse abdominis muscle at the level of the anterior superior iliac spine. The most common causes of compression of the ilioinguinal nerve at this anatomic location involve injury to the nerve induced by trauma, including direct blunt trauma to the nerve, as well as damage during inguinal herniorrhaphy and pelvic surgery. Rarely, ilioinguinal neuralgia will occur spontaneously.

SIGNS AND SYMPTOMS

Ilioinguinal neuralgia presents as paresthesias, burning pain, and occasionally numbness over the lower abdomen that radiates into the scrotum or labia and occasionally into the inner upper thigh. The pain does not radiate below the knee. The pain of ilioinguinal neuralgia is made worse by extension of the lumbar spine, which puts traction on the nerve. Patients suffering from ilioinguinal neuralgia will often assume a bent-forward novice skier's position (Fig. 47–1). If the condition remains untreated, progressive motor deficit consisting of bulging of the anterior abdominal wall muscles may occur. This bulging may be confused with inguinal hernia.

Physical findings include sensory deficit in the inner thigh, scrotum, or labia in the distribution of the ilioinguinal nerve. Weakness of the anterior abdominal wall musculature may be present. Tinel's sign may be elicited by tapping over the ilioinguinal nerve at the point at which it pierces the transverse abdomi-

nal muscle. As mentioned, the patient may assume a bent-forward novice skiers' position.

TESTING

Electromyography will help distinguish ilioinguinal nerve entrapment from lumbar plexopathy, lumbar radiculopathy, and diabetic polyneuropathy. Plain radiographs of the hip and pelvis are indicated for all patients who present with ilioinguinal neuralgia to rule out occult bony pathology. Based on the patient's clinical presentation, additional testing, including complete blood count, uric acid, sedimentation rate, and antinuclear antibody testing, may be indicated. Magnetic resonance imaging of the lumbar plexus is indicated if tumor or hematoma is suspected. The injection technique described here will serve as both a diagnostic and therapeutic maneuver.

DIFFERENTIAL DIAGNOSIS

It should be remembered that lesions of the lumbar plexus from trauma, hematoma, tumor, diabetic neuropathy, or inflammation can mimic the pain, numbness, and weakness of ilioinguinal neuralgia and must be included in the differential diagnosis. Furthermore, there is significant intrapatient variability in the anatomy of the ilioinguinal nerve that can result in significant variation in the patient's clinical presentation. The ilioinguinal nerve is a branch of the L1 nerve root with contribution from T12 in some patients. The nerve follows a curvilinear course that takes it from its origin of the L1 and occasionally T12 somatic nerves to inside the concavity of the ileum. The ilioinguinal nerve continues anteriorly to perforate the transverse abdominis muscle at the level of the anterior superior iliac spine. The nerve may interconnect with the iliohypogastric nerve as it continues to pass along its course medially and inferiorly where

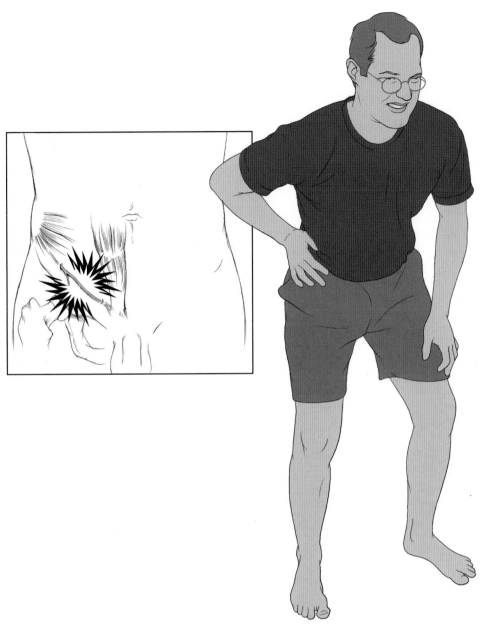

Figure 47–1. The patient suffering from ilioinguinal neuralgia will often bend forward in the novice skier's position to relieve the pain.

it accompanies the spermatic cord through the inguinal ring and into the inguinal canal. The distribution of the sensory innervation of the ilioinguinal nerves varies from patient to patient because there may be considerable overlap with the iliohypogastric nerve. In general, the ilioinguinal nerve provides sensory innervation to the upper portion of the skin of the inner thigh and the root of the penis and upper scrotum in men or the mons pubis and lateral labia in women.

TREATMENT

Pharmacologic management of ilioinguinal neuralgia is usually disappointing, and general nerve block will be required to provide pain relief. Initial treatment of ilioinguinal neuralgia should consist of treatment with simple analgesics, nonsteroidal anti-inflammatory drugs, or cyclooxygenase-2 inhibitors. Avoidance of repetitive activities thought to exacerbate the symptoms of ilioinguinal neuralgia (e.g., squatting or sitting for prolonged periods) will also help ameliorate the patient's symptoms. If the patient fails to respond to these conservative measures, a next reasonable step is ilioinguinal nerve block with local anesthetic and steroid.

Ilioinguinal nerve block is performed by placing the patient in the supine position with a pillow under the knees, if lying with the legs extended increases the patient's pain due to traction on the nerve. The anterior superior iliac spine is identified by palpation. A point 2 inches medial and 2 inches inferior to the anterior superior iliac spine is then identified and prepped with antiseptic solution. A 1½-inch 25-gauge needle is then advanced at an oblique angle toward the pubic symphysis (Fig. 47–2). From 5 to 7 mL of 1.0% preservative-free lidocaine in solution with 40 mg of methylprednisolone is injected in a fanlike manner as the needle pierces the fascia of the external oblique muscle. Care must be taken not to place the needle too deep and enter the peritoneal cavity and perforate the abdominal viscera.

Because of overlapping innervation of the ilioinguinal and iliohypogastric nerve, it is not unusual to block branches of each nerve when performing ilioinguinal nerve block. After injection of the solution, pressure is applied to the injection site to decrease the incidence of postblock ecchymosis and hematoma formation, which can be quite dramatic, especially in the anticoagulated patient.

COMPLICATIONS AND PITFALLS

The clinician should be aware that due to the anatomy of the ilioinguinal nerve, damage to or entrapment of the nerve anywhere along its course can produce a similar clinical syndrome. This means that a careful search for pathology at the T12-L1 spinal segments and along the path of the nerve in the pelvis is mandatory in all patients who present with ilioinguinal neuralgia without a history of inguinal surgery or trauma to the region.

The major side effect of ilioinguinal nerve block is postblock ecchymosis and hematoma formation. If needle placement is too deep and enters the peritoneal cavity, perforation of the colon may result in the formation of intra-abdominal abscess and fistula formation. Early detection of infection is crucial to avoid potentially life-threatening sequelae.

CLINICAL PEARLS

Ilioinguinal neuralgia is a common cause of lower abdominal and pelvic pain. Ilioinguinal nerve block is a simple technique that can produce dramatic relief for patients suffering from ilioinguinal neuralgia. As mentioned, pressure should be maintained on the injection site after the block to avoid ecchymosis and hematoma formation. For patients who do not rapidly respond to ilioinguinal nerve block, consideration should be given to epidural steroid injection of the T12-L1 segments.

If a patient presents with pain suggestive of ilioinguinal neuralgia and does not respond to ilioinguinal nerve blocks, a diagnosis of lesions more proximal in the lumbar plexus or an L1 radiculopathy should be considered. Such patients will often respond to epidural steroid blocks. Electromyography and magnetic resonance imaging of the lumbar plexus are indicated in this patient population to help rule out other causes of ilioinguinal pain, including malignancy invading the lumbar plexus or epidural or vertebral metastatic disease at T12-L1.

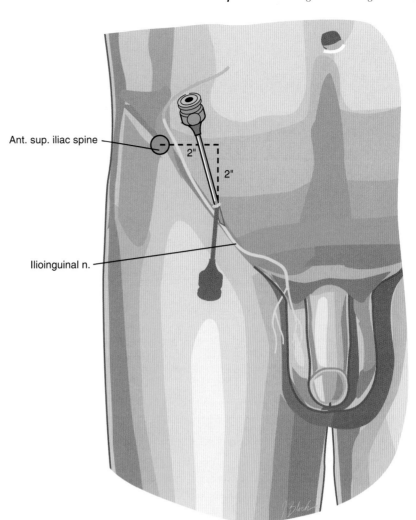

Ant. sup. iliac spine

2"

2"

Ilioinguinal n.

Figure 47–2. Correct needle placement for ilioinguinal nerve block. (From Waldman SD: Atlas of Interventional Pain Management. Philadelphia, WB Saunders, 1998, p 285.)

48

Genitofemoral Neuralgia

ICD-9 CODE 355.8

THE CLINICAL SYNDROME

Genitofemoral neuralgia is one of the most common causes of lower abdominal and pelvic pain encountered in clinical practice. Genitofemoral neuralgia may be caused by compression of or damage to the genitofemoral nerve anywhere along its path. The genitofemoral nerve arises from fibers of the L1 and L2 nerve roots. The genitofemoral nerve passes through the substance of the psoas muscle, where it divides into a genital and a femoral branch. The femoral branch passes beneath the inguinal ligament along with the femoral artery and provides sensory innervation to a small area of skin on the inside of the thigh. The genital branch passes through the inguinal canal to provide innervation to the round ligament of the uterus and labia majora in women. In men, the genital branch of the genitofemoral nerve passes with the spermatic cord to innervate the cremasteric muscles and provide sensory innervation to the bottom of the scrotum.

The most common causes of genitofemoral neuralgia involve injury to the nerve induced by trauma, including direct blunt trauma to the nerve, as well as damage during inguinal herniorrhaphy and pelvic surgery. Rarely, genitofemoral neuralgia will occur spontaneously.

SIGNS AND SYMPTOMS

Genitofemoral neuralgia presents as paresthesias, burning pain, and occasionally numbness over the lower abdomen that radiates into inner thigh in both men and women and into the labia majora in women and the bottom of the scrotum and cremasteric muscles in men. The pain does not radiate below the knee. The pain of genitofemoral neuralgia is made worse by extension of the lumbar spine, which puts traction on the nerve. Patients suffering from genitofemoral neuralgia will often assume a bent-forward novice skiers' position (Fig. 48–1).

Physical findings include sensory deficit in the inner thigh, base of the scrotum, or labia majora in the distribution of the genitofemoral nerve. Weakness of the anterior abdominal wall musculature may occasionally be present. Tinel's sign may be elicited by tapping over the genitofemoral nerve at the point it passes beneath the inguinal ligament. As mentioned, the patient may assume a bent-forward novice skiers' position.

TESTING

Electromyography will help distinguish genitofemoral nerve entrapment from lumbar plexopathy, lumbar radiculopathy, and diabetic polyneuropathy. Plain radiographs of the hip and pelvis are indicated for all patients who present with genitofemoral neuralgia to rule out occult bony pathology. Based on the patient's clinical presentation, additional testing, including complete blood count, uric acid, sedimentation rate, and antinuclear antibody testing, may be indicated. Magnetic resonance imaging of the lumbar plexus is indicated if tumor or hematoma is suspected. The injection technique described here will serve as both a diagnostic and therapeutic maneuver.

DIFFERENTIAL DIAGNOSIS

It should be remembered that lesions of the lumbar plexus from trauma, hematoma, tumor, diabetic neuropathy, or inflammation can mimic the pain, numbness, and weakness of genitofemoral neuralgia and must be included in the differential diagnosis. Furthermore, there is significant intrapatient variability in the anatomy of the genitofemoral nerve that can re-

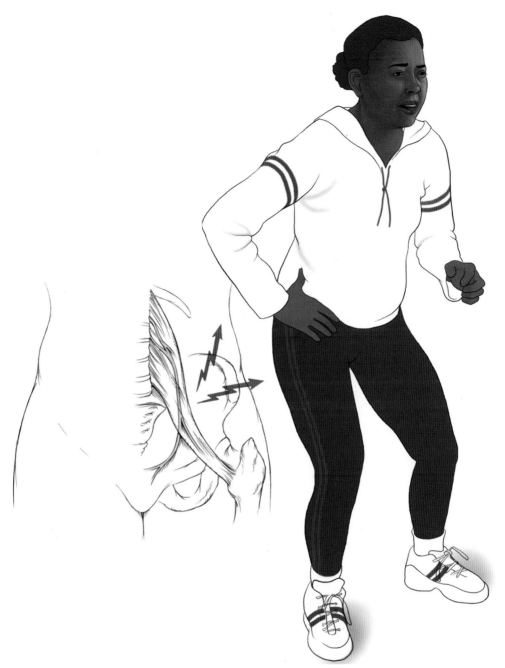

Figure 48–1. The pain of genitofemoral neuralgia will radiate into the inner thigh of men and women and into the labia majora in women and inferior scrotum in men.

sult in significant variation in the patient's clinical presentation.

TREATMENT

Pharmacologic management of genitofemoral neuralgia is usually disappointing, and nerve block will often be required to provide pain relief. Initial treatment of genitofemoral neuralgia should consist of simple analgesics, nonsteroidal anti-inflammatory drugs, or cyclooxygenase-2 inhibitors. Avoidance of repetitive activities thought to exacerbate the symptoms of genitofemoral neuralgia (e.g., squatting or sitting for prolonged periods) will also help ameliorate the patient's symptoms. If the condition fails to respond to these conservative measures, a next reasonable step is genitofemoral nerve block with local anesthetic and steroid.

Genitofemoral nerve block is performed by placing the patient in supine position with a pillow under the knees, if lying with the legs extended increases the patient's pain due to traction on the nerve. The genital branch of the genitofemoral nerve is blocked as follows. The pubic tubercle is identified by palpation. A point just lateral to the pubic tubercle is then identified and prepped with antiseptic solution. A 1½-inch 25-gauge needle is then advanced at an oblique angle toward the pubic symphysis (Fig. 48–2). From 3 to 5 mL of 1.0% preservative-free lidocaine in solution with 80 mg methylprednisolone is injected in a fanlike manner as the needle pierces the inguinal ligament. Care must be taken not to place the needle deep enough to enter the peritoneal cavity and perforate the abdominal viscera.

The femoral branch of the genitofemoral nerve is blocked by identifying the middle third of the inguinal ligament. After preparation of the skin with antiseptic solution, 3 to 5 mL of 1.0% lidocaine is infiltrated subcutaneously just below the ligament (see Fig. 48–2). Care must be taken not to enter the femoral artery or vein or inadvertently block the femoral nerve. The needle must be kept subcutaneous, because too deep placement may allow the needle to enter the peritoneal cavity and perforate the abdominal viscera. If there is an inflammatory component to the pain, the local anesthetic is combined with 80 mg methylprednisolone and is injected in incremental doses. Subsequent daily nerve blocks are carried out in a similar manner substituting 40 mg methylprednisolone for the initial 80-mg dose.

Because of overlapping innervation of the ilioin-guinal and iliohypogastric nerve, it is not unusual to block branches of each nerve when performing genitofemoral nerve block. After injection of the solution, pressure is applied to the injection site to decrease the incidence of postblock ecchymosis and hematoma formation, which can be quite dramatic, especially in the anticoagulated patient.

COMPLICATIONS AND PITFALLS

The clinician should be aware that due to the anatomy of the genitofemoral nerve, damage to or entrapment of the nerve anywhere along its course can produce a similar clinical syndrome. This means that a careful search for pathology at the L1-2 spinal segments and along the path of the nerve in the pelvis is mandatory in all patients who present with genitofemoral neuralgia without a history of inguinal surgery or trauma to the region.

The major side effect of genitofemoral nerve block is postblock ecchymosis and hematoma formation. If needle placement is too deep and the needle enters the peritoneal cavity, perforation of the colon may result in the formation of intra-abdominal abscess and fistula formation. Early detection of infection is crucial to avoid potentially life-threatening sequelae.

CLINICAL PEARLS

Genitofemoral neuralgia is a common cause of lower abdominal and pelvic pain. Genitofemoral nerve block is a simple technique that can produce dramatic relief for patients suffering from genitofemoral neuralgia. As mentioned, pressure should be maintained on the injection site after the block to avoid ecchymosis and hematoma formation. For patients who do not rapidly respond to genitofemoral nerve block, consideration should be given to epidural steroid injection of the L1-2 segments.

If a patient presents with pain suggestive of genitofemoral neuralgia and does not respond to genitofemoral nerve blocks, a diagnosis of lesions more proximal in the lumbar plexus or an L1 radiculopathy should be considered. Such patients will often respond to epidural steroid blocks. Electromyography and magnetic resonance imaging of the lumbar plexus are indicated in this patient population to help rule out other causes of genitofemoral pain, including malignancy invading the lumbar plexus or epidural or vertebral metastatic disease at T12-L1.

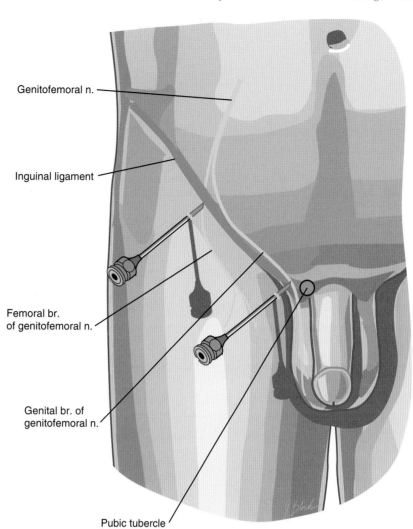

Genitofemoral n.

Inguinal ligament

Femoral br.
of genitofemoral n.

Genital br. of
genitofemoral n.

Pubic tubercle

Figure 48–2. Correct needle placement
for genitofemoral nerve block. (From Waldman SD: Atlas of Interventional Pain Management. Philadelphia, WB Saunders, 1998,
p 365.)

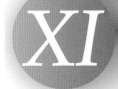

XI Lumbar Spine and Sacroiliac Joint Pain Syndromes

49

Lumbar Radiculopathy

ICD-9 CODE 724.4

THE CLINICAL SYNDROME

Lumbar radiculopathy is a constellation of symptoms consisting of neurogenic back and lower extremity pain emanating from the lumbar nerve roots. In addition to the pain, the patient with lumbar radiculopathy may experience associated numbness, weakness, and loss of reflexes. The causes of lumbar radiculopathy include herniated disc, foraminal stenosis, tumor, osteophyte formation, and rarely infection. Many patients and their physicians will refer to the constellation of symptoms that comprise lumbar radiculopathy as sciatica.

SIGNS AND SYMPTOMS

The patient suffering from lumbar radiculopathy will complain of pain, numbness, tingling, and paresthesias in the distribution of the affected nerve root or roots (Table 49–1). Patients may also note weakness and lack of coordination in the affected extremity. Muscle spasms and back pain as well as pain referred into the buttocks are common (Fig. 49–1). Decreased sensation, weakness, and reflex changes are demonstrated on physical examination. Patients with lumbar radiculopathy will commonly experience

a reflex shifting of the trunk to one side. This reflex shifting is called *list*. Occasionally, a patient suffering from lumbar radiculopathy will experience compression of the lumbar spinal nerve roots and cauda equina, resulting in myelopathy or cauda equina syndrome. Lumbar myelopathy is most commonly due to midline herniated lumbar disc, spinal stenosis, tumor, or rarely infection. Patients suffering from lumbar myelopathy or cauda equina syndrome will experience varying degrees of lower extremity weakness and bowel and bladder symptomatology. This represents a neurosurgical emergency and should be treated as such.

TESTING

Magnetic resonance imaging (MRI) of the lumbar spine will provide the clinician with the best information regarding the lumbar spine and its contents. MRI is highly accurate and will help identify abnormalities that may put the patient at risk for the development of lumbar myelopathy. In patients who cannot undergo MRI (e.g., patients with pacemakers), computed tomography (CT) or myelography is a reasonable second choice. Radionucleotide bone scanning and plain radiography are indicated if fracture or bony abnormality such as metastatic disease is being considered.

Although MRI, CT, and myelography can supply useful neuroanatomic information, electromyography and nerve conduction velocity testing will provide the clinician with neurophysiologic information that can

Table 49–1. Clinical Features of Lumbar Radiculopathy

Lumbar Root	Pain	Sensory Changes	Weakness	Reflex Changes
L4	Back, shin, thigh, and leg	Shin numbness	Ankle dorsiflexors	Knee jerk
L5	Back, posterior thigh, and leg	Numbness of top of foot and first web space	Extensor hallucis longus	None
S1	Back, posterior calf, and leg	Numbness of lateral foot	Gastrocnemeus and soleus	Ankle jerk

delineate the actual status of each individual nerve root and the lumbar plexus. Screening laboratory testing consisting of complete blood count, erythrocyte sedimentation rate, and automated blood chemistry testing should be performed if the diagnosis of lumbar radiculopathy is in question.

DIFFERENTIAL DIAGNOSIS

Lumbar radiculopathy is a clinical diagnosis that is supported by a combination of clinical history, physical examination, radiography, and MRI. Pain syndromes that may mimic lumbar radiculopathy include low back strain, lumbar bursitis, lumbar fibromyositis, inflammatory arthritis, and disorders of the lumbar spinal cord, roots, plexus, and nerves. MRI of the lumbar spine should be carried out for all patients suspected of suffering from lumbar radiculopathy. Screening laboratory testing consisting of complete blood count, erythrocyte sedimentation rate, antinuclear antibody testing, HLA B-27 antigen screening, and automated blood chemistry testing should be performed if the diagnosis of lumbar radiculopathy is in question to help rule out other causes of the patient's pain.

TREATMENT

Lumbar radiculopathy is best treated with a multimodality approach. Physical therapy, including heat modalities and deep sedative massage, combined with nonsteroidal anti-inflammatory drugs and skeletal muscle relaxants represent a reasonable starting point. The addition of caudal or lumbar steroid epidural nerve blocks is a reasonable next step. Caudal or lumbar epidural blocks with local anesthetic and steroid have been shown to be extremely effective in the treatment of lumbar radiculopathy. Underlying sleep disturbance and depression are best treated with a tricylic antidepressant compound such as nortriptyline, which can be started at a single bedtime dose of 25 mg.

COMPLICATIONS AND PITFALLS

The failure to accurately diagnosis lumbar radiculopathy may put the patient at risk for the development of lumbar myelopathy, which if untreated may progress to paraparesis or paraplegia. Electromyography will help sort out plexopathy from radiculopathy and also help identify coexistent entrapment neuropathy such as tarsal tunnel syndrome that may confuse the diagnosis.

CLINICAL PEARLS

Tarsal syndrome should also be differentiated from lumbar radiculopathy involving the lumbar nerve roots, which may at times mimic tibial nerve compression. Furthermore, it should be remembered that lumbar radiculopathy and tibial nerve entrapment may coexist in the "double crush" syndrome. The double crush syndrome is seen most commonly with median nerve entrapment at the wrist or carpal tunnel syndrome.

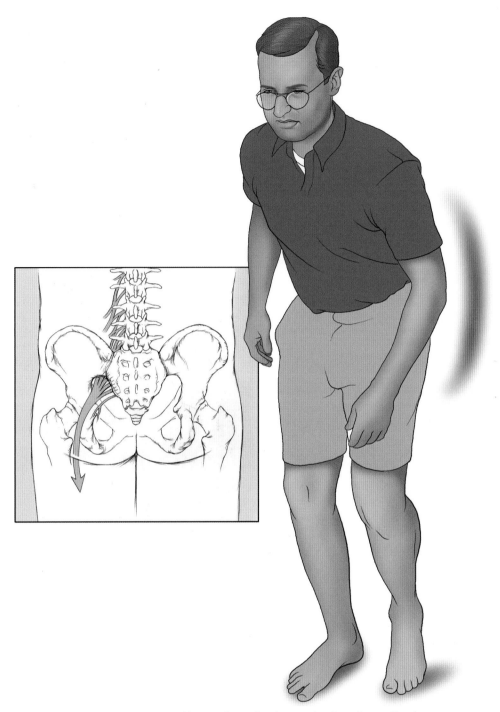

Figure 49–1. The patient suffering from lumbar radiculopathy will often assume an unnatural posture in an attempt to take pressure off the affected nerve root and relieve pain.

50 *Spinal Stenosis*

ICD-9 Code 724.02

THE CLINICAL SYNDROME

Spinal stenosis is the result of a congenital or an acquired narrowing of the spinal canal. Clinically, the pain of spinal stenosis usually presents in a characteristic manner as pain and weakness in the legs and calves when walking. This neurogenic pain is called *pseudoclaudication* or *neurogenic claudication*. These symptoms are usually accompanied by lower extremity pain emanating from the lumbar nerve roots. In addition to the pain, the patient with spinal stenosis may experience associated numbness, weakness, and loss of reflexes. The causes of spinal stenosis include bulging or herniated disc, facet arthropathy, and thickening and buckling of the interlaminar ligaments. All of these inciting factors tend to worsen with age.

SIGNS AND SYMPTOMS

The patient suffering from spinal stenosis will complain of calf and leg pain and fatigue with walking, standing, or lying supine. This fatigue and pain will disappear if the patient flexes the lumbar spine or assumes the sitting position. Extension of the spine may also cause an increase in symptoms. Patients will also complain of pain, numbness, tingling, and paresthesias in the distribution of the affected nerve root or roots. Patients may also note weakness and lack of coordination in the affected extremity. Muscle spasms and back pain as well as pain referred into the trapezius and intrascapular region are common (Fig. 50–1). Decreased sensation, weakness, and reflex changes are demonstrated on physical examination.

Occasionally, a patient suffering from spinal stenosis will experience compression of the lumbar spinal nerve roots and cauda equina resulting in myelopathy or cauda equina syndrome. Patients suffering from lumbar myelopathy or cauda equina syndrome will experience varying degrees of lower extremity weakness and bowel and bladder symptomatology. This represents a neurosurgical emergency and should be treated as such, although the onset of symptoms is often insidious.

TESTING

Magnetic resonance imaging (MRI) of the lumbar spine will provide the clinician with the best information regarding the lumbar spine and its contents. MRI is highly accurate and will help identify abnormalities that may put the patient at risk for the development of lumbar myelopathy. In patients who cannot undergo MRI (e.g., patients with pacemakers), computed tomography (CT) or myelography are reasonable second choices. Radionucleotide bone scanning and plain radiography are indicated if coexistent fracture or bony abnormality such as metastatic disease is being considered.

Although MRI, CT, and myelography can supply useful neuroanatomic information, electromyography and nerve conduction velocity testing will provide the clinician with neurophysiologic information that can delineate the actual status of each individual nerve root and the lumbar plexus. Screening laboratory testing consisting of complete blood count, erythrocyte sedimentation rate, and automated blood chemistry testing should be performed if the diagnosis of spinal stenosis is in question.

DIFFERENTIAL DIAGNOSIS

Spinal stenosis is a clinical diagnosis that is supported by a combination of clinical history, physical examination, radiography, and MRI. Pain syndromes that may mimic spinal stenosis include low back

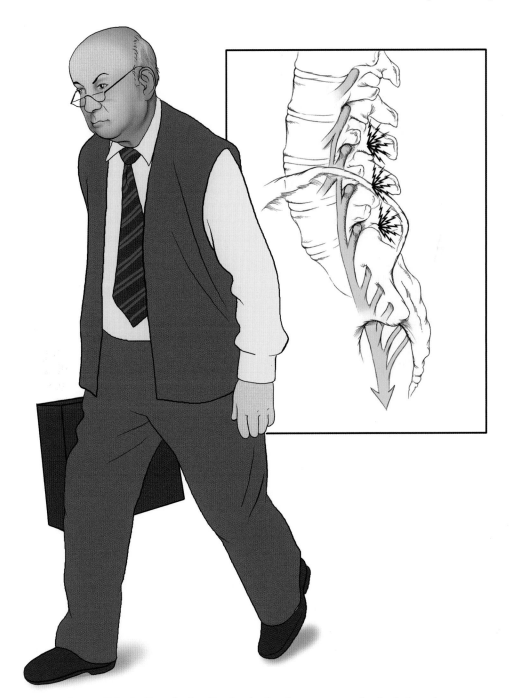

Figure 50–1. Pseudoclaudication is the sine qua non of spinal stenosis.

strain, lumbar bursitis, lumbar fibromyositis, inflammatory arthritis, and disorders of the lumbar spinal cord, roots, plexus, and nerves including diabetic femoral neuropathy. MRI of the lumbar spine should be carried out on all patients suspected of suffering from spinal stenosis. Screening laboratory testing consisting of complete blood count, erythrocyte sedimentation rate, antinuclear antibody testing, HLA B-27 antigen screening, and automated blood chemistry testing should be performed if the diagnosis of spinal stenosis is in question to help rule out other causes of the patient's pain.

TREATMENT

Spinal stenosis is best treated with a multimodality approach. Physical therapy, including heat modalities and deep sedative massage, combined with nonsteroidal anti-inflammatory drugs and skeletal muscle relaxants represents a reasonable starting point. The addition of caudal or lumbar steroid epidural nerve blocks is a reasonable next step. Caudal epidural blocks with local anesthetic and steroid have been shown to be extremely effective in the treatment of spinal stenosis. Underlying sleep disturbance and depression are best treated with a tricylic antidepressant compound such as nortriptyline, which can be started at a single bedtime does of 25 mg.

COMPLICATIONS AND PITFALLS

The failure to accurately diagnosis spinal stenosis may put the patient at risk for the development of lumbar myelopathy or cauda equina syndrome, which if untreated may progress to paraparesis or paraplegia. Electromyography will help sort out plexopathy from radiculopathy and also help identify co-existent entrapment neuropathy such as tarsal tunnel syndrome that confuses the diagnosis.

CLINICAL PEARLS

Spinal stenosis is a common cause of back and lower extremity pain. The finding of pseudoclaudication should point the clinician toward this diagnosis. It should be remembered that this syndrome worsens with age and that the onset of lumbar myelopathy or cauda equina syndrome may be insidious and can be missed without careful questioning and physical examination.

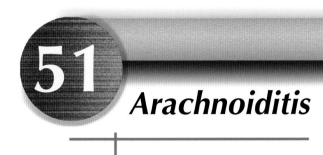

51

Arachnoiditis

ICD-9 CODE 322.9

THE CLINICAL SYNDROME

Arachnoiditis is a term used to describe thickening, scarring, and inflammation of the arachnoid membrane. These abnormalities may be self-limited or may lead to compression of the nerve roots and spinal cord. In addition to pain, the patient with arachnoiditis may experience associated numbness, weakness, loss of reflexes, and bowel and bladder symptomatology. The cause of arachnoiditis is unknown but may include herniated disc, infection, tumor, myelography, spine surgery, or intrathecal administration of drugs. Anecdotal reports of arachnoiditis after epidural and subarachnoid administration of methylprednisolone acetate preparations have surfaced.

SIGNS AND SYMPTOMS

The patient suffering from arachnoiditis will complain of pain, numbness, tingling, and paresthesias in the distribution of the affected nerve root or roots (Table 51–1). Patients may also note weakness and lack of coordination in the affected extremity. Muscle spasms and back pain as well as pain referred into the buttocks are common (Fig. 51–1). Decreased sensation, weakness, and reflex changes are demonstrated on physical examination. Occasionally, a patient suffering from arachnoiditis will experience compression of the lumbar spinal cord, nerve roots, and cauda equina resulting in myelopathy or cauda equina syndrome. Patients suffering from lumbar myelopathy or cauda equina syndrome due to arachnoiditis will experience varying degrees of lower extremity weakness and bowel and bladder symptomatology.

TESTING

Magnetic resonance imaging (MRI) of the lumbar spine will provide the clinician with the best information regarding the lumbar spine and its contents. MRI is highly accurate and will help identify abnormalities that may put the patient at risk for the development of lumbar myelopathy or cauda equina syndrome. In patients who cannot undergo MRI (e.g., patients with pacemakers), computed tomography (CT) or myelography are reasonable second choices. Radionucleotide bone scanning and plain radiography are indicated if fracture or bony abnormality such as metastatic disease is being considered.

Although MRI, CT, and myelography can supply useful neuroanatomic information, electromyography and nerve conduction velocity testing will provide the clinician with neurophysiologic information that can delineate the actual status of each individual nerve root and the lumbar plexus. Screening laboratory testing consisting of complete blood count, erythrocyte

Table 51–1. Clinical Features of Arachnoiditis

Lumbar Root	Pain	Sensory Changes	Weakness	Reflex Changes
L4	Back, shin, thigh, and leg	Shin numbness	Ankle dorsiflexors	Knee jerk
L5	Back, posterior thigh, and leg	Numbness of top of foot and first web space	Extensor hallucis longus	None
S1	Back, posterior calf, and leg	Numbness of lateral foot	Gastrocnemeus and soleus	Ankle jerk

sedimentation rate, and automated blood chemistry testing should be performed if the diagnosis of arachnoiditis is in question.

DIFFERENTIAL DIAGNOSIS

Arachnoiditis is a clinical diagnosis that is supported by a combination of clinical history, physical examination, radiography, and MRI. Pain syndromes that may mimic arachnoiditis include tumor, infection, and disorders of the lumbar spinal cord, roots, plexus, and nerves. MRI of the lumbar spine should be carried out on all patients suspected of suffering from arachnoiditis. Screening laboratory testing consisting of complete blood count, erythrocyte sedimentation rate, antinuclear antibody testing, HLA B-27 antigen screening, and automated blood chemistry testing should be performed if the diagnosis of arachnoiditis is in question to help rule out other causes of the patient's pain.

TREATMENT

There is little consensus as to how best treat the patient suffering from arachnoiditis, and most efforts are aimed at decompressing nerve roots and spinal cord and/or treating the inflammatory component of the disease. Epidural neurolysis and/or caudal administration of steroids may help decompress nerve roots if the pathology is localized. More generalized cases of arachnoiditis will often require surgical de-

compressive laminectomy. The results of all modalities are disappointing at best. Underlying sleep disturbance and depression are best treated with a tricylic antidepressant compound such as nortriptyline, which can be started at a single bedtime does of 25 mg. Neuropathic pain associated with arachnoiditis may respond to gabapentin. Spinal cord stimulation may also help provide symptomatic relief. Opioid analgesics should be used with caution if at all.

COMPLICATIONS AND PITFALLS

The failure to accurately diagnosis arachnoiditis may put the patient at risk for the development of lumbar myelopathy or cauda equina syndrome, which if untreated may progress to paraparesis or paraplegia. Electromyography will help sort out plexopathy from arachnoiditis and also help identify coexistent entrapment neuropathy such as tarsal tunnel syndrome that confuse the diagnosis.

CLINICAL PEARLS

Arachnoiditis is a potentially devastating disease that may be erroneously attributed to the clinician's efforts to diagnose and treat low back and lower extremity pain. For this reason, MRI and electromyography should be obtained sooner rather than later in patients without a clear etiology as to the pathology responsible for their symptomatology.

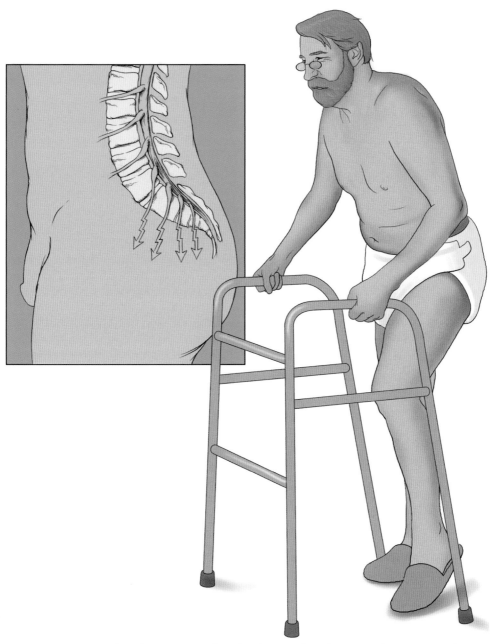

Figure 51–1. Arachnoiditis may result in lumbar myelopathy or cauda equina syndrome.

52

Sacroiliac Joint Pain

ICD-9 CODE 724.6

THE CLINICAL SYNDROME

Pain emanating from the sacroiliac joint commonly occurs after the patient lifts while in an awkward position, putting strain on the joint and supporting ligaments and soft tissues. The sacroiliac joint is also susceptible to the development of arthritis from a variety of conditions that have in common the ability to damage the joint cartilage. Osteoarthritis of the joint is the most common form of arthritis that results in sacroiliac joint pain. However, rheumatoid arthritis and posttraumatic arthritis are also common causes of sacroiliac pain secondary to arthritis. Less common causes of arthritis-induced sacroiliac pain include the collagen vascular diseases, such as ankylosing spondylitis, infection, and Lyme disease. The collagen vascular diseases will generally present as a polyarthropathy rather than as a monoarthropathy limited to the sacroiliac joint, although sacroiliac pain secondary to the collagen vascular disease ankylosing spondylitis responds exceedingly well to the intra-articular injection technique described here. Occasionally, the clinician will encounter patients with iatrogenically induced sacroiliac joint dysfunction due to overaggressive bone graft harvesting for spinal fusions.

SIGNS AND SYMPTOMS

The majority of patients presenting with sacroiliac pain secondary to strain or arthritis will present with the complaint of pain that is localized around the sacroiliac joint and upper leg. The pain of sacroiliac joint strain or arthritis radiates into the posterior buttocks and the back of the legs. The pain does not radiate below the knees. Activity makes the pain worse, with rest and heat providing some relief. The pain is constant and characterized as aching in nature. The pain may interfere with sleep. On physical examination, there will be tenderness to palpation of the affected sacroiliac joint. The patient will often favor the affected leg and exhibit a list to the unaffected side (Fig. 52–1). Spasm of the lumbar paraspinal musculature is often present, as is limitation of range of motion of the lumbar spine in the erect position that improves in the sitting position due to relaxation of the hamstring muscles. Patients with pain emanating from the sacroiliac joint will exhibit a positive pelvic rock test. The pelvic rock test is performed by placing the hands on the iliac crests and the thumbs on the anterior superior iliac spines and then forcibly compressing the pelvis toward the midline. A positive test is indicated by the production of pain around the sacroiliac joint.

TESTING

Plain radiography is indicated in all patients who present with sacroiliac pain. Based on the patient's clinical presentation, additional testing including complete blood count, sedimentation rate, HLA B-27 antigen screening, and antinuclear antibody testing may be indicated.

DIFFERENTIAL DIAGNOSIS

Pain emanating from the sacroiliac joint can often be confused with low back strain, lumbar bursitis, lumbar fibromyositis, inflammatory arthritis, and disorders of the lumbar spinal cord, roots, plexus, and nerves. Plain radiographs of the lumbar spine and sacroiliac joints should be obtained for all patients thought to be suffering from sacroiliac joint pain. Magnetic resonance imaging of the lumbar spine and sacroiliac joint should be carried out on those patients suspected of suffering from sacroiliac joint pain whose cause is not clearly defined. Radionucleotide

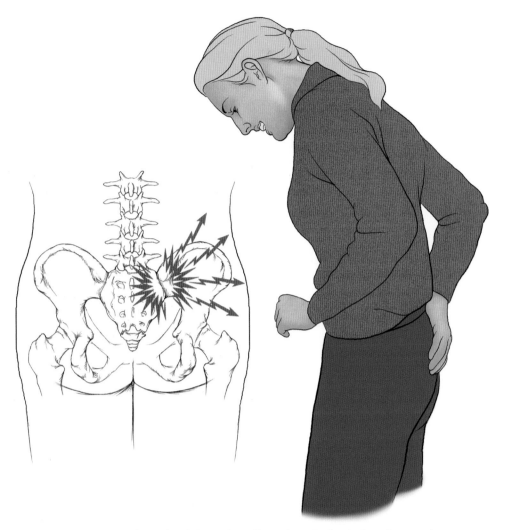

Figure 52–1. Sacroiliac joint pain radiates into the buttock and upper leg.

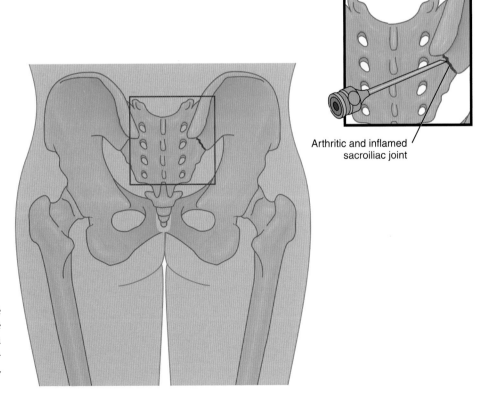

Arthritic and inflamed
sacroiliac joint

Figure 52–2. Correct needle placement for injection of the sacroiliac joint. (From Waldman SD: Atlas of Pain Management Injection Techniques. Philadelphia, WB Saunders, 2000, p 227.)

bone scanning should also be considered in such patients to rule out tumor and unsuspected insufficiency fractures that may be missed on conventional radiographs. Screening laboratory testing consisting of complete blood count, erythrocyte sedimentation rate, antinuclear antibody testing, HLA B-27 antigen screening, and automated blood chemistry testing should be performed if the diagnosis is in question to help rule out other causes of the patient's pain.

TREATMENT

Initial treatment of the pain and functional disability associated with sacroiliac joint pain should include a combination of the nonsteroidal anti-inflammatory drugs or cyclooxygenase-2 inhibitors and physical therapy. The local application of heat and cold may also be beneficial. For patients who do not respond to these treatment modalities, the following injection technique with local anesthetic and steroid may be a reasonable next step.

Injection of the sacroiliac joint is carried out by placing the patient in the supine position and properly preparing the skin overlying the affected sacroiliac joint space with antiseptic solution. A sterile syringe containing 4.0 mL of 0.25% preservative-free bupivacaine and 40 mg methylprednisolone is attached to a 25-gauge needle using strict aseptic technique. With strict aseptic technique, the posterior superior spine of the ilium is identified. At this point, the needle is carefully advanced through the skin and subcutaneous tissues at a 45-degree angle toward the affected sacroiliac joint (Fig. 52–2). If bone is encountered, the needle is withdrawn into the subcutaneous tissues and redirected superiorly and slightly more lateral. After the joint space is entered, the contents of the syringe are gently injected. There should be little resistance to injection. If resistance is encountered, the needle is probably in a ligament and should be advanced slightly into the joint space until the injection proceeds without significant resistance. The needle is then removed, and a sterile pressure dressing and ice pack are placed at the injection site.

COMPLICATIONS AND PITFALLS

The major complication of intra-articular injection of the sacroiliac is infection. This complication should be exceedingly rare if strict aseptic technique is followed. Approximately 25% of patients will complain of a transient increase in pain after intra-articular injection of the sacroiliac joint and should be warned of such. Care must be taken to avoid injection too laterally or the needle may traumatize the sciatic nerve.

CLINICAL PEARLS

Disorders of the sacroiliac joint can be distinguished from pain emanating from the lumbar spine by having the patient bend forward while seated. Patients with sacroiliac pain can bend forward with relative ease due to relaxation of the hamstring muscles in the seated position. Patients with lumbar spine pain will experience an exacerbation of pain when bending forward while seated.

The above injection technique is extremely effective in the treatment of sacroiliac joint pain. Coexistent bursitis and tendinitis may also contribute to sacroiliac pain and may require additional treatment with more localized injection of local anesthetic and methylprednisolone acetate. This technique is a safe procedure if careful attention is paid to the clinically relevant anatomy in the areas to be injected. Care must be taken to use sterile technique to avoid infection, and universal precautions to avoid risk to the operator. The incidence of ecchymosis and hematoma formation can be decreased if pressure is placed on the injection site immediately after injection. The use of physical modalities including local heat as well as gentle range of motion exercises should be introduced several days after the patient undergoes this injection technique for sacroiliac pain. Vigorous exercises should be avoided as they will exacerbate the patient's symptomatology.

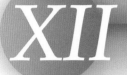

XII Pelvic Pain Syndromes

53

Osteitis Pubis

ICD-9 CODE 733.5

THE CLINICAL SYNDROME

Osteitis pubis is a constellation of symptoms consisting of a localized tenderness over the symphysis pubis, pain radiating into the inner thigh, and a waddling gait. Characteristic radiographic changes consisting of erosion, sclerosis, and widening of the symphysis pubis are pathognomonic for osteitis pubis (Fig. 53–1). A disease of the second through fourth decade, osteitis pubis affects females more frequently than males. Osteitis pubis occurs most commonly after bladder, inguinal, or prostate surgery and is thought to be due to hematogenous spread of infection to the relatively avascular symphysis pubis. Osteitis pubis can appear without an obvious inciting factor or infection.

SIGNS AND SYMPTOMS

On physical examination, the patient will exhibit point tenderness over the symphysis pubis. The patient may be tender over the anterior pelvis and may note that the pain radiates into the inner thigh with palpation of the symphysis pubis. Patients may adopt a waddling gait in order to avoid movement of the symphysis pubis. This dysfunctional gait may result in lower extremity bursitis and tendinitis, which may confuse the clinical picture and further increase the patient's pain and disability.

TESTING

Plain radiography is indicated in all patients who present with pain thought to be emanating from the symphysis pubis to rule out occult bony pathology and tumor. Based on the patient's clinical presentation, additional testing including complete blood count, prostate specific antigen, sedimentation rate, serum protein electrophoresis, and antinuclear antibody testing may be indicated. Magnetic resonance imaging of the pelvis is indicated if occult mass or tumor is suspected. Radionucleotide bone scanning may be useful to rule out stress fractures not seen on plain radiographs. The following injection technique will serve as both a diagnostic and therapeutic maneuver.

DIFFERENTIAL DIAGNOSIS

A pain syndrome clinically similar to osteitis pubis can be seen in patients suffering from rheumatoid arthritis and ankylosing spondylitis but without the characteristic radiographic changes of osteitis pubis. Multiple myeloma and metastatic tumors may also mimic the pain and radiographic changes of osteitis pubis. Insufficiency fractures of the pubic rami should also be considered if generalized osteoporosis is present.

TREATMENT

Initial treatment of the pain and functional disability associated with osteitis pubis should include a combination of the nonsteroidal anti-inflammatory drugs or cyclooxygenase-2 inhibitors and physical therapy. The local application of heat and cold may also be beneficial. For patients who do not respond to these treatment modalities, the following injection technique with local anesthetic and steroid may be a reasonable next step.

Injection for osteitis pubis is carried out by placing the patient in the supine position. The midpoints of pubic bones and the symphysis pubis are identified by palpation. Proper preparation with antiseptic solution of the skin overlying this point is then carried out. A syringe containing 2.0 mL of 0.25% preservative-free bupivacaine and 40 mg methylprednisolone is attached to a 3½-inch 25-gauge needle.

The needle is then carefully advanced through the previously identified point at a right angle to the skin directly toward the center of the pubic symphysis. The needle is advanced very slowly until the needle impinges on the fibroelastic cartilage of the joint. The needle is then withdrawn slightly out of the joint, and after careful aspiration for blood and if no paresthesia is present, the contents of the syringe are then gently injected. There should be minimal resistance to injection.

COMPLICATIONS AND PITFALLS

The proximity to the pelvic contents makes it imperative that this procedure be carried out only by those well versed in the regional anatomy and experienced in performing injection techniques. Many patients will also complain of a transient increase in pain after this injection technique. Reactivation of latent infection, although rare, can occur, and careful attention to sterile technique is mandatory.

CLINICAL PEARLS

Osteitis pubis should be suspected in patients presenting with pain over the pubic symphysis in the absence of trauma. The above injection technique is extremely effective in the treatment of osteitis pubis. This technique is a safe procedure if careful attention is paid to the clinically relevant anatomy in the areas to be injected. Care must be taken to use sterile technique to avoid infection, and universal precautions to avoid risk to the operator. Most side effects of this injection technique are related to needle-induced trauma to the injection site and underlying tissues. The incidence of ecchymosis and hematoma formation can be decreased if pressure is placed on the injection site immediately after injection.

The use of physical modalities, including local heat, as well as gentle stretching exercises, should be introduced several days after the patient undergoes this injection technique. Vigorous exercises should be avoided as they will exacerbate the patient's symptomatology. Simple analgesics, nonsteroidal anti-inflammatory drugs, and antimyotonic agents such as tizanidine may be used concurrently with this injection technique.

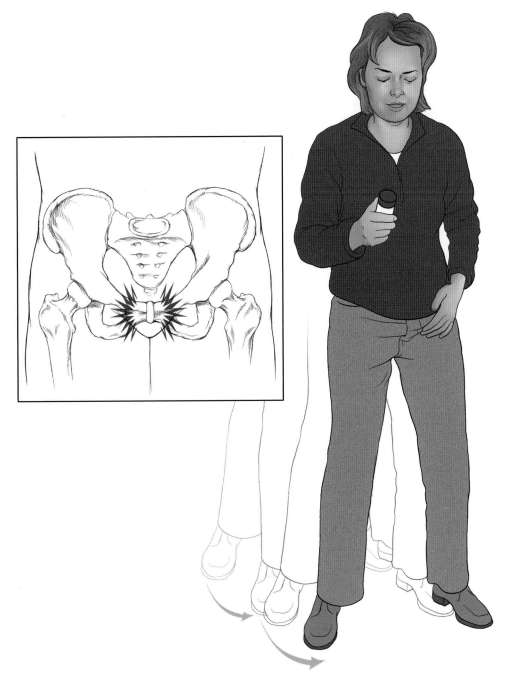

Figure 53–1. Patients with osteitus pubis will often develop a waddling gait.

54 *Piriformis Syndrome*

ICD-9 CODE 355.9

THE CLINICAL SYNDROME

Piriformis syndrome is an entrapment neuropathy that presents as pain, numbness, paresthesias, and associated weakness in the distribution of the sciatic nerve. Piriformis syndrome is caused by compression of the sciatic nerve by the piriformis muscle as it passes through the sciatic notch. The piriformis muscle's primary function is to externally rotate the femur at the hip joint. The piriformis muscle is innervated by the sacral plexus. With internal rotation of the femur, the tendinous insertion and belly of the muscle can compress the sciatic nerve and, if this persists, cause entrapment of the sciatic nerve. These symptoms often begin as severe pain in the buttocks that may radiate into the lower extremity and foot. Patients suffering from piriformis syndrome may develop altered gait, which may result in the development of coexistent sacroiliac, back, and hip pain, which may confuse the clinical picture. If the condition remains untreated, progressive motor deficit of the gluteal muscles and lower extremity can result. The onset of symptoms of piriformis syndrome usually occurs after direct trauma to the sacroiliac and gluteal region and occasionally as a result of repetitive hip and lower extremity motions or repeated pressure on the piriformis muscle and underlying sciatic nerve.

SIGNS AND SYMPTOMS

Physical findings include tenderness over the sciatic notch. A positive Tinel's sign over the sciatic nerve as it passes beneath the piriformis muscle is often present. A positive straight leg raising test is suggestive of sciatic nerve entrapment, which may be due to piriformis syndrome. Palpation of the piriformis muscle will reveal tenderness and a swollen, indurated muscle belly. Lifting or bending at the waist and hips will increase the pain symptomatology in most patients suffering from piriformis syndrome (Fig. 54–1). Weakness of affected gluteal muscles and lower extremity, and ultimately muscle wasting, are often seen in advanced untreated piriformis syndrome.

TESTING

Electromyography will help distinguish lumbar radiculopathy from piriformis syndrome. Plain radiographs of the back, hip, and pelvis are indicated in all patients who present with piriformis syndrome to rule out occult bony pathology. Based on the patient's clinical presentation, additional testing including complete blood count, uric acid, sedimentation rate, and antinuclear antibody testing may be indicated. Magnetic resonance imaging of the back is indicated if herniated disc, spinal stenosis, or a space-occupying lesion is suspected. Injection in the region of the sciatic nerve at this level will serve as both a diagnostic and therapeutic maneuver.

DIFFERENTIAL DIAGNOSIS

Piriformis syndrome is often misdiagnosed as lumbar radiculopathy or attributed to primary hip pathology. Radiographs of the hip and electromyography will help distinguish piriformis syndrome from radiculopathy of pain emanating from the hip. Most patients suffering from a lumbar radiculopathy will have back pain associated with reflex, motor and sensory changes, whereas patients with piriformis syndrome will have only secondary back pain and no reflex changes. The motor and sensory changes of piriformis syndrome will be limited to the distribution of the sciatic nerve below the sciatic notch. It should be remembered that lumbar radiculopathy

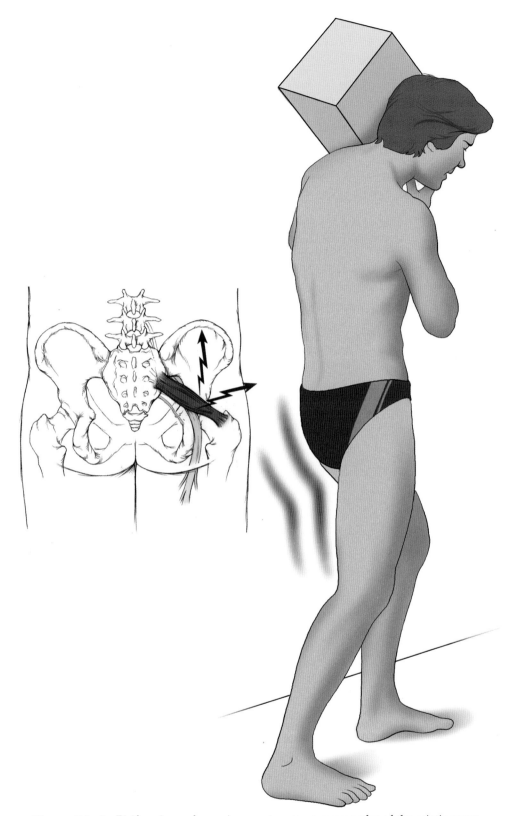

Figure 54–1. Piriformis syndrome is an entrapment neuropathy of the sciatic nerve.

and sciatic nerve entrapment may coexist as the "double crush" syndrome. As mentioned, piriformis syndrome causes alteration of gait that may result in secondary back and radicular symptomatology, which may coexist with this entrapment neuropathy.

TREATMENT

Initial treatment of the pain and functional disability associated with piriformis syndrome should include a combination of the nonsteroidal anti-inflammatory drugs or cyclooxygenase-2 inhibitors and physical therapy. The local application of heat and cold may also be beneficial. Any repetitive activity that may exacerbate the patient's symptomatology should be avoided. Nighttime splinting of the affected extremity by placing a pillow between the legs if the patient sleeps on his or her side may be beneficial. If the patient is suffering from significant paresthesias, gabapentin may be added. For patients who do not respond to these treatment modalities, injection of local anesthetics in combination with methlyprednisolone acetate in the region of the sciatic nerve at the level of the piriformis muscle may be a reasonable next step. Rarely, surgical release of the entrapment is required to provide relief.

COMPLICATIONS AND PITFALLS

The main side effect of injection in the region of the sciatic nerve is postblock ecchymosis and hematoma. Because a paresthesia is elicited with this technique, the potential for needle-induced trauma to the sciatic nerve remains a possibility. By advancing the needle slowly and withdrawing the needle slightly away from the nerve, needle-induced trauma to the sciatic nerve can be avoided.

CLINICAL PEARLS

Patients suffering from piriformis syndrome may develop altered gait that may result in the development of coexistent sacroiliac, back, and hip pain, which may confuse the clinical picture. Careful physical examination combined with the aforementioned testing should help the clinician sort out the diagnostic possibilities.

55

Ischiogluteal Bursitis

ICD-9 CODE 726.5

THE CLINICAL SYNDROME

The ischial bursa lies between the gluteus maximus muscle and the bone of the ischial tuberosity. It may exist as a single bursal sac or, in some patients, as a multisegmented series of sacs that may be loculated in nature. The ischial bursa is vulnerable to injury from both acute trauma and repeated microtrauma. Acute injuries frequently take the form of direct trauma to the bursa from falls onto the buttocks and from overuse such as prolonged riding of horses or bicycles. Running on uneven or soft surfaces such as sand may also cause ischial bursitis (Fig. 55–1). If the inflammation of the ischial bursa becomes chronic, calcification of the bursa may occur.

SIGNS AND SYMPTOMS

The patient suffering from ischial bursitis will frequently complain of pain at the base of the buttock with resisted extension off the lower extremity. The pain is localized to the area over the ischial tuberosity with referred pain noted into the hamstring muscle, which may also develop coexistent tendinitis. Often, the patient will be unable to sleep on the affected hip and may complain of a sharp, catching sensation when extending and flexing the hip, especially on first awakening. Physical examination may reveal point tenderness over the ischial tuberosity. Passive straight leg raising and active resisted extension of the affected lower extremity will reproduce the pain. Sudden release of resistance during this maneuver will markedly increase the pain.

TESTING

Plain radiographs of the hip may reveal calcification of the bursa and associated structures consistent with chronic inflammation. Magnetic resonance imaging is indicated if disruption of the hamstring musculotendinous unit is suspected. The injection technique described here will serve as both a diagnostic and therapeutic maneuver and will also treat hamstring tendinitis. Screening laboratory testing consisting of a complete blood count, erythrocyte sedimentation rate, and antinuclear antibody testing is indicated if collagen vascular disease is suspected. Plain radiography and radionucleotide bone scanning are indicated in the presence of trauma or if tumor is a possibility.

DIFFERENTIAL DIAGNOSIS

Although the diagnosis of ischiogluteal bursitis is usually straightforward, this painful condition can occasionally be confused with sciatica, primary pathology of the hip, insufficiency fractures of the pelvis, and tendinitis of the hamstrings. Tumors of the hip and pelvis may be overlooked and should be considered in the differential diagnosis of ischiogluteal bursitis.

TREATMENT

Initial treatment of the pain and functional disability associated with ischiogluteal bursitis should include a combination of the nonsteroidal anti-inflammatory drugs or cyclooxygenase-2 inhibitors and physical therapy. The local application of heat and cold may also be beneficial. Any repetitive activity that may exacerbate the patient's symptomatology should be avoided. For patients who do not respond to these treatment modalities, the following injection technique may be a reasonable next step.

To inject the ischiogluteal bursa, the patient is placed in the lateral position with the affected side up and the affected leg flexed at the knee. Proper preparation of the skin overlying the ischial tuberosity with antiseptic solution is then carried out. A syringe containing 4.0 mL of 0.25% preservative-free bupivacaine and 40 mg methylprednisolone is attached to a 1½-inch 25-gauge needle. The ischial tuberosity is then identified with a sterilely gloved finger. Before needle placement, the patient should be advised to say "there" immediately if he or she feels a paresthesia into the lower extremity, indicating that the needle has impinged on the sciatic nerve. Should a paresthesia occur, the needle should be immediately withdrawn and repositioned more medially. The needle is then carefully advanced at that point through the skin, subcutaneous tissues, muscle, and tendon until it impinges on the bone of the ischial tuberosity. Care must be taken to keep the needle in the midline and to not advance it laterally, or it could impinge on the sciatic nerve. After careful aspiration and if no paresthesia is present, the contents of the syringe are then gently injected into the bursa.

COMPLICATIONS AND PITFALLS

If the patient continues the repetitive activities responsible for the evolution of ischiogluteal bursitis, improvement will be limited and the patient should be warned of such. The proximity to the sciatic nerve makes it imperative that this procedure be carried out only by those well versed in the regional anatomy and experienced in performing injection techniques. Many patients will also complain of a transient increase in pain after injection of the affected bursa and tendons.

CLINICAL PEARLS

Although the treatments are the same, ischial bursitis can be distinguished from hamstring tendinitis by the facts that ischial bursitis will present with point tenderness over the ischial bursa and that the tenderness of hamstring tendinitis is more diffuse over the upper muscle and tendons of the hamstring. This injection technique is extremely effective in the treatment of ischial bursitis and hamstring tendinitis. The technique is a safe procedure if careful attention is paid to the clinically relevant anatomy in the areas to be injected.

The use of physical modalities including local heat as well as gentle stretching exercises should be introduced several days after the patient undergoes this injection technique. Vigorous exercises should be avoided, as they will exacerbate the patient's symptomatology. Simple analgesics, nonsteroidal anti-inflammatory drugs, and antimyotonic agents such as tizanidine may be used concurrently with this injection technique.

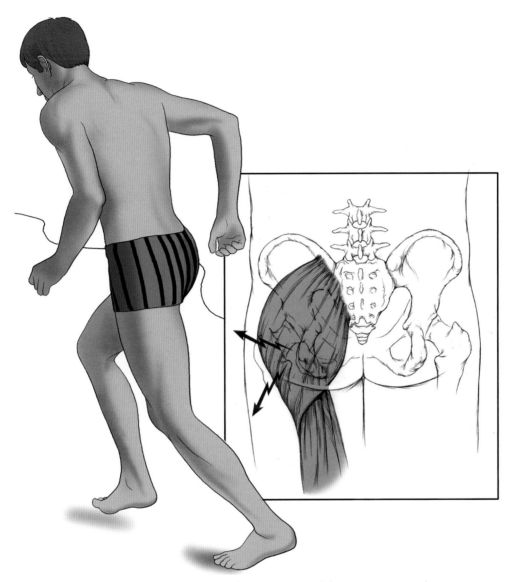

Figure 55–1. Ischiogluteal bursitis is often perpetuated by running on soft, uneven surfaces and will present clinically as point tenderness over the initial tuberosity.

56

Coccydynia

ICD-9 CODE 724.79

THE CLINICAL SYNDROME

Coccydynia is a common pain syndrome that is characterized by pain localized to the tailbone that radiates into the lower sacrum and perineum. Coccydynia affects females more frequently than males. Coccydynia occurs most commonly after direct trauma to the coccyx from a kick or a fall directly onto the coccyx. Coccydynia can also occur after difficult vaginal delivery. The pain of coccydynia is thought to be the result of strain of the sacrococcygeal ligament or occasionally due to fracture of the coccyx. Less commonly, arthritis of the sacrococcygeal joint can result in coccydynia.

SIGNS AND SYMPTOMS

On physical examination, the patient will exhibit point tenderness over the coccyx with the pain being increased with movement of the coccyx. Movement of the coccyx may also cause sharp paresthesias into the rectum, which can be quite distressing to the patient. On rectal examination, the levator ani, piriformis, and coccygeus muscles may feel indurated, and palpation of these muscles may induce severe spasm. Sitting may exacerbate the pain of coccydynia, and the patient may attempt to sit on one buttock to avoid pressure on the coccyx (Fig. 56–1).

TESTING

Plain radiography is indicated in all patients who present with pain thought to be emanating from the coccyx to rule out occult bony pathology and tumor. Based on the patient's clinical presentation, additional testing including complete blood count, prostate specific antigen, sedimentation rate, and antinuclear antibody testing may be indicated. Magnetic resonance imaging of the pelvis is indicated if occult mass or tumor is suspected. Radionucleotide bone scanning may be useful to rule out stress fractures not seen on plain radiographs. The injection technique described below will serve as both a diagnostic and therapeutic maneuver.

DIFFERENTIAL DIAGNOSIS

Primary pathology of the rectum and anus may occasionally be confused with the pain of coccydynia. Primary tumors or metastatic lesions of the sacrum and/or coccyx may also present as coccydynia. Proctalgia fugax may also mimic the pain of coccydynia but can be distinguished because movement of the coccyx will not reproduce the pain. Insufficiency fractures of the pelvis and sacrum may on occasion also mimic coccydynia, as can pathology of the sacroiliac joints.

TREATMENT

A short course of conservative therapy consisting of simple analgesics, nonsteroidal anti-inflammatory drugs or cyclooxygenase-2 inhibitors, and a foam donut to prevent further irritation to the sacrococcygeal ligament is a reasonable first step in the treatment of patients suffering from coccydynia. If the patient does not experience rapid improvement, the following injection technique is a reasonable next step.

To treat the pain of coccydynia, the patient is placed in the prone position. The legs and heels are abducted to prevent tightening of the gluteal muscles, which can make identification of the sacrococcygeal joint more difficult. Preparation of a wide area of skin

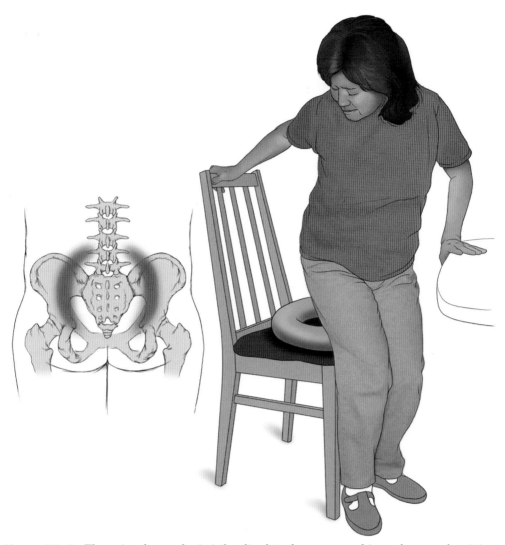

Figure 56–1. The pain of coccydynia is localized to the coccyx and is made worse by sitting.

with antiseptic solution is then carried out so that all of the landmarks can be palpated aseptically. A fenestrated sterile drape is placed to avoid contamination of the palpating finger. The middle finger of the nondominant hand is placed over the sterile drape into the natal cleft with the fingertip palpating the sacrococcygeal joint at the base of the sacrum. After location of the sacrococcygeal joint, a 1½-inch 25-gauge needle is inserted through the skin at a 45-degree angle into the region of the sacrococcygeal joint and ligament.

If the sacrococcygeal ligament is penetrated, a "pop" will be felt and the needle should be withdrawn back through the ligament. If contact with the bony wall of the sacrum occurs, the needle should be withdrawn slightly. This will disengage the needle tip from the periosteum. When the needle is satisfactorily positioned, a syringe containing 5 mL of 1.0% preservative-free lidocaine and 40 mg methylprednisolone is attached to the needle.

Gentle aspiration is carried out to identify cerebrospinal fluid or blood. If the aspiration test is negative, the contents of the syringe are slowly injected. There should be little resistance to injection. Any significant pain or sudden increase in resistance during injection suggests incorrect needle placement, and the clinician should stop injecting immediately and reassess the position of the needle. The needle is then removed, and a sterile pressure dressing and ice pack are placed at the injection site.

COMPLICATIONS AND PITFALLS

Coccydynia should be considered a diagnosis of exclusion in the absence of trauma to the coccyx and its ligaments. Failure to diagnose underlying tumor can have disastrous consequences. This injection technique is safe if careful attention to technique is observed. The major complication of the injection technique is infection due to proximity to the rectum. This complication should be exceedingly rare if strict aseptic technique is followed. Approximately 25% of patients will complain of a transient increase in pain after this injection technique and should be warned of such.

CLINICAL PEARLS

The use of a foam donut along with the treatment modalities discussed may provide symptomatic relief and allow the sacrococcygeal ligament to heal. The injection technique is extremely effective in the treatment of coccydynia. Coexistent sacroiliitis may contribute to coccygeal pain and may require additional treatment with more localized injection of local anesthetic and methylprednisolone acetate. This technique is a safe procedure if careful attention is paid to the clinically relevant anatomy in the areas to be injected. Care must be taken to use sterile technique to avoid infection, as well as universal precautions to avoid risk to the operator. The incidence of ecchymosis and hematoma formation can be decreased if pressure is placed on the injection site immediately after injection. The use of physical modalities including local heat as well as gentle range of motion exercises and rectal massage of the affected muscles should be introduced several days after the patient undergoes this injection technique for coccygeal pain. Vigorous exercises should be avoided as they will exacerbate the patient's symptomatology. Simple analgesics and nonsteroidal anti-inflammatory drugs may be used concurrently with this injection technique.

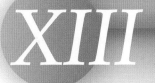

XIII Hip and Lower Extremity Pain Syndromes

57

Arthritis Pain of the Hip

ICD-9 CODE 715.95

THE CLINICAL SYNDROME

Arthritis of the hip is a common painful condition encountered in clinical practice. The hip joint is susceptible to the development of arthritis from a variety of conditions that have in common the ability to damage the joint cartilage. Osteoarthritis of the joint is the most common form of arthritis that results in hip joint pain. However, rheumatoid arthritis and post-traumatic arthritis are also common causes of hip pain secondary to arthritis. Less common causes of arthritis-induced hip pain include the collagen vascular diseases, infection, villonodular synovitis, and Lyme disease. Acute infectious arthritis will usually be accompanied by significant systemic symptoms, including fever and malaise, and should be easily recognized by the astute clinician and treated appropriately with culture and antibiotics, rather than with injection therapy. The collagen vascular diseases will generally present as a polyarthropathy rather than a monoarthropathy limited to the hip joint, although hip pain secondary to collagen vascular disease responds exceedingly well to the treatment modalities described here.

SIGNS AND SYMPTOMS

The majority of patients presenting with hip pain secondary to arthritis of the hip joint will present with the complaint of pain that is localized around the hip and upper leg (Fig. 57–1). The pain may initially present as ill-defined pain in the groin and occasionally is localized to the buttocks. Activity makes the pain worse, with rest and heat providing some relief. The pain is constant and characterized as aching in nature. The pain may interfere with sleep.

Some patients will complain of a grating or popping sensation with use of the joint, and crepitus may be present on physical examination.

In addition to the pain, patients suffering from arthritis of the hip joint will often experience a gradual decrease in functional ability, with decreasing hip range of motion making simple everyday tasks such as walking, climbing stairs, and getting in and out of automobiles quite difficult. With continued disuse, muscle wasting may occur and a "frozen hip" due to adhesive capsulitis may develop.

TESTING

Plain radiography is indicated in all patients who present with hip pain. Based on the patient's clinical presentation, additional testing including complete blood count, sedimentation rate, and antinuclear antibody testing may be indicated. Magnetic resonance imaging of the hip is indicated if aseptic necrosis or occult mass or tumor is suspected.

DIFFERENTIAL DIAGNOSIS

Lumbar radiculopathy may mimic the pain and disability associated with arthritis of the hip. In such patients, the hip examination should be negative. Entrapment neuropathies such as meralgia paresthetica may also confuse the diagnosis, as may trochanteric bursitis, both of which may coexist with arthritis of the hip. Primary and metastatic tumors of the hip and spine may also present in a manner analogous to arthritis of the hip.

TREATMENT

Initial treatment of the pain and functional disability associated with arthritis of the hip should include a combination of the nonsteroidal anti-inflammatory drugs or cyclooxygenase-2 inhibitors and physical therapy. The local application of heat and cold may also be beneficial. For patients who do not respond to these treatment modalities, an intra-articular injection of local anesthetic and steroid may be a reasonable next step.

Intra-articular injection of the hip is performed by placing the patient in the supine position. The skin overlying the hip, subacromial region, and joint space is prepared. A sterile syringe containing 4.0 mL of 0.25% preservative-free bupivacaine and 40 mg methylprednisolone is attached to a 2-inch 25-gauge needle using strict aseptic technique. With strict aseptic technique, the femoral artery is identified. At a point approximately 2 inches lateral to the femoral artery just below the inguinal ligament, the hip joint space is identified. The needle is then carefully advanced through the skin and subcutaneous tissues through the joint capsule into the joint. If bone is encountered, the needle is withdrawn into the subcutaneous tissues and redirected superiorly and slightly more medial. After the joint space is entered, the contents of the syringe are gently injected. There should be little resistance to injection. If resistance is encountered, the needle is probably in a ligament or tendon and should be advanced slightly into the joint space until the injection proceeds without significant resistance. The needle is then removed, and a sterile pressure dressing and ice pack are placed at the injection site.

SIDE EFFECTS AND COMPLICATIONS

Failure to identify primary or metastatic tumor of the hip or spine that is responsible for the patient's pain may yield disastrous results. The major complication of intra-articular injection of the hip is infection. This complication should be exceedingly rare if strict aseptic technique is followed. Approximately 25% of patients will complain of a transient increase in pain after intra-articular injection of the hip joint and should be warned of such.

CLINICAL PEARLS

Coexistent bursitis and tendinitis may also contribute to hip pain and may require additional treatment with more localized injection of local anesthetic and methylprednisolone acetate. The injection technique described is extremely effective in the treatment of pain secondary to the aforementioned causes of arthritis of the hip joint. This technique is a safe procedure if careful attention is paid to the clinically relevant anatomy in the areas to be injected. Care must be taken to use sterile technique to avoid infection, as well as the use of universal precautions to avoid risk to the operator. The incidence of ecchymosis and hematoma formation can be decreased if pressure is placed on the injection site immediately after injection. The use of physical modalities, including local heat as well as gentle range of motion exercises, should be introduced several days after the patient undergoes this injection technique for hip pain. Vigorous exercises should be avoided as they will exacerbate the patient's symptomatology.

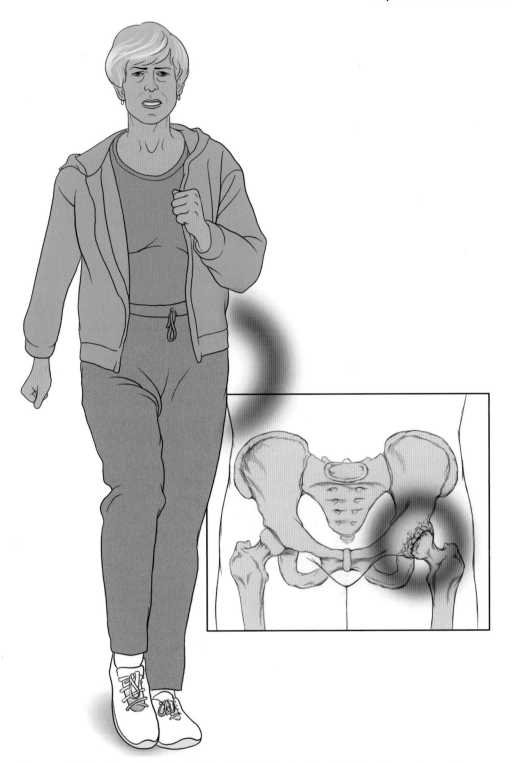

Figure 57–1. The pain of arthritis of the hip is localized to the hip, groin, and upper leg and is made worse with weight-bearing exercise.

58

Meralgia Paresthetica

ICD-9 CODE 355.1

THE CLINICAL SYNDROME

Meralgia paresthetica is caused by compression of the lateral femoral cutaneous nerve by the inguinal ligament. This entrapment neuropathy presents as pain, numbness, and dysesthesias in the distribution of the lateral femoral cutaneous nerve. These symptoms often begin as a burning pain in the lateral thigh with associated cutaneous sensitivity. Patients suffering from meralgia paresthetica note that sitting, squatting, or wearing wide belts that compress the lateral femoral cutaneous nerve will cause the symptoms of meralgia paresthetica to worsen (Fig. 58–1). Although traumatic lesions to the lateral femoral cutaneous nerve have been implicated in the onset of meralgia paresthetica, in most patients, no obvious antecedent trauma can be identified.

SIGNS AND SYMPTOMS

Physical findings include tenderness over the lateral femoral cutaneous nerve at the origin of the inguinal ligament at the anterior superior iliac spine. A positive Tinel's sign over the lateral femoral cutaneous nerve as it passes beneath the inguinal ligament may be present. Careful sensory examination of the lateral thigh will reveal a sensory deficit in the distribution of the lateral femoral cutaneous nerve. No motor deficit should be present. Sitting or the wearing of tight waistbands or wide belts that compress the lateral femoral cutaneous nerve may exacerbate the symptoms of meralgia paresthetica.

TESTING

Electromyography will help distinguish lumbar radiculopathy and diabetic femoral neuropathy from meralgia paresthetica. Plain radiographs of the back, hip, and pelvis are indicated in all patients who present with meralgia paresthetica to rule out occult bony pathology. Based on the patient's clinical presentation, additional testing, including complete blood count, uric acid, sedimentation rate, and antinuclear antibody testing, may be indicated. Magnetic resonance imaging of the back is indicated if herniated disc, spinal stenosis, or a space-occupying lesion is suspected. The injection technique described here will serve as both a diagnostic and therapeutic maneuver.

DIFFERENTIAL DIAGNOSIS

Meralgia paresthetica is often misdiagnosed as lumbar radiculopathy or trochanteric bursitis or is attributed to primary hip pathology. Radiographs of the hip and electromyography will help distinguish meralgia paresthetica from radiculopathy or pain emanating from the hip. Most patients suffering from a lumbar radiculopathy will have back pain associated with reflex, motor, and sensory changes, whereas patients with meralgia paresthetica will have no back pain and no motor or reflex changes. The sensory changes of meralgia paresthetica will be limited to the distribution of the lateral femoral cutaneous nerve and should not extend below the knee. It should be remembered that lumbar radiculopathy and lateral femoral cutaneous nerve entrapment may coexist as the "double crush" syndrome. Occasionally, diabetic femoral neuropathy may produce anterior thigh pain, which may confuse the diagnosis.

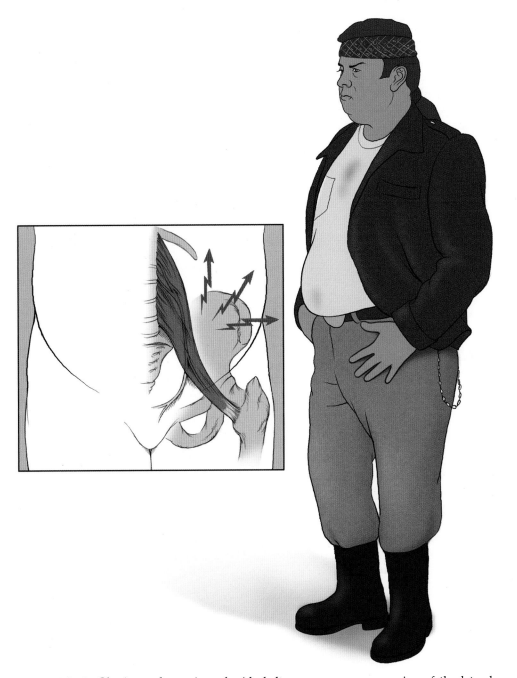

Figure 58–1. Obesity and wearing of wide belts may cause compression of the lateral femoral cutaneous nerve and cause meralgia paresthetica.

TREATMENT

The patient suffering from meralgia paresthetica should be instructed in avoidance techniques to help reduce the unpleasant symptoms and pain associated with this entrapment neuropathy. A short course of conservative therapy consisting of simple analgesics, nonsteroidal anti-inflammatory drugs, or cyclooxygenase-2 inhibitors is a reasonable first step in the treatment of patients suffering from meralgia paresthetica. If the patient does not experience rapid improvement, the following injection technique is a reasonable next step.

To treat the pain of meralgia paresthetica, the patient is placed in the supine position with a pillow under the knees if lying with the legs extended increases the patient's pain due to traction on the nerve. The anterior superior iliac spine is identified by palpation. A point 1 inch medial to the anterior superior iliac spine and just inferior to the inguinal ligament is then identified and prepped with antiseptic solution (Fig. 58–2). A 1½-inch 25-gauge needle is then advanced perpendicular to the skin slowly until the needle is felt to pop through the fascia. A paresthesia is often elicited. After careful aspiration, 5 to 7 mL of 1.0% preservative-free lidocaine and 40 mg methylprednisolone are injected in a fanlike pattern as the needle pierces the fascia of the external oblique muscle. Care must be taken to not place the needle deep enough to enter the peritoneal cavity and perforate the abdominal viscera. After injection of the solution, pressure is applied to the injection site to decrease the incidence of postblock ecchymosis and hematoma formation, which can be quite dramatic, especially in the anticoagulated patient.

COMPLICATIONS AND PITFALLS

Care must be taken to rule out other conditions that may mimic the pain of meralgia paresthetica. The main side effect of the described nerve block is post-block ecchymosis and hematoma. If needle placement is too deep and it enters the peritoneal cavity, perforation of the colon may result in the formation of an intra-abdominal abscess and a fistula. Early detection of infection is crucial to avoid potentially life-threatening sequelae. If the needle is placed too medial, blockade of the femoral nerve may occur and make ambulation difficult.

CLINICAL PEARLS

Meralgia paresthetica is a common pain complaint encountered in clinical practice. It is often misdiagnosed as lumbar radiculopathy. The described nerve block is a simple technique that can produce dramatic relief for patients suffering from meralgia paresthetica.

If a patient presents with pain suggestive of lateral femoral cutaneous neuralgia and does not respond to lateral femoral cutaneous nerve blocks, a diagnosis of lesions more proximal in the lumbar plexus or an L2-3 radiculopathy should be considered. Such patients will often respond to epidural steroid blocks. Electromyography and magnetic resonance imaging of the lumbar plexus are indicated in this patient population to help rule out other causes of lateral femoral cutaneous pain, including malignancy invading the lumbar plexus or epidural or vertebral metastatic disease at L2-3.

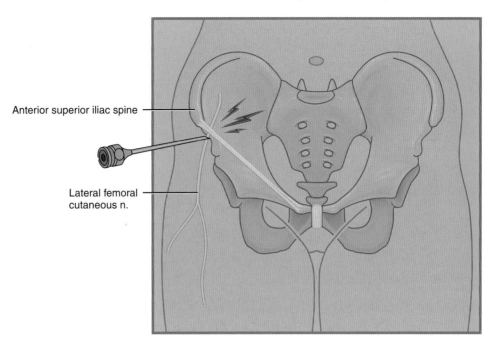

Anterior superior iliac spine

Lateral femoral
cutaneous n.

Figure 58–2. Correct needle placement for injection of the lateral femoral cutaneous nerve to treat meralgia paresthetica. (From Waldman SD: Atlas of Pain Management Injection Techniques. Philadelphia, WB Saunders, 2000, p 241.)

59 Phantom Limb Pain

ICD-9 CODE 053.19

THE CLINICAL SYNDROME

Almost all patients who undergo amputation experience the sensation that the absent body part is still present. This sensation is often painful and quite distressing to the patient. The genesis of this phenomenon is not fully understood, but it is thought to be mediated in large part at the spinal cord level. Congenitally absent limbs do not seem to be subject to the same phenomenon. Patients with phantom limb pain will often describe the limb in vivid detail, albeit with the limb distorted or in abnormal position. In many patients, the sensation of a phantom limb will fade with time, but in some, phantom pain remains a distressing part of their daily life. The pain of phantom limb pain is often described as a constant unpleasant, dysesthetic pain that may be exacerbated by movement or stimulation of the affected cutaneous regions. There may be sharp, shooting neuritic pain superimposed on the constant dysesthetic symptoms. Some patients suffering from phantom limb pain will also note a burning component reminiscent of reflex sympathetic dystrophy. Some investigators report that severe limb pain before amputation increases the incidence of phantom limb pain, but other investigators have failed to prove this correlation.

SIGNS AND SYMPTOMS

The phantom limb pain may take multiple forms. It most often takes the form of dysesthetic pain. Additionally, the patient with phantom limb pain may experience abnormal kinesthetic sensation (i.e., the limb is in an abnormal position). The patient may also experience abnormal kinetic sensation (i.e., feeling that the phantom limb is moving). It has been re-

ported that many patients with phantom limb pain experience a telescoping phenomenon, in which the proximal part of the absent limb is missing (Fig. 59-1). When this occurs, that patient may report that the phantom foot feels like it is attached directly to the proximal thigh. Phantom limb pain may fade over time, with younger patients more likely to experience a diminution of phantom limb symptomatology. Due to the unusual nature of phantom limb sensation and pain, a behavioral component to the pain is invariably present.

TESTING

In most instances, the diagnosis of phantom limb pain roots is easily made on clinical grounds. Testing is generally used to identify other treatable coexisting diseases, such as radiculopathy. Such testing should include basic screening laboratory testing, examination of the stump for neuroma, tumor, or occult infection, and plain radiographs and radionucleotide bone scanning if fracture or osteomyelitis is suspected.

DIFFERENTIAL DIAGNOSIS

Careful initial evaluation, including a thorough history and physical examination, is indicated in all patients suffering from phantom limb pain if the possibility of infection or fracture is present. If the amputation was necessitated due to malignancy, the possibility of occult tumor remains ever present. Other causes of pain in the distribution of the innervation of the affected limb, including radiculopathy and peripheral neuropathy, should be considered.

TREATMENT

The first step for all clinicians caring for patients with phantom limb pain is to reassure the patient

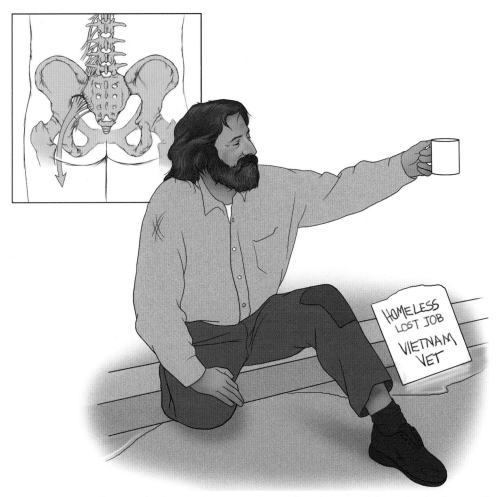

Figure 59–1. Phantom limb pain is present in varying degrees of intensity in almost all patients who undergo amputation of a body part.

that phantom sensations and/or pain after the loss of a limb is normal and that these sensations are real, not imagined. This alone will often reduce the anxiety and suffering of the patient. It is the consensus of most pain specialists that the earlier in the natural course of a painful disease that may lead to amputation, such as peripheral vascular insufficiency, that treatment is initiated, the less likely it is that the patient will develop phantom limb pain. In fact, many pain specialists recommend preemptive analgesia if the viability of a limb is in doubt before surgical amputation whenever possible. The following treatments have been shown to be useful in the palliation of phantom limb pain.

Adjuvant Analgesics

The anticonvulsant *gabapentin* represents a first-line treatment in the palliation of phantom limb pain. Treatment with gabapentin should begin early in the course of the disease, and this drug may be used concurrently with neural blockade, opioid analgesics, and other adjuvant analgesics, including the antidepressant compounds, if care is taken to avoid central nervous system side effects. Gabapentin is started at a bedtime dose of 300 mg and is titrated upward in 300-mg increments to a maximum dose of 3600 mg given in divided doses as side effects allow.

Carbamazepine should be considered in patients suffering from severe neuritic pain who have not responded to nerve blocks and gabapentin. If this drug is used, rigid monitoring for hematologic parameters is indicated, especially in patients receiving chemotherapy or radiation therapy. *Phenytoin* may also be beneficial in the treatment of neuritic pain but should not be used in patients with lymphoma because the drug may induce a pseudolymphoma-like state that is difficult to distinguish from the actual lymphoma itself.

Antidepressants

Antidepressant compounds may also be useful adjuncts in the initial treatment of the patient suffering from phantom limb pain. On an acute basis, these drugs will help alleviate the significant sleep disturbance that is commonly seen in this setting. In addition, the antidepressants may be valuable in helping ameliorate the neuritic component of the pain, which is treated less effectively with narcotic analgesics. After several weeks of treatment, the antidepressants may exert a mood-elevating effect that may be desirable in some patients. Care must be taken to observe closely for central nervous system side effects in this

patient population. These drugs may cause urinary retention and constipation.

Nerve Blocks

Sympathetic neural blockade with local anesthetic and steroid via either epidural nerve block or blockade of the sympathetic nerves subserving the painful area appears to be a reasonable next step if the aforementioned pharmacologic modalities fail to control the pain of phantom limb pain. The exact mechanism of pain relief from neural blockade in the treatment of phantom limb pain is unknown, but it may be related to modulation of pain transmission at the spinal cord level. In general, neurodestructive procedures have a very low success rate and should be used only after all other treatments have been optimized, if at all.

Opioid Analgesics

Opioid analgesics have a limited role in the management of phantom limb pain, and in the experience of this author, they frequently do more harm than good. Careful administration of potent, long-acting narcotic analgesics (e.g., oral morphine elixir or methadone) on a time-contingent rather than PRN basis may represent a beneficial adjunct to the pain relief provided by sympathetic neural blockade. Because many patients suffering from phantom limb pain are elderly or have severe multisystem disease, close monitoring for the potential side effects of potent narcotic analgesics (e.g., confusion or dizziness, which may cause a patient to fall) is warranted. Daily dietary fiber supplementation and use of milk of magnesia should be started along with opioid analgesics to prevent the side effect of constipation.

Adjunctive Treatments

The application of ice packs to the area affected with phantom limb pain may provide relief in some patients. The application of heat will increase pain in most patients, presumably because of increased conduction of small fibers, but it is beneficial in an occasional patient and may be worth trying if the application of cold is ineffective. Transcutaneous electrical nerve stimulation and vibration may also be effective in a limited number of patients. The favorable risk-to-benefit ratio of all these modalities makes them reasonable alternatives for patients who cannot or will not undergo sympathetic neural blockade or tolerate pharmacologic interventions. The topical application of capsaicin may be beneficial in some patients suffering from phantom limb pain. However, the burning associated with this drug when applied to the painful area often limits the usefulness of this intervention.

COMPLICATIONS

Although there are no complications specifically associated with phantom limb pain itself, the consequences of the unremitting pain are devastating. Failure to aggressively treat the pain of phantom limb pain and the associated symptoms of sleep disturbance and depression can result in suicide.

CLINICAL PEARLS

Because the pain of phantom limb pain is so devastating, the clinician must endeavor to rapidly and aggressively treat it. If phantom limb pain develops, aggressive treatment as outlined with special attention to the insidious onset of severe depression should be undertaken. If serious depression occurs, hospitalization with suicide precautions is mandatory.

60 Trochanteric Bursitis

ICD-9 CODE 726.5

THE CLINICAL SYNDROME

Trochanteric bursitis is a commonly encountered pain complaint in clinical practice. The patient suffering from trochanteric bursitis will frequently complain of pain in the lateral hip that can radiate down the leg, mimicking sciatica. The pain is localized to the area over the trochanter. Often, the patient will be unable to sleep on the affected hip and may complain of a sharp, catching sensation with range of motion of the hip, especially on first arising (Fig. 60–1). The patient may note that walking upstairs is becoming increasingly more difficult. Trochanteric bursitis often coexists with arthritis of the hip joint, back and sacroiliac joint disease, and gait disturbance.

The trochanteric bursa lies between the greater trochanter and the tendon of the gluteus medius and the iliotibial tract. This bursa may exist as a single bursal sac or, in some patients, as a multisegmented series of sacs that may be loculated in nature. The trochanteric bursa is vulnerable to injury from both acute trauma and repeated microtrauma. Acute injuries frequently take the form of direct trauma to the bursa via falls directly onto the greater trochanter or previous hip surgery as well as from overuse injuries, including running on soft or uneven surfaces. If the inflammation of the trochanteric bursa becomes chronic, calcification of the bursa may occur.

SIGNS AND SYMPTOMS

Physical examination of the patient suffering from trochanteric bursitis will reveal point tenderness in the lateral thigh just over the greater trochanter. Passive adduction and abduction as well as active resisted abduction of the affected lower extremity will reproduce the pain. Sudden release of resistance during this maneuver will markedly increase the pain. There should be no sensory deficit in the distribution of the lateral femoral cutaneous nerve as seen with meralgia paresthetica, which is often confused with trochanteric bursitis.

TESTING

Plain radiographs of the hip may reveal calcification of the bursa and associated structures consistent with chronic inflammation. Magnetic resonance imaging is indicated if occult mass or tumor of the hip or groin is suspected. Complete blood count and erythrocyte sedimentation rate are useful if infection is suspected. Electromyography will help distinguish trochanteric bursitis from meralgia paresthetica and sciatica. The injection technique described here will serve as both a diagnostic and therapeutic maneuver.

DIFFERENTIAL DIAGNOSIS

Trochanteric bursitis frequently coexists with arthritis of the hip, which may require specific treatment to provide palliation of pain and return of function. Occasionally, trochanteric bursitis can be confused with meralgia paresthetica as both present with pain in the lateral thigh. The two syndromes can be distinguished in that patients suffering from meralgia paresthetica will not have pain on palpation over the greater trochanter. Electromyography will help sort out confusing clinical presentations. The clinician must consider the potential for primary or secondary tumors of the hip in the differential diagnosis of trochanteric bursitis.

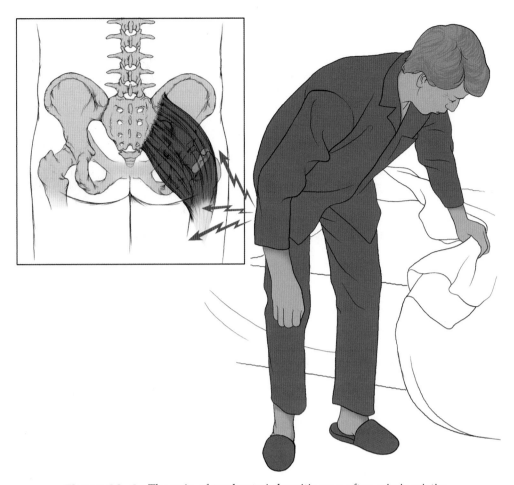

Figure 60-1. The pain of trochanteric bursitis may often mimic sciatica.

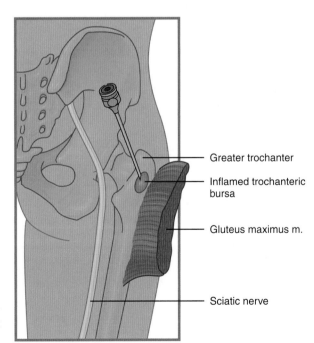

Greater trochanter

Inflamed trochanteric bursa

Gluteus maximus m.

Sciatic nerve

Figure 60-2. Correct needle placement for injection of the tro-chanteric bursa. (From Waldman SD: Atlas of Pain Management Injection Techniques. Philadelphia, WB Saunders, 2000, p 221.)

TREATMENT

A short course of conservative therapy consisting of simple analgesics, nonsteroidal anti-inflammatory drugs or cyclooxygenase-2 inhibitors is a reasonable first step in the treatment of patients suffering from trochanteric bursitis. The patient should be instructed to avoid repetitive activity that may be responsible for the development of trochanteric bursitis, such as running on sand. If the patient does not experience rapid improvement, the following injection technique is a reasonable next step.

Injection of the trochanteric bursa can be carried out by placing the patient in the lateral decubitus position with the affected side up. The midpoint of the greater trochanter is identified. Proper preparation of the skin overlying this point is then carried out with antiseptic solution (Fig. 60–2). A syringe containing 2.0 mL of 0.25% preservative-free bupivacaine and 40 mg methylprednisolone is attached to a 3½-inch 25-gauge needle.

Before needle placement, the patient should be advised to say "there" immediately if he or she feels a paresthesia into the lower extremity, indicating that the needle has impinged on the sciatic nerve. If a paresthesia occurs, the needle should be immediately withdrawn and repositioned more laterally. The needle is then carefully advanced through the previously identified point at a right angle to the skin directly toward the center of the greater trochanter. The needle is advanced very slowly to avoid trauma to the sciatic nerve until it hits the bone. The needle is then withdrawn out of the periosteum, and after careful aspiration for blood and if no paresthesia is present, the contents of the syringe are then gently injected into the bursa. There should be minimal resistance to injection.

COMPLICATIONS AND PITFALLS

Care must be taken to rule out other conditions that may mimic the pain of trochanteric bursitis. The main pitfall of the described nerve block is proximity to the sciatic nerve, which makes it imperative that this procedure be carried out only by those well versed in the regional anatomy and experienced in performing injection techniques. Many patients will also complain of a transient increase in pain after injection of the bursa. Infection, although rare, can occur, and careful attention to sterile technique is mandatory.

CLINICAL PEARLS

Trochanteric bursitis frequently coexists with arthritis of the hip, which may require specific treatment to provide palliation of pain and return of function. This injection technique is extremely effective in the treatment of trochanteric bursitis. This technique is a safe procedure if careful attention is paid to the clinically relevant anatomy in the areas to be injected. Most side effects of this injection technique are related to needle-induced trauma to the injection site and underlying tissues. Special care must be taken to avoid trauma to the sciatic nerve.

The use of physical modalities including local heat as well as gentle stretching exercises should be introduced several days after the patient undergoes this injection technique. Vigorous exercises should be avoided as they will exacerbate the patient's symptomatology. Simple analgesics, nonsteroidal anti-inflammatory drugs, and antimyotonic agents may be used concurrently with this injection technique.

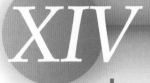

XIV Knee Pain Syndromes

61 Arthritis Pain of the Knee

ICD-9 CODE 715.96

THE CLINICAL SYNDROME

Arthritis of the knee is a painful condition commonly encountered in clinical practice. The knee joint is susceptible to the development of arthritis from a variety of conditions that have in common the ability to damage the joint cartilage. Osteoarthritis of the joint is the most common form of arthritis that results in knee joint pain. However, rheumatoid arthritis and post-traumatic arthritis are also common causes of knee pain secondary to arthritis. Less common causes of arthritis-induced knee pain include the collagen vascular diseases, infection, villonodular synovitis, and Lyme disease. Acute infectious arthritis will usually be accompanied by significant systemic symptoms, including fever and malaise, and should be easily recognized by the astute clinician and treated appropriately with culture and antibiotics, rather than with injection therapy. The collagen vascular diseases will generally present as a polyarthropathy rather than as a monoarthropathy limited to the knee joint, although knee pain secondary to collagen vascular disease responds exceedingly well to the treatment modalities described here.

SIGNS AND SYMPTOMS

The majority of patients presenting with knee pain secondary to osteoarthritis and post-traumatic arthritis pain will present with the complaint of pain that is localized around the knee and distal femur. Activity makes the pain worse, with rest and heat providing some relief. The pain is constant and characterized as aching in nature. The pain may interfere with sleep. Some patients will complain of a grating or popping sensation with use of the joint, and crepitus may be present on the physical examination.

In addition to the described pain, patients suffering from arthritis of the knee joint will often experience a gradual decrease in functional ability with decreasing knee range of motion, making simple everyday tasks such as walking, climbing stairs, and getting in and out of cars quite difficult (Fig. 61–1). With continued disuse, muscle wasting may occur, and a "frozen knee" due to adhesive capsulitis may develop.

TESTING

Plain radiographs are indicated for all patients who present with knee pain. Based on the patient's clinical presentation, additional testing, including complete blood count, sedimentation rate, and antinuclear antibody testing, may be indicated. Magnetic resonance imaging of the knee is indicated if aseptic necrosis or occult mass or tumor is suspected.

DIFFERENTIAL DIAGNOSIS

Lumbar radiculopathy may mimic the pain and disability associated with arthritis of the knee. In such patients, the knee examination should be negative. Entrapment neuropathies such as meralgia paresthetica may also confuse the diagnosis, as may bursitis of the knee; both of these conditions may coexist with arthritis of the knee. Primary and metastatic tumors of the femur and spine may also present in a manner analogous to arthritis of the knee.

TREATMENT

Initial treatment of the pain and functional disability associated with arthritis of the knee should include a combination of the nonsteroidal anti-inflammatory drugs or cyclooxygenase-2 inhibitors and

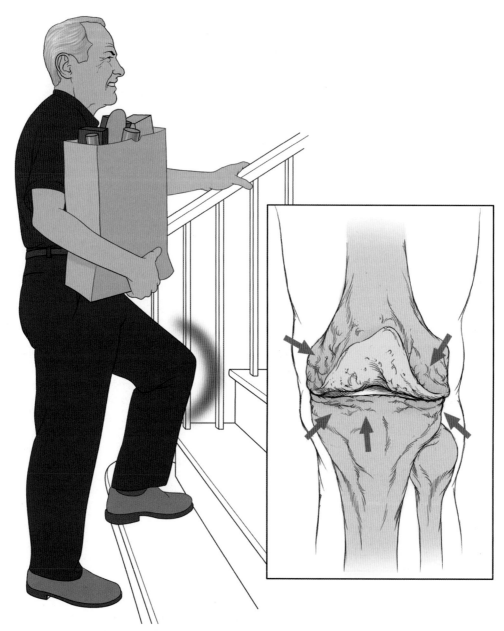

Figure 61–1. The pain of arthritis of the knee is made worse with weight-bearing activities.

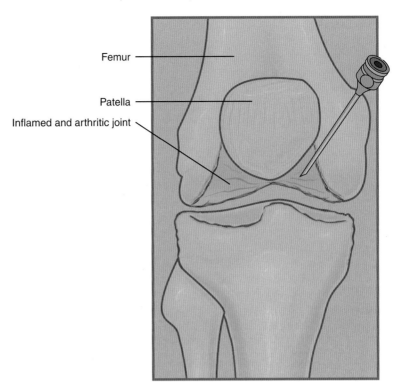

Femur

Patella

Inflamed and arthritic joint

Figure 61-2. Proper needle placement for intra-articular injection of the knee. (From Waldman SD: Atlas of Pain Management Injection Techniques. Philadelphia, WB Saunders, 2000, p 251.)

physical therapy. The local application of heat and cold may also be beneficial. For patients who do not respond to these treatment modalities, an intra-articular injection of local anesthetic and steroid may be a reasonable next step.

For intra-articular injection of the knee, the patient is placed in the supine position with a rolled blanket underneath the knee to gently flex the joint. The skin overlying the medial joint is prepped with antiseptic solution. A sterile syringe containing 5.0 mL of 0.25% preservative-free bupivacaine and 40 mg methylprednisolone is attached to a 1½-inch 25-gauge needle using strict aseptic technique. With strict aseptic technique, the joint space is identified. The clinician places his or her thumb on the lateral margin of the patella and pushes it medially. At a point at the middle of the medial edge of the patella, the needle is inserted between the patella and femoral condyles. The needle is then carefully advanced through the skin and subcutaneous tissues through the joint capsule into the joint (Fig. 61–2). If bone is encountered, the needle is withdrawn into the subcutaneous tissues and redirected superiorly. After the joint space is entered, the contents of the syringe are gently injected. There should be little resistance to injection. If resistance is encountered, the needle is probably in a ligament or tendon and should be advanced slightly into the joint space until the injection proceeds without significant resistance. The needle is then removed, and a sterile pressure dressing and ice pack are placed at the injection site.

SIDE EFFECTS AND COMPLICATIONS

Failure to identify primary or metastatic tumor of the knee or spine that is responsible for the patient's pain may yield disastrous results. The major complication of intra-articular injection of the knee is infection. This complication should be exceedingly rare if strict aseptic technique is followed. Approximately 25% of patients will complain of a transient increase in pain after intra-articular injection of the knee joint and should be warned of such.

CLINICAL PEARLS

Coexistent bursitis and tendinitis may also contribute to knee pain and may require additional treatment with more localized injection of local anesthetic and methylprednisolone acetate. The described injection technique is extremely effective in the treatment of pain secondary to the aforementioned causes of arthritis of the knee joint. This technique is a safe procedure if careful attention is paid to the clinically relevant anatomy in the areas to be injected. Care must be taken to use sterile technique to avoid infection as well as the use of universal precautions to avoid risk to the operator. The incidence of ecchymosis and hematoma formation can be decreased if pressure is placed on the injection site immediately after the injection. The use of physical modalities including local heat as well as gentle range of motion exercises should be introduced several days after the patient undergoes this injection technique for knee pain. Vigorous exercises should be avoided as they will exacerbate the patient's symptomatology.

62

Medial Collateral Ligament Syndrome

ICD-9 CODE 717.82

THE CLINICAL SYNDROME

Patients with medial collateral ligament syndrome will present with pain over the medial joint and increased pain on passive valgus and external rotation of the knee. Activity, especially involving flexion and external rotation of the knee, will make the pain worse, with rest and heat providing some relief. The pain is constant and characterized as aching in nature. The patient with injury to the medial collateral ligament may complain of locking or popping with flexion of the affected knee. The pain may interfere with sleep. Coexistent bursitis, tendinitis, arthritis, and/or internal derangement of the knee may confuse the clinical picture after trauma to the knee joint.

The medial collateral ligament syndrome is characterized by pain at the medial aspect of the knee joint. It is usually the result of trauma to the medial collateral ligament from falls with the leg in valgus and externally rotated, typically during snow skiing accidents or football clipping injuries (Fig. 62–1). The medial collateral ligament is a broad, flat bandlike ligament that runs from the medial condyle of the femur to the medial aspect of the shaft of the tibia, where it attaches just above the groove where the semimembranous muscle attaches. It also attaches to the edge of the medial semilunar cartilage. The ligament is susceptible to strain at the joint line or avulsion at its origin or insertion.

SIGNS AND SYMPTOMS

Patients with injury of the medial collateral ligament will exhibit tenderness along the course of the ligament from the medial femoral condyle to its tibial insertion. If the ligament is avulsed from its bony insertions, tenderness may be localized to the proximal or distal ligaments, whereas patients suffering from strain of the ligament will exhibit more diffuse tenderness. Patients with severe injury to the ligament may exhibit laxity of the joint when valgus and varus stress are placed on the affected knee. Because pain may produce muscle guarding, magnetic resonance imaging (MRI) of the knee may be necessary to confirm the clinician's clinical impression. Joint effusion and swelling may be present with injury to the medial collateral ligament but also are suggestive of intra-articular damage. Again, MRI will help confirm the diagnosis.

TESTING

Plain radiographs are indicated for all patients who present with medial collateral ligament syndrome pain. Based on the patient's clinical presentation, additional testing, including complete blood count, sedimentation rate, and antinuclear antibody testing, may be indicated. MRI of the knee is indicated if internal derangement or occult mass or tumor is suspected. Bone scan may be useful to identify occult stress fractures involving the joint, especially if trauma has occurred.

TREATMENT

Initial treatment of the pain and functional disability associated with injury to the medial collateral ligament should include a combination of the nonsteroidal anti-inflammatory drugs or cyclooxygenase-2 inhibitors and physical therapy. The local application of heat and cold may also be beneficial. Any repetitive activity that may exacerbate the patient's symptomatology should be avoided. For patients who do not respond to these treatment modalities and do not have a lesion that will require surgical repair, the following injection technique may be a reasonable next step.

Injection of the medial collateral ligament is carried out by placing the patient in the supine position with a rolled blanket underneath the knee to gently flex the joint. The skin overlying the lateral aspect of the knee joint is prepped with antiseptic solution. A sterile syringe containing 2.0 mL of 0.25% preservative-free bupivacaine and 40 mg methylprednisolone is attached to a 1½-inch 25-gauge needle using strict aseptic technique. With strict aseptic technique, the most tender portion of the ligament is identified. At this point, the needle is inserted at a 45-degree angle to the skin. The needle is then carefully advanced through the skin and subcutaneous tissues into proximity with the medial collateral ligament. If bone is encountered, the needle is withdrawn into the subcutaneous tissues and redirected superiorly. The contents of the syringe are then gently injected. There should be little resistance to injection. If resistance is encountered, the needle is probably in a ligament or tendon and should be advanced or withdrawn slightly until the injection proceeds without significant resistance. The needle is then removed, and a sterile pressure dressing and ice pack are placed at the injection site.

SIDE EFFECTS AND COMPLICATIONS

MRI should be carried out on all patients with injury to the medial collateral ligament who fail to respond to conservative therapy or who exhibit joint instability on clinical examination. The major complication of the described injection technique is infection. This complication should be exceedingly rare if strict aseptic technique is followed. Approximately 25% of patients will complain of a transient increase in pain after injection of the medial collateral ligament of the knee and should be warned of such.

CLINICAL PEARLS

Patients with injury to the medial collateral ligament are best examined with the knee in the slightly flexed position. The clinician may want to examine the non-painful knee first to reduce the patient's anxiety and to ascertain what the normal examination is like. The described injection technique is extremely effective in the treatment of pain secondary to the aforementioned causes of medial collateral ligament syndrome. Coexistent bursitis, tendinitis, arthritis, and internal derangement of the knee may also contribute to the patient's pain and may require additional treatment with more localized injection of local anesthetic and methylprednisolone acetate.

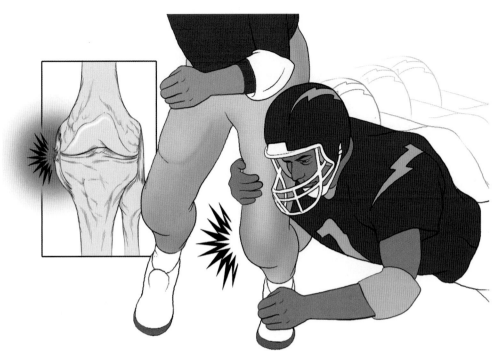

Figure 62–1. Medial collateral ligament syndrome is characterized by medial joint pain that is made worse with flexion or external rotation of the knee.

63 *Suprapatellar Bursitis*

ICD-9 CODE 726.69

THE CLINICAL SYNDROME

The suprapatellar bursa is vulnerable to injury from both acute trauma and repeated microtrauma. The suprapatellar bursa extends superiorly from beneath the patella under the quadriceps femoris muscle. This bursa may exist as a single bursal sac or, in some patients, as a multisegmented series of sacs that may be loculated in nature. Acute injuries frequently take the form of direct trauma to the bursa via falls directly onto the knee or from patellar fractures, as well as from overuse injuries, including running on soft or uneven surfaces, or from jobs that require crawling on the knees, such as carpet laying. If the inflammation of the suprapatellar bursa becomes chronic, calcification of the bursa may occur.

The patient suffering from suprapatellar bursitis will frequently complain of pain in the anterior knee above the patella that can radiate superiorly into the distal anterior thigh. Often, the patient will be unable to kneel or walk down stairs (Fig. 63–1). The patient may also complain of a sharp, catching sensation with range of motion of the knee, especially on first arising. Suprapatellar bursitis often coexists with arthritis and tendinitis of the knee joint, and these other pathological processes may confuse the clinical picture.

SIGNS AND SYMPTOMS

Physical examination may reveal point tenderness in the anterior knee just above the patella. Passive flexion as well as active resisted extension of the knee will reproduce the pain. Sudden release of resistance during this maneuver will markedly increase the pain. There may be swelling in the suprapatellar re-

gion with a boggy feeling to palpation. Occasionally, the suprapatellar bursa may become infected with resulting systemic symptoms, including fever and malaise, as well as local symptoms, including rubor, color, and dolor.

TESTING

Plain radiographs of the knee may reveal calcification of the bursa and associated structures including the quadriceps tendon consistent with chronic inflammation. Magnetic resonance imaging is indicated if internal derangement, occult mass, or tumor of the knee is suspected. Electromyography will help distinguish suprapatellar bursitis from femoral neuropathy, lumbar radiculopathy, and plexopathy. The following injection technique will serve as both a diagnostic and therapeutic maneuver. Complete blood count, automated chemistry profile including uric acid, sedimentation rate, and antinuclear antibody testing are indicated if collagen vascular disease is suspected. If infection is considered, aspiration, Gram stain, and culture of bursal fluid are indicated on an emergency basis.

DIFFERENTIAL DIAGNOSIS

Due to the unique anatomy of the region, not only the suprapatellar bursa but also the associated tendons and other bursae of the knee can become inflamed and confuse the diagnosis. The suprapatellar bursa extends superiorly from beneath the patella under the quadriceps femoris muscle and its tendon. The bursa is held in place by a small portion of the vastus intermedius muscle called the *articularis genus muscle*. Both the quadriceps tendon and the suprapatellar bursa are subject to the development of inflammation after overuse, misuse, or direct trauma. The quadriceps tendon is made up of fibers from the four muscles that compose the quadriceps muscle: the vas-

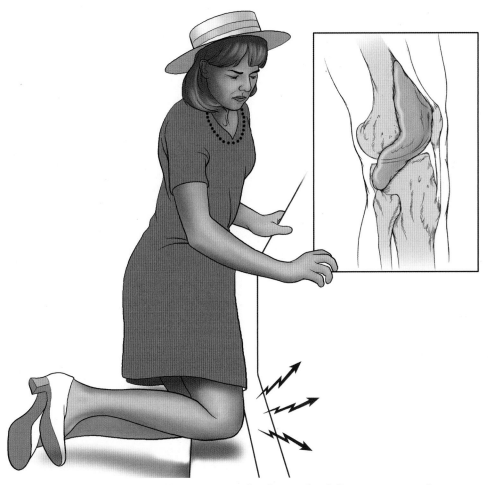

Figure 63–1. Suprapatellar bursitis is usually the result of direct trauma to the suprapatellar bursa from either acute injury or repeated microtrauma.

tus lateralis, the vastus intermedius, the vastus medialis, and the rectus femoris. These muscles are the primary extensors of the lower extremity at the knee. The tendons of these muscles converge and unite to form a single exceedingly strong tendon. The patella functions as a sesamoid bone within the quadriceps tendon, with fibers of the tendon expanding around the patella to form the medial and lateral patella retinacula, which help strengthen the knee joint. These fibers are called *expansions* and are vulnerable to strain, and the tendon proper is subject to the development of tendinitis. The suprapatellar, infrapatellar, and prepatellar bursae may also concurrently become inflamed with dysfunction of the quadriceps tendon. It should be remembered that anything that alters the normal biomechanics of the knee can result in inflammation of the suprapatellar bursa.

TREATMENT

A short course of conservative therapy consisting of simple analgesics, nonsteroidal anti-inflammatory drugs, or cyclooxygenase-2 inhibitors and a knee brace to prevent further trauma is a reasonable first step in the treatment of patients suffering from suprapatellar bursitis. If the patient does not experience rapid improvement, the following injection technique is a reasonable next step. The goals of this injection technique are explained to the patient. The patient is placed in the supine position with a rolled blanket underneath the knee to gently flex the joint. The skin overlying the medial aspect of the knee joint is prepped with antiseptic solution. A sterile syringe containing 2.0 mL of 0.25% preservative-free bupivacaine and 40 mg methylprednisolone is attached to a 1½-inch 25-gauge needle using strict aseptic technique. With strict aseptic technique, the superior margin of the medial patella is identified. Just above this point, the needle is inserted horizontally to slide just beneath the quadriceps tendon. If the needle strikes the femur, it is then withdrawn slightly and redirected in a more anterior trajectory. When the needle

is in position just below the quadriceps tendon, the contents of the syringe are then gently injected. There should be little resistance to injection. If resistance is encountered, the needle is probably in a ligament or tendon and should be advanced or withdrawn slightly until the injection proceeds without significant resistance. The needle is then removed, and a sterile pressure dressing and ice pack are placed at the injection site.

COMPLICATIONS AND PITFALLS

Failure to identify primary or metastatic tumor of the distal femur or joint that is responsible for the patient's pain may yield disastrous results. The major complication of this injection technique is infection. This complication should be exceedingly rare if strict aseptic technique is followed. Approximately 25% of patients will complain of a transient increase in pain after injection of the suprapatellar bursa of the knee and should be warned of such.

CLINICAL PEARLS

Coexistent bursitis, tendinitis, arthritis, and internal derangement of the knee may also contribute to the patient's pain and may require additional treatment with more localized injection of local anesthetic and methylprednisolone acetate. The described injection technique is extremely effective in the treatment of pain secondary to suprapatellar bursitis. This technique is a safe procedure if careful attention is paid to the clinically relevant anatomy in the areas to be injected. The use of physical modalities including local heat as well as gentle range of motion exercises should be introduced several days after the patient undergoes this injection technique for suprapatellar bursitis pain. Vigorous exercises should be avoided as they will exacerbate the patient's symptomatology. Simple analgesics and nonsteroidal anti-inflammatory drugs may be used concurrently with this injection technique.

64

Prepatellar Bursitis

ICD-9 CODE 726.65

THE CLINICAL SYNDROME

The prepatellar bursa is vulnerable to injury from both acute trauma and repeated microtrauma. The prepatellar bursa lies between the subcutaneous tissues and the patella. This bursa may exist as a single bursal sac or, in some patients, as a multisegmented series of sacs that may be loculated in nature. Acute injuries frequently take the form of direct trauma to the bursa via falls directly onto the knee or from patellar fractures, as well as from overuse injuries, including running on soft or uneven surfaces. Prepatellar bursitis may also result from jobs that require crawling or kneeling on the knees, such as carpet laying or scrubbing floors, hence the other name for prepatellar bursitis: housemaid's knee (Fig. 64–1). If the inflammation of the prepatellar bursa becomes chronic, calcification of the bursa may occur.

SIGNS AND SYMPTOMS

The patient suffering from prepatellar bursitis will frequently complain of pain and swelling in the anterior knee over the patella that can radiate superiorly and inferiorly into the area surrounding the knee. Often, the patient will be unable to kneel or to walk down stairs. The patient may also complain of a sharp, catching sensation with range of motion of the knee, especially on first arising. Prepatellar bursitis often coexists with arthritis and tendinitis of the knee joint and these other pathological processes may confuse the clinical picture.

TESTING

Plain radiographs of the knee may reveal calcification of the bursa and associated structures, including the quadriceps tendon, consistent with chronic inflammation. Magnetic resonance imaging is indicated if internal derangement, occult mass, or tumor of the knee is suspected. Electromyography will help distinguish prepatellar bursitis from femoral neuropathy, lumbar radiculopathy, and plexopathy. The following injection technique will serve as a diagnostic and therapeutic maneuver. Antinuclear antibody testing is indicated if collagen vascular disease is suspected. If infection is considered, aspiration, Gram stain, and culture of bursal fluid are indicated on an emergency basis.

DIFFERENTIAL DIAGNOSIS

Due to the unique anatomy of the region, not only the prepatellar bursa but also the associated tendons and other bursae of the knee can become inflamed and confuse the diagnosis. The prepatellar bursa lies between the subcutaneous tissues and the patella. The bursa is held in place by ligamentum patellae. Both the quadriceps tendon and the prepatellar bursa are subject to the development of inflammation after overuse, misuse, or direct trauma. The quadriceps tendon is made up of fibers from the four muscles that compose the quadriceps muscle: the vastus lateralis, the vastus intermedius, the vastus medialis, and the rectus femoris. These muscles are the primary extensors of the lower extremity at the knee. The tendons of these muscles converge and unite to form a single, exceedingly strong tendon. The patella functions as a sesamoid bone within the quadriceps tendon, with fibers of the tendon expanding around the patella to form the medial and lateral patella retinacula, which help strengthen the knee joint. These fibers are called *expansions* and are vulnerable to strain, and the tendon proper is subject to the development of tendinitis. The suprapatellar, infrapatellar, and prepatellar bursae may also concurrently become inflamed with dysfunction of the quadriceps tendon. It should be remembered that anything that alters the normal biomechanics of the knee can result in inflammation of the prepatellar bursa.

TREATMENT

A short course of conservative therapy consisting of simple analgesics, nonsteroidal anti-inflammatory drugs, or cyclooxygenase-2 inhibitors and a knee brace to prevent further trauma is a reasonable first step in the treatment of patients suffering from prepatellar bursitis. If the patient does not experience rapid improvement, the following injection technique is a reasonable next step. The patient is placed in the supine position with a rolled blanket underneath the knee to gently flex the joint. The skin overlying the patella is prepped with antiseptic solution. A sterile syringe containing 2.0 mL of 0.25% preservative-free bupivacaine and 40 mg methylprednisolone is attached to a 1½-inch 25-gauge needle using strict aseptic technique. With strict aseptic technique, the center of the medial patella is identified (Fig. 64–2). Just above this point, the needle is inserted horizontally to slide subcutaneously into the prepatellar bursa. If the needle strikes the patella, it is then withdrawn slightly and redirected in a more anterior trajectory. When the needle is in position in proximity to the prepatellar bursa, the contents of the syringe are then gently injected. There should be little resistance to injection. If resistance is encountered, the needle is probably in a ligament or tendon and should be advanced or withdrawn slightly until the injection proceeds without significant resistance. The needle is then removed, and a sterile pressure dressing and ice pack are placed at the injection site.

COMPLICATIONS AND PITFALLS

Failure to identify primary or metastatic tumor of the distal femur or joint that is responsible for the patient's pain may yield disastrous results. The major complication of this injection technique is infection. This complication should be exceedingly rare if strict aseptic technique is followed. Approximately 25% of patients will complain of a transient increase in pain after injection of the suprapatellar bursa of the knee and should be warned of such.

CLINICAL PEARLS

Coexistent bursitis, tendinitis, arthritis, and internal derangement of the knee may also contribute to the patient's pain and may require additional treatment with more localized injection of local anesthetic and methylprednisolone acetate. This injection technique is extremely effective in the treatment of pain secondary to prepatellar bursitis. This technique is a safe procedure if careful attention is paid to the clinically relevant anatomy in the areas to be injected. The use of physical modalities including local heat as well as gentle range of motion exercises should be introduced several days after the patient undergoes this injection technique for prepatellar bursitis pain. Vigorous exercises should be avoided as they will exacerbate the patient's symptomatology. Simple analgesics and nonsteroidal anti-inflammatory drugs may be used concurrently with this injection technique.

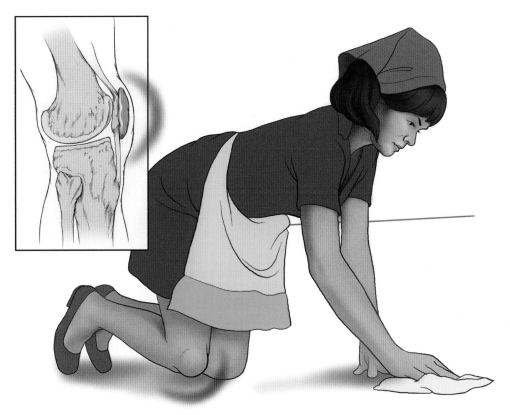

Figure 64–1. Prepatellar bursitis is also known as housemaid's knee because of its prevalence in people whose work requires prolonged crawling or kneeling.

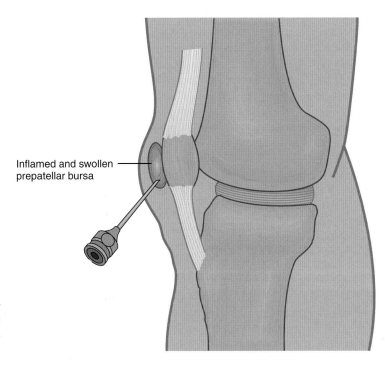

Inflamed and swollen prepatellar bursa

Figure 64–2. Correct needle placement for injection of the prepatellar bursa. (From Waldman SD: Atlas of Pain Management Injection Techniques. Philadelphia, WB Saunders, 2000, p 272.)

65

Superficial Infrapatellar Bursitis

ICD-9 CODE 726.69

THE CLINICAL SYNDROME

The superficial infrapatellar bursa is vulnerable to injury from both acute trauma and repeated microtrauma. The superficial infrapatellar bursa lies between the subcutaneous tissues and the upper part of the ligamentum patellae. The deep infrapatellar bursa lies between the ligamentum patellae and the tibia. These bursae may exist as single bursal sacs or, in some patients, as a multisegmented series of sacs that may be loculated in nature. Acute injuries frequently take the form of direct trauma to the bursa via falls directly onto the knee or from patellar fractures, as well as from overuse injuries, including running on soft or uneven surfaces. Superficial infrapatellar bursitis may also result from jobs that require crawling or kneeling on the knees, such as carpet laying or scrubbing floors (Fig. 65–1). If the inflammation of the superficial infrapatellar bursa becomes chronic, calcification of the bursa may occur.

SIGNS AND SYMPTOMS

The patient suffering from superficial infrapatellar bursitis will frequently complain of pain and swelling in the anterior knee over the patella that can radiate superiorly and inferiorly into the area surrounding the knee. Often, the patient will be unable to kneel or to walk down stairs. The patient may also complain of a sharp, catching sensation with range of motion of the knee, especially on first arising. Superficial infrapatellar bursitis often coexists with arthritis and tendinitis of the knee joint, and these other pathological processes may confuse the clinical picture.

TESTING

Plain radiographs of the knee may reveal calcification of the bursa and associated structures, including the quadriceps tendon, consistent with chronic inflammation. Magnetic resonance imaging is indicated if internal derangement, occult mass, or tumor of the knee is suspected. Electromyography will help distinguish superficial infrapatellar bursitis from femoral neuropathy, lumbar radiculopathy, and plexopathy. The following injection technique will serve as a diagnostic and therapeutic maneuver. Antinuclear antibody testing is indicated if collagen vascular disease is suspected. If infection is considered, aspiration, Gram stain, and culture of bursal fluid are indicated on an emergency basis.

DIFFERENTIAL DIAGNOSIS

Due to the unique anatomy of the region, not only the superficial infrapatellar bursa but also the associated tendons and other bursae of the knee can become inflamed and confuse the diagnosis. Both the quadriceps tendon and the superficial infrapatellar bursa are subject to the development of inflammation after overuse, misuse, or direct trauma. The quadriceps tendon is made up of fibers from the four muscles that compose the quadriceps muscle: the vastus lateralis, the vastus intermedius, the vastus medialis, and the rectus femoris. These muscles are the primary extensors of the lower extremity at the knee. The tendons of these muscles converge and unite to form a single, exceedingly strong tendon. The patella functions as a sesamoid bone within the quadriceps tendon, with fibers of the tendon expanding around the patella to form the medial and lateral patella retinacula, which help strengthen the knee joint. These fibers are called *expansions,* and are vulnerable to strain, and the tendon proper is subject to the development

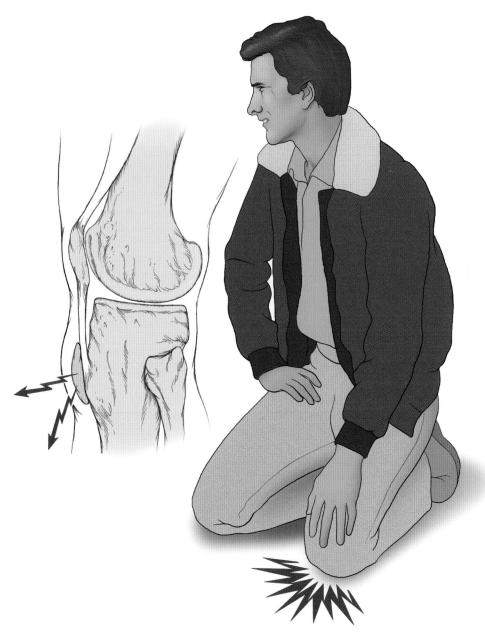

Figure 65–1. Infrapatellar bursitis is a common cause of inferior knee pain.

of tendinitis. The suprapatellar, infrapatellar, and superficial infrapatellar bursae may also concurrently become inflamed with dysfunction of the quadriceps tendon. It should be remembered that anything that alters the normal biomechanics of the knee can result in inflammation of the superficial infrapatellar bursa.

TREATMENT

A short course of conservative therapy consisting of simple analgesics, nonsteroidal anti-inflammatory drugs, or cyclooxygenase-2 inhibitors and a knee brace to prevent further trauma is a reasonable first step in the treatment of patients suffering from superficial infrapatellar bursitis. If the patient does not experience rapid improvement, the following injection technique is a reasonable next step.

To inject the superficial infrapatellar bursa, the patient is placed in the supine position with a rolled blanket underneath the knee to gently flex the joint. The skin overlying the patella is prepped with antiseptic solution. A sterile syringe containing 2.0 mL of 0.25% preservative-free bupivacaine and 40 mg methylprednisolone is attached to a 1½-inch 25-gauge needle using strict aseptic technique. With strict aseptic technique, the center of the lower pole of the patella is identified. Just below this point, the needle is inserted at a 45-degree angle to slide subcutaneously into the superficial infrapatellar bursa. If the needle strikes the patella, it is then withdrawn slightly and redirected in a more inferior trajectory. When the needle is in position in proximity to the superficial infrapatellar bursa, the contents of the syringe are then gently injected. There should be little resistance to injection. If resistance is encountered, the needle is probably in a ligament or tendon and should be advanced or withdrawn slightly until the injection proceeds without significant resistance. The needle is then removed, and a sterile pressure dressing and ice pack are placed at the injection site.

COMPLICATIONS AND PITFALLS

Failure to identify primary or metastatic tumor of the distal femur or joint that is responsible for the patient's pain may yield disastrous results. The major complication of this injection technique is infection. This complication should be exceedingly rare if strict aseptic technique is followed. Approximately 25% of patients will complain of a transient increase in pain after injection of the suprapatellar bursa of the knee and should be warned of such.

CLINICAL PEARLS

Coexistent bursitis, tendinitis, arthritis, and internal derangement of the knee may also contribute to the patient's pain and may require additional treatment with more localized injection of local anesthetic and methylprednisolone acetate. The described injection technique is extremely effective in the treatment of pain secondary to superficial infrapatellar bursitis. This technique is a safe procedure if careful attention is paid to the clinically relevant anatomy in the areas to be injected. The use of physical modalities including local heat as well as gentle range of motion exercises should be introduced several days after the patient undergoes this injection technique for infrapatellar bursitis pain. Vigorous exercises should be avoided as they will exacerbate the patient's symptomatology. Simple analgesics and nonsteroidal anti-inflammatory drugs may be used concurrently with this injection technique.

66

Deep Infrapatellar Bursitis

ICD-9 CODE 726.69

THE CLINICAL SYNDROME

The deep infrapatellar bursa is vulnerable to injury from both acute trauma and repeated microtrauma. The superficial infrapatellar bursa lies between the subcutaneous tissues and the upper part of the ligamentum patellae. The deep infrapatellar bursa lies between the ligamentum patellae and the tibia. These bursae may exist as single bursal sacs or, in some patients, as a multisegmented series of sacs that may be loculated in nature. Acute injuries frequently take the form of direct trauma to the bursa via falls directly onto the knee (Fig. 66–1) or from patellar fractures, as well as from overuse injuries, including running on soft or uneven surfaces. Deep infrapatellar bursitis may also result from jobs requiring crawling and kneeling on the knees, such as carpet laying or scrubbing floors. If the inflammation of the superficial infrapatellar bursa becomes chronic, calcification of the bursa may occur.

SIGNS AND SYMPTOMS

The patient suffering from deep infrapatellar bursitis will frequently complain of pain and swelling in the anterior knee below the patella that can radiate inferiorly into the area surrounding the knee. Often, the patient will be unable to kneel or to walk down stairs. The patient may also complain of a sharp, catching sensation with range of motion of the knee, especially on first arising. Infrapatellar bursitis often coexists with arthritis and tendinitis of the knee joint, and these other pathological processes may confuse the clinical picture.

Physical examination may reveal point tenderness in the anterior knee just below the patella. Swelling and fluid accumulation surrounding the lower patella are often present. Passive flexion as well as active resisted extension of the knee will reproduce the pain. Sudden release of resistance during this maneuver will markedly increase the pain. The deep infrapatellar bursa is not as susceptible to infection as the superficial infrapatellar bursa.

TESTING

Plain radiographs of the knee may reveal calcification of the bursa and associated structures, including the quadriceps tendon, consistent with chronic inflammation. Magnetic resonance imaging is indicated if internal derangement, occult mass, or tumor of the knee is suspected. Electromyography will help distinguish deep and superficial infrapatellar bursitis from femoral neuropathy, lumbar radiculopathy, and plexopathy. The following injection technique will serve as a diagnostic and therapeutic maneuver. Antinuclear antibody testing is indicated if collagen vascular disease is suspected. If infection is considered, aspiration, Gram stain, and culture of bursal fluid are indicated on an emergency basis.

DIFFERENTIAL DIAGNOSIS

Due to the unique anatomy of the region, not only the deep infrapatellar bursa but also the associated tendons and other bursae of the knee can become inflamed and confuse the diagnosis. Both the quadriceps tendon and the deep and superficial infrapatellar bursae are subject to the development of inflammation after overuse, misuse, or direct trauma. The quadriceps tendon is made up of fibers from the four muscles that compose the quadriceps muscle: the vastus lateralis, the vastus intermedius, the vastus medialis, and the rectus femoris. These muscles are the primary extensors of the lower extremity at the knee. The tendons of these muscles converge and unite to form a single exceedingly strong tendon. The patella functions as a sesamoid bone within the quadriceps tendon, with fibers of the tendon expanding around the patella to form the medial and lateral patella retinacula, which help strengthen the knee joint. These fibers are called *expansions* and are vulnerable to strain, and the tendon proper is subject to the development of tendinitis. The suprapatellar, prepatellar, and superficial infrapatellar bursae may also concurrently become inflamed with dysfunction of the quadriceps tendon. It should be remembered that anything that alters the normal biomechanics of the knee can result in inflammation of the deep infrapatellar bursa.

TREATMENT

A short course of conservative therapy consisting of simple analgesics, nonsteroidal anti-inflammatory drugs, or cyclooxygenase-2 inhibitors and a knee brace to prevent further trauma is a reasonable first step in the treatment of patients suffering from deep infrapatellar bursitis. If the patient does not experience rapid improvement, the following injection technique is a reasonable next step.

To inject the deep infrapatellar bursa, the patient is placed in the supine position with a rolled blanket underneath the knee to gently flex the joint. The skin overlying the medial portion of the lower margin of the patella is prepped with antiseptic solution. A sterile syringe containing 2.0 mL of 0.25% preservative-free bupivacaine and 40 mg methylprednisolone is attached to a 1½-inch 25-gauge needle using strict aseptic technique. With strict aseptic technique, the medial lower margin of the patella is identified. Just below this point, the needle is inserted at a right angle to the patella to slide beneath the ligamentum patellar into the deep infrapatellar bursa. If the needle strikes the patella, it is then withdrawn slightly and redirected in a more inferior trajectory. When the needle is in position in proximity to the deep infrapatellar bursa, the contents of the syringe are then gently injected. There should be little resistance to injection. If resistance is encountered, the needle is probably in a ligament or tendon and should be advanced or withdrawn slightly until the injection proceeds without significant resistance. The needle is then removed, and a sterile pressure dressing and ice pack are placed at the injection site.

COMPLICATIONS AND PITFALLS

Failure to identify primary or metastatic tumor of the distal femur or joint that is responsible for the patient's pain may yield disastrous results. The major complication of this injection technique is infection. This complication should be exceedingly rare if strict aseptic technique is followed. Approximately 25% of patients will complain of a transient increase in pain after injection of the infrapatellar bursa of the knee and should be warned of such.

CLINICAL PEARLS

Coexistent bursitis, tendinitis, arthritis, and internal derangement of the knee may also contribute to the patient's pain and may require additional treatment with more localized injection of local anesthetic and methylprednisolone acetate. The described injection technique is extremely effective in the treatment of pain secondary to deep infrapatellar bursitis. This technique is a safe procedure if careful attention is paid to the clinically relevant anatomy in the areas to be injected. The use of physical modalities including local heat as well as gentle range of motion exercises should be introduced several days after the patient undergoes this injection technique for infrapatellar bursitis pain. Vigorous exercises should be avoided as they will exacerbate the patient's symptomatology. Simple analgesics and nonsteroidal anti-inflammatory drugs may be used concurrently with this injection technique.

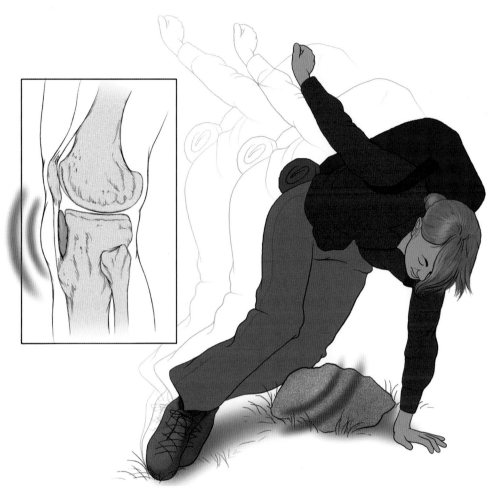

Figure 66–1. Deep infrapatellar bursitis commonly presents as inferior knee pain accompanied by a catching sensation, especially on rising from a sitting position.

67

Baker's Cyst of the Knee

ICD-9 CODE 727.51

THE CLINICAL SYNDROME

A common finding on physical examination of the knee, Baker's cyst is the result of an abnormal accumulation of synovial fluid in the medial aspect of the popliteal fossa. Overproduction of synovial fluid from the knee joint results in the formation of a cystic sac. This sac often communicates with the knee joint, with a one-way valve effect causing a gradual expansion of the cyst. Often, a tear of the medial meniscus or tendinitis of the medial hamstring tendon is the inciting factor responsible for the development of a Baker's cyst. Patients suffering from rheumatoid arthritis are especially susceptible to the development of Baker's cysts.

SIGNS AND SYMPTOMS

Patients with Baker's cysts will complain of a feeling of fullness behind the knee. Often, they will notice a lump behind the knee that becomes more apparent when they flex the affected knee. The cyst may continue to enlarge and may dissect inferiorly into the calf (Fig. 67-1). Patients suffering from rheumatoid arthritis are prone to this phenomenon, and the pain associated with dissection into the calf may be confused with thrombophlebitis and inappropriately treated with anticoagulants. Occasionally, the Baker's cyst may spontaneously rupture, usually after frequent squatting.

On physical examination, the patient suffering from Baker's cyst will have a cystic swelling in the medial aspect of the popliteal fossa. Baker's cysts can become quite large, especially in patients suffering from rheumatoid arthritis. Activity that includes squatting or walking makes the pain of Baker's cyst worse, with

rest and heat providing some relief. The pain is constant and characterized as aching in nature. The pain may interfere with sleep. Baker's cysts may spontaneously rupture, and there may be rubor and color in the calf that may mimic thrombophlebitis. Homan's sign will be negative, and no cords will be palpable.

TESTING

Plain radiographs are indicated for all patients who present with Baker's cyst. Based on the patient's clinical presentation, additional testing, including complete blood count, sedimentation rate, and antinuclear antibody testing, may be indicated. Magnetic resonance imaging of the knee is indicated if internal derangement or occult mass or tumor is suspected and is also useful in confirming the presence of a Baker's cyst.

DIFFERENTIAL DIAGNOSIS

As mentioned, Baker's cyst may rupture spontaneously and may be misdiagnosed as thrombophlebitis. Occasionally, tendinitis of the medial hamstring tendon may be confused with Baker's cyst, as may injury to the medial meniscus. Primary or metastatic tumors in the region, although rare, must be considered in the differential diagnosis.

TREATMENT

Although surgery is often required to successfully treat Baker's cyst, conservative therapy consisting of an elastic bandage combined with a short trial of nonsteroidal anti-inflammatory drugs or cyclooxygenase-2 inhibitors is warranted. It these conservative treatments fail, the following injection technique represents a reasonable next step.

To inject a Baker's cyst, the patient is placed in the prone position with the anterior ankle resting on a

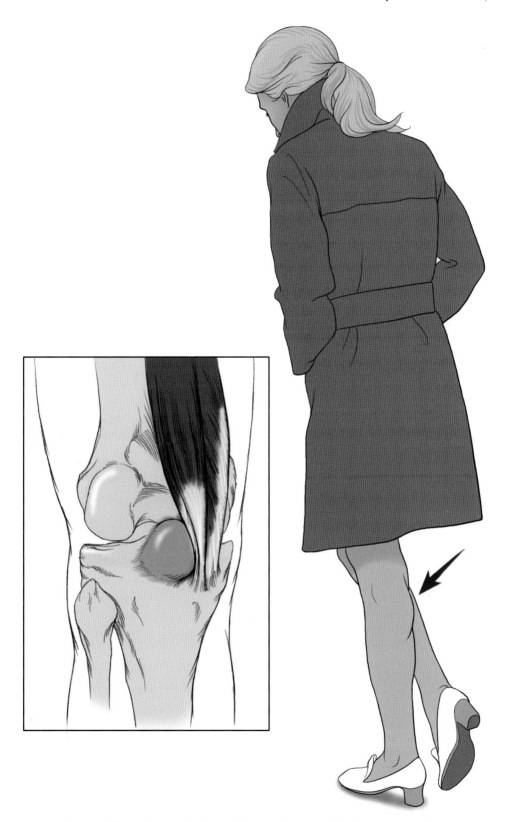

Figure 67–1. The patient suffering with Baker's cyst will often complain of a sensation of fullness or a lump behind the knee.

folded towel to slightly flex the knee. The middle of the popliteal fossa is identified, and at a point two fingers medial and two fingers below the popliteal crease, the skin is prepped with antiseptic solution. A syringe containing 2.0 mL of 0.25% preservative-free bupivacaine and 40 mg methylprednisolone is attached to a 2-inch 22-gauge needle.

The needle is then carefully advanced through the previously identified point at a 45-degree angle from the medial border of the popliteal fossa directly toward the Baker's cyst. While the clinician continuously aspirates, the needle is advanced very slowly to avoid trauma to the tibial nerve or popliteal artery or vein.

When the cyst is entered, synovial fluid will suddenly aspirate into the syringe. At this point, if there is no paresthesia in the distribution of the common peroneal or tibial nerve, the contents of the syringe are then gently injected. There should be minimal resistance to injection. A pressure dressing is then placed over the cyst to prevent fluid reaccumulation.

COMPLICATIONS AND PITFALLS

Failure to diagnose primary knee pathology, such as tears of the medial meniscus, may lead to further pain and disability. Magnetic resonance imaging should help identify internal derangement of the knee. The proximity to the common peroneal and tibial nerve as well as the popliteal artery and vein makes it imperative that this procedure be carried out only by those well versed in the regional anatomy and experienced in performing injection techniques. Many patients will also complain of a transient increase in pain after this injection technique. Although rare, infection may occur if careful attention to sterile technique is not followed.

CLINICAL PEARLS

When bursae become inflamed, they may overproduce synovial fluid, which can become trapped in saclike cysts due to a one-way valve phenomenon. This occurs commonly in the medial aspect of the popliteal fossa and is called a Baker's cyst. The aforementioned injection technique is extremely effective in the treatment of pain and swelling secondary to Baker's cyst. Coexistent semimembranosus bursitis, medial hamstring tendinitis, and/or internal derangement of the knee may also contribute to knee pain and may require additional treatment with more localized injection of local anesthetic and methylprednisolone acetate.

68

Pes Anserine Bursitis

ICD-9 CODE 726.61

THE CLINICAL SYNDROME

The pes anserine bursa lies beneath the pes anserine tendon, which is the insertional tendon of the sartorius, gracilis, and semitendinous muscles to the medial side of the tibia. This bursa may exist as single bursal sacs or, in some patients, as a multisegmented series of sacs that may be loculated in nature. Patients with pes anserine bursitis will present with pain over the medial knee joint and increased pain on passive valgus and external rotation of the knee. Activity, especially involving flexion and external rotation of the knee, will make the pain worse, with rest and heat providing some relief. Often, the patient will be unable to kneel or to walk down stairs (Fig. 68–1).

SIGNS AND SYMPTOMS

The pain of pes anserine bursitis is constant and characterized as aching in nature. The pain may interfere with sleep. Coexistent bursitis, tendinitis, arthritis, and/or internal derangement of the knee may confuse the clinical picture after trauma to the knee joint. Frequently, the medial collateral ligament is also involved if the patient has sustained trauma to the medial knee joint. If the inflammation of the pes anserine bursae becomes chronic, calcification of the bursae may occur.

Physical examination may reveal point tenderness in the anterior knee just below the medial knee joint at the tendinous insertion of the pes anserine. Swelling and fluid accumulation surrounding the bursa are often present. Active resisted flexion of the knee will reproduce the pain. Sudden release of resistance during this maneuver will markedly increase the pain. Rarely, the pes anserine bursa will become infected in a manner analogous to infection of the prepatellar bursa.

TESTING

Plain radiographs of the knee may reveal calcification of the bursa and associated structures, including the pes anserine tendon, consistent with chronic inflammation. Magnetic resonance imaging is indicated if internal derangement, occult mass, or tumor of the knee is suspected. Electromyography will help distinguish pes anserine bursitis from neuropathy, lumbar radiculopathy, and plexopathy. The following injection technique will serve as a diagnostic and therapeutic maneuver.

DIFFERENTIAL DIAGNOSIS

The pes anserine bursa is prone to the development of inflammation after overuse, misuse, or direct trauma. The medial collateral ligament is often also involved if the medial knee has been subjected to trauma. The medial collateral ligament is a broad, flat bandlike ligament that runs from the medial condyle of the femur to the medial aspect of the shaft of the tibia, where it attaches just above the groove of the semimembranosus muscle. It also attaches to the edge of the medial semilunar cartilage. The medial collateral ligament is crossed at its lower part by the tendons of the sartorius, gracilis, and semitendinosus muscles. Because of the unique anatomic relationships of the medial knee, it is often difficult on clinical grounds to accurately diagnose which anatomic structure is responsible for the patient's pain. Magnetic resonance imaging will help sort things out and rule out lesions such as tears of the medial meniscus that may require surgical intervention. It should be remembered that anything that alters the normal biomechanics of the knee can result in inflammation of the pes anserine bursa.

TREATMENT

A short course of conservative therapy consisting of simple analgesics, nonsteroidal anti-inflammatory drugs, or cyclooxygenase-2 inhibitors and a knee brace to prevent further trauma is a reasonable first step in the treatment of patients suffering from pes anserine bursitis. If the patient does not experience rapid improvement, the following injection technique is a reasonable next step.

To inject the pes anserine bursa, the patient is placed in the supine position with a rolled blanket underneath the knee to gently flex the joint. The skin just below the medial knee joint is prepped with antiseptic solution. A sterile syringe containing 2.0 mL of 0.25% preservative-free bupivacaine and 40 mg methylprednisolone is attached to a 1½-inch 25-gauge needle using strict aseptic technique. With strict aseptic technique, the pes anserine tendon is identified by having the patient strongly flex his or her leg against resistance. The point distal to the medial joint space at which the pes anserine tendon attaches to the tibia is the location of the pes anserine bursa. The bursa will usually be identified by point tenderness at that spot. At this point, the needle is inserted at a 45-degree angle to the tibia to pass through the skin and subcutaneous tissues into the pes anserine bursa. If the needle strikes the tibia, it is then withdrawn slightly into the substance of the bursa. When the needle is in position in proximity to the pes anserine bursa, the contents of the syringe are then gently injected. There should be little resistance to injection. If resistance is encountered, the needle is probably in a ligament or tendon and should be advanced or withdrawn slightly until the injection proceeds without significant resistance. The needle is then removed, and a sterile pressure dressing and ice pack are placed at the injection site.

COMPLICATIONS AND PITFALLS

Failure to identify primary or metastatic tumor of the distal femur or joint that is responsible for the patient's pain may yield disastrous results. The major complication of this injection technique is infection. This complication should be exceedingly rare if strict aseptic technique is followed. Approximately 25% of patients will complain of a transient increase in pain after injection of the pes anserine bursa of the knee and should be warned of such.

CLINICAL PEARLS

Coexistent bursitis, tendinitis, arthritis, and internal derangement of the knee may also contribute to the patient's pain and may require additional treatment with more localized injection of local anesthetic and methylprednisolone acetate. The described injection technique is extremely effective in the treatment of pain secondary to pes anserine bursitis. This technique is a safe procedure if careful attention is paid to the clinically relevant anatomy in the areas to be injected. The use of physical modalities including local heat as well as gentle range of motion exercises should be introduced several days after the patient undergoes this injection technique for pes anserine bursitis pain. Vigorous exercises should be avoided because they will exacerbate the patient's symptomatology. Simple analgesics and nonsteroidal anti-inflammatory drugs may be used concurrently with this injection technique. The major complication of this injection technique is infection. This complication should be exceedingly rare if strict aseptic technique is followed. Approximately 25% of patients will complain of a transient increase in pain after injection of the pes anserine bursa of the knee and should be warned of such.

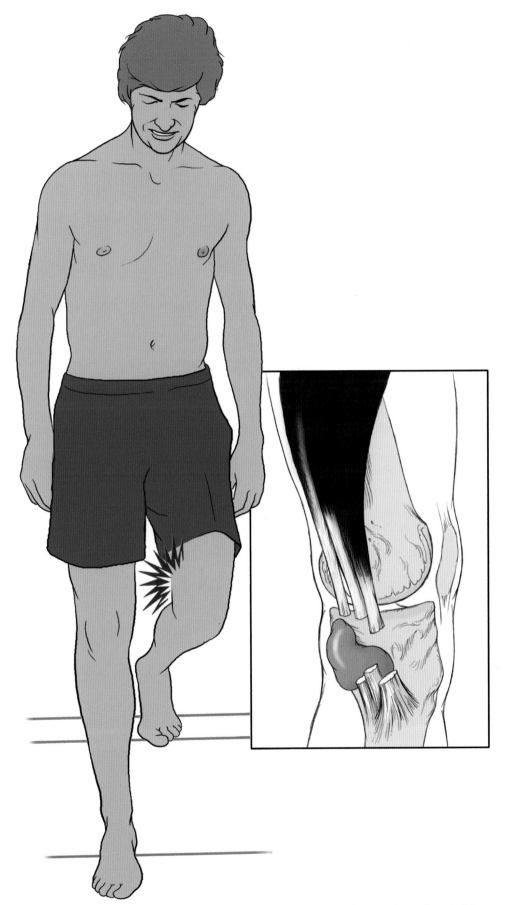

Figure 68–1. Patients with pes anserine bursitis will frequently complain of medial knee pain that is made worse with kneeling or walking down stairs.

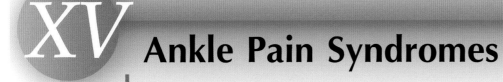

XV Ankle Pain Syndromes

69

Arthritis Pain of the Ankle

ICD-9 CODE 715.97

THE CLINICAL SYNDROME

Arthritis of the ankle is a common painful condition encountered in clinical practice. The ankle joint is susceptible to the development of arthritis from a variety of conditions that have in common the ability to damage the joint cartilage. Osteoarthritis of the joint is the most common form of arthritis that results in ankle joint pain. However, rheumatoid arthritis and post-traumatic arthritis are also common causes of ankle pain secondary to arthritis. Less common causes of arthritis-induced ankle pain include the collagen vascular diseases, infection, villonodular synovitis, and Lyme disease. Acute infectious arthritis will usually be accompanied by significant systemic symptoms, including fever and malaise, and should be easily recognized by the astute clinician and treated appropriately with culture and antibiotics, rather than with injection therapy. The collagen vascular diseases will generally present as a polyarthropathy rather than a monoarthropathy limited to the ankle joint, although ankle pain secondary to collagen vascular disease responds exceedingly well to the treatment modalities described here.

SIGNS AND SYMPTOMS

The majority of patients presenting with ankle pain secondary to arthritis will present with the complaint of pain that is localized around the ankle and distal lower extremity. Activity makes the pain worse, with rest and heat providing some relief. The pain is constant and characterized as aching in nature. The pain may interfere with sleep. Some patients will complain of a grating or popping sensation with use of the joint, and crepitus may be present on physical examination.

In addition to the aforementioned pain, patients suffering from arthritis of the ankle joint will often experience a gradual decrease in functional ability with decreasing ankle range of motion, making simple everyday tasks such as walking and climbing stairs and ladders quite difficult (Fig. 69–1). With continued disuse, muscle wasting may occur, and a "frozen ankle" due to adhesive capsulitis may develop.

TESTING

Plain radiographs are indicated in all patients who present with ankle pain. Based on the patient's clinical presentation, additional testing, including complete blood count, sedimentation rate, and antinuclear antibody testing, may be indicated. Magnetic resonance imaging of the ankle is indicated if aseptic necrosis or occult mass or tumor is suspected.

DIFFERENTIAL DIAGNOSIS

Lumbar radiculopathy may mimic the pain and disability associated with arthritis of the ankle. In such patients, the ankle examination should be negative. Entrapment neuropathies such as tarsal tunnel syndrome may also confuse the diagnosis, as may bursitis of the ankle, both of which may coexist with arthritis of the ankle. Primary and metastatic tumors of the distal tibia and fibula and spine may also present in a manner analogous to arthritis of the ankle, as may occult fractures.

TREATMENT

Initial treatment of the pain and functional disability associated with arthritis of the ankle should include a combination of the nonsteroidal anti-inflammatory drugs or cyclooxygenase-2 inhibitors and physical therapy. The local application of heat and cold may also be beneficial. Avoidance of repetitive activities that aggravate the patient's symptomatology, as well as short-term immobilization of the ankle joint, may also provide relief. For patients who do not respond to these treatment modalities, an intra-articular injection of local anesthetic and steroid may be a reasonable next step.

To perform intra-articular injection of the ankle, the patient is placed in the supine position, and the skin overlying the ankle joint is properly prepared with antiseptic solution. A sterile syringe containing 2.0 mL of 0.25% preservative-free bupivacaine and 40 mg methylprednisolone is attached to a 1½-inch 25-gauge needle using strict aseptic technique. With the foot in neutral position, the junction of the tibia and fibula just above the talus is identified. At this point, a triangular indentation indicating the joint space will be easily palpable. The needle is then carefully advanced through the skin and subcutaneous tissues through the joint capsule into the joint. If bone is encountered, the needle is withdrawn into the subcutaneous tissues and redirected superiorly and slightly more medial. After the joint space is entered, the contents of the syringe are gently injected. There should be little resistance to injection. If resistance is encountered, the needle is probably in a ligament or tendon and should be advanced slightly into the joint space until the injection proceeds without significant resistance. The needle is then removed, and a sterile pressure dressing and ice pack are placed at the injection site.

SIDE EFFECTS AND COMPLICATIONS

Failure to identify primary or metastatic tumor of the ankle or spine that is responsible for the patient's pain may yield disastrous results. The major complication of intra-articular injection of the ankle is infection. This complication should be exceedingly rare if strict aseptic technique is followed. Approximately 25% of patients will complain of a transient increase in pain after intra-articular injection of the ankle joint and should be warned of such.

CLINICAL PEARLS

Coexistent bursitis and tendinitis may also contribute to ankle pain and may require additional treatment with more localized injection of local anesthetic and methylprednisolone acetate. The described injection technique is extremely effective in the treatment of pain secondary to the causes of arthritis of the ankle joint. This technique is a safe procedure if careful attention is paid to the clinically relevant anatomy in the areas to be injected. The use of physical modalities including local heat as well as gentle range of motion exercises should be introduced several days after the patient undergoes this injection technique for ankle pain. Vigorous exercises should be avoided because they will exacerbate the patient's symptomatology.

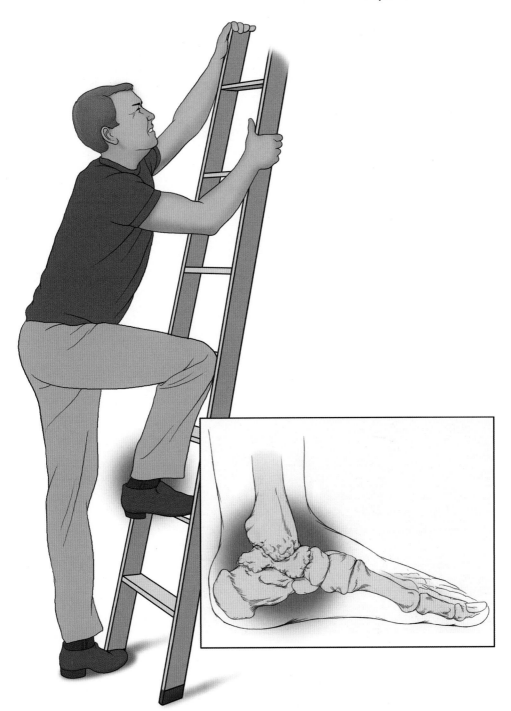

Figure 69–1. Arthritis of the ankle is a common cause of ankle pain, which is often made worse with activity.

70

Arthritis Pain of the Midtarsal Joints

ICD-9 CODE 715.97

THE CLINICAL SYNDROME

Arthritis of the midtarsal joints is a common painful condition encountered in clinical practice. The midtarsal joints are susceptible to the development of arthritis from a variety of conditions that have in common the ability to damage the joint cartilage. Osteoarthritis of the joint is the most common form of arthritis that results in midtarsal joint pain. However, rheumatoid arthritis and post-traumatic arthritis are also common causes of midtarsal pain secondary to arthritis. Less common causes of arthritis-induced midtarsal pain include the collagen vascular diseases, infection, and Lyme disease. Acute infectious arthritis will usually be accompanied by significant systemic symptoms, including fever and malaise, and should be easily recognized by the astute clinician and treated appropriately with culture and antibiotics, rather than with injection therapy. The collagen vascular diseases will generally present as a polyarthropathy rather than a monoarthropathy limited to the midtarsal joints, although midtarsal pain secondary to collagen vascular disease responds exceedingly well to the treatment modalities described here.

SIGNS AND SYMPTOMS

The majority of patients presenting with midtarsal joint pain secondary to osteoarthritis and post-traumatic arthritis pain will present with the complaint of pain that is localized to the dorsum of the foot. Activity, especially inversion and adduction of the midtarsal joints, makes the pain worse, with rest and heat providing some relief. The pain is constant and characterized as aching in nature. The pain may interfere with sleep. Some patients will complain of a grating or popping sensation with use of the joints, and crepitus may be present on physical examination. In addition to this pain, patients suffering from arthritis of the midtarsal joint will often experience a gradual decrease in functional ability with decreasing midtarsal range of motion, making simple everyday tasks such as walking and climbing stairs quite difficult (Fig. 70–1).

TESTING

Plain radiographs are indicated for all patients who present with midtarsal pain (Fig. 70–2). Based on the patient's clinical presentation, additional testing, including complete blood count, sedimentation rate, and antinuclear antibody testing, may be indicated. Magnetic resonance imaging of the midtarsal joints is indicated if aseptic necrosis or occult mass or tumor is suspected.

DIFFERENTIAL DIAGNOSIS

Primary pathology of the foot, including gout and occult fractures, may mimic the pain and disability associated with arthritis of the midtarsal. Entrapment neuropathies such as tarsal tunnel syndrome may also confuse the diagnosis, as may bursitis and plantar fasciitis of the foot, both of which may coexist with arthritis of the midtarsal joints. Primary and metastatic tumors of the foot may also present in a manner analogous to arthritis of the midtarsal joints.

TREATMENT

Initial treatment of the pain and functional disability associated with arthritis of the midtarsal joints should include a combination of the nonsteroidal

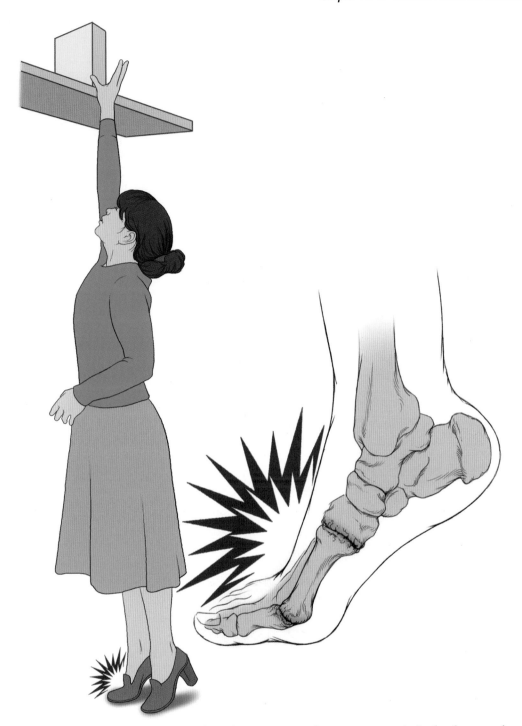

Figure 70–1. Arthritis of the midtarsal joints commonly presents as pain in the dorsum of the foot that is made worse with inversion and adduction of the affected joints.

anti-inflammatory drugs or cyclooxygenase-2 inhibitors and physical therapy. The local application of heat and cold may also be beneficial. Avoidance of repetitive activities that aggravate the patient's symptomatology as well as short-term immobilization of the midtarsal joint may also provide relief. For patients who do not respond to these treatment modalities, an intra-articular injection of local anesthetic and steroid may be a reasonable next step.

The goals of this injection technique are explained to the patient. The patient is placed in the supine position, and the skin overlying the most tender midtarsal joint is properly prepared with antiseptic solution. A sterile syringe containing 2.0 mL of 0.25% preservative-free bupivacaine and 40 mg methylprednisolone is attached to a ⅝-inch 25-gauge needle using strict aseptic technique. With strict aseptic technique, the affected joint space is identified. At this point, the needle is carefully advanced at a right angle to the dorsal aspect of the ankle through the skin and subcutaneous tissues through the joint capsule into the joint. If bone is encountered, the needle is withdrawn into the subcutaneous tissues and redirected superiorly. After the joint space is entered, the contents of the syringe are gently injected. There should be little resistance to injection. If resistance is encountered, the needle is probably in a ligament or tendon and should be advanced slightly into the joint space until the injection proceeds without significant resistance. The needle is then removed, and a sterile pressure dressing and ice pack are placed at the injection site.

SIDE EFFECTS AND COMPLICATIONS

Failure to identify primary or metastatic tumor of the midtarsal joints that is responsible for the patient's pain may yield disastrous results. The major complication of intra-articular injection of the midtarsal joint is infection. This complication should be exceedingly rare if strict aseptic technique is followed. Approximately 25% of patients will complain of a transient increase in pain after intra-articular injection of the midtarsal joint and should be warned of such.

CLINICAL PEARLS

Coexistent bursitis and tendinitis may also contribute to midtarsal joint pain and may require additional treatment with more localized injection of local anesthetic and methlyprednisolone acetate. The described injection technique is extremely effective in the treatment of pain secondary to the aforementioned causes of arthritis of the midtarsal joints. This technique is a safe procedure if careful attention is paid to the clinically relevant anatomy in the areas to be injected. The use of physical modalities including local heat as well as gentle range of motion exercises should be introduced several days after the patient undergoes this injection technique for midtarsal pain. Vigorous exercises should be avoided because they will exacerbate the patient's symptomatology.

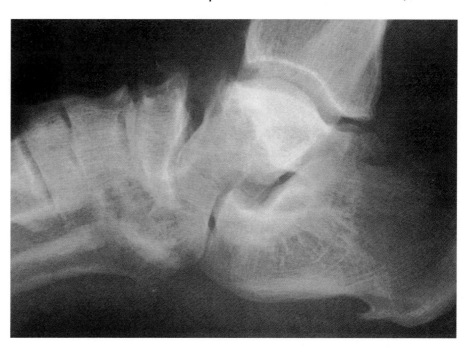

Figure 70-2. Lateral view of the tarsal bones showing osteoarthritis secondary to a vertical talus. (From Brower AC, Flemming DJ: Arthritis in Black and White, 2nd ed. Philadelphia, WB Saunders, 1997, p 281.)

71

Deltoid Ligament Strain

ICD-9 CODE 845.01

THE CLINICAL SYNDROME

The deltoid ligament is susceptible to strain from acute injury due to sudden overpronation of the ankle or to repetitive microtrauma to the ligament from overuse or misuse, such as long distance running on soft or uneven surfaces. The deltoid ligament is exceptionally strong and is not as subject to strain as the anterior talofibular ligament. The deltoid ligament has two layers; both attach above to the medial malleolus. A deep layer attaches below to the medial body of the talus, with the superficial fibers attaching to the medial talus and the sustentaculum tali of the calcaneus and the navicular tuberosity.

SIGNS AND SYMPTOMS

Patients with strain of the deltoid ligament will complain of pain just below the medial malleolus (Fig. 71–1). Plantar flexion and eversion of the ankle joint will exacerbate the pain. Often, patients with injury to the deltoid ligament will note a "pop" followed by significant swelling and the inability to walk.

On physical examination, there will be point tenderness over the medial malleolus. With acute trauma, ecchymosis over the ligament may be noted. Passive eversion and plantar flexion of the ankle joint will exacerbate the pain. Coexistent bursitis and arthritis of the ankle and subtalar joint may also be present and confuse the clinical picture.

TESTING

Plain radiographs are indicated for all patients who present with ankle pain. Based on the patient's clini-cal presentation, additional testing, including complete blood count, sedimentation rate, and antinuclear antibody testing, may be indicated. Magnetic resonance imaging of the ankle is indicated if disruption of the deltoid ligament or joint instability, occult mass, or tumor is suspected. Radionuclide bone scanning should be used if occult fracture is suspected.

DIFFERENTIAL DIAGNOSIS

Avulsion fractures of the calcaneus, tallus, medial malleolus, and the base of the fifth metatarsal can mimic the pain of injury to the deltoid ligament. Bursitis and tendinitis as well as gout of the midtarsal joints may coexist with deltoid ligament strain and may confuse the diagnosis. Tarsal tunnel syndrome may occur after ankle trauma and may further confuse the clinical picture.

TREATMENT

Initial treatment of the pain and functional disability associated with deltoid ligament strain should include a combination of the nonsteroidal anti-inflammatory drugs or cyclooxygenase-2 inhibitors and physical therapy. The local application of heat and cold may also be beneficial. Avoidance of repetitive activities that aggravate the patient's symptomatology, as well as short-term immobilization of the ankle joint, may also provide relief. For patients who do not respond to these treatment modalities, the following injection technique may be a reasonable next step.

To perform deltoid ligament injection, the patient is placed in the supine position, and the skin overlying the area of the medial malleolus is properly prepared with antiseptic solution. A sterile syringe containing 2.0 mL of 0.25% preservative-free bupivacaine and 40 mg methylprednisolone is attached to a 1½-inch 25-gauge needle using strict aseptic technique. With

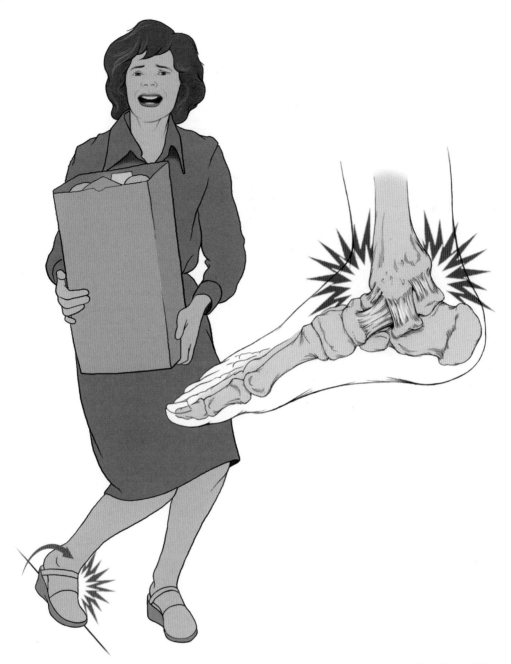

Figure 71–1. With deltoid ligament strain, patients may notice a "pop" followed by significant swelling.

strict aseptic technique, with the lower extremity slightly abducted, the lower margin of the medial malleolus is identified. At this point, the needle is carefully advanced at a 30-degree angle to the ankle through the skin and subcutaneous tissues to impinge on the lower margin of the medial malleolus. The needle is then withdrawn slightly, and the contents of the syringe are gently injected. There will be slight resistance to injection. If significant resistance is encountered, the needle is probably in the ligament and should be withdrawn slightly until the injection proceeds without significant resistance. The needle is then removed, and a sterile pressure dressing and ice pack are placed at the injection site.

COMPLICATIONS AND PITFALLS

Failure to identify occult fractures of the ankle and foot may result in significant morbidity. Radionuclide bone scanning and magnetic resonance imaging of the ankle should be performed on all patients experiencing unexplained ankle and foot pain, especially if trauma is present. The major complication of the described injection technique is infection. This complication should be exceedingly rare if strict aseptic technique is followed. Approximately 25% of pa-

tients will complain of a transient increase in pain after injection of the deltoid ligament and should be warned of such. Injection around strained ligaments should always be done gently to avoid further damage to the already compromised ligament.

CLINICAL PEARLS

It is estimated that approximately 25,000 people will sprain an ankle every day. Although viewed as benign by the lay public, ankle sprains can result in significant permanent pain and disability. The described injection technique is extremely effective in the treatment of pain secondary to the deltoid ligament strain. Coexistent arthritis, bursitis, and tendinitis may also contribute to medial ankle pain and may require additional treatment with more localized injection of local anesthetic and methylprednisolone acetate. The use of physical modalities including local heat as well as gentle range of motion exercises should be introduced several days after the patient undergoes this injection technique for ankle pain. Vigorous exercises should be avoided because they will exacerbate the patient's symptomatology. Simple analgesics and nonsteroidal anti-inflammatory drugs may be used concurrently with this injection technique.

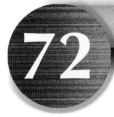

Anterior Tarsal Tunnel Syndrome

ICD-9 CODE 355.5

THE CLINICAL SYNDROME

Anterior tarsal tunnel syndrome is caused by compression of the deep peroneal nerve as it passes beneath the superficial fascia of the ankle. The most common cause of compression of the deep peroneal nerve at this anatomic location is trauma to the dorsum of the foot. Severe, acute plantar flexion of the foot has been implicated in anterior tarsal tunnel syndrome, as has the wearing of overly tight shoes or squatting and bending forward, as when planting flowers (Fig. 72–1). Anterior tarsal tunnel syndrome is much less common than posterior tarsal tunnel syndrome.

SIGNS AND SYMPTOMS

This entrapment neuropathy presents primarily as pain, numbness, and paresthesias of the dorsum of the foot that radiates into the first dorsal web space. These symptoms may also radiate proximal to the entrapment into the anterior ankle. There is no motor involvement unless the distal lateral division of the deep peroneal nerve is involved. Nighttime foot pain analogous to the nocturnal pain of carpal tunnel syndrome is often present. The patient may report that holding the foot in the everted position decreases the pain and paresthesias of anterior tarsal tunnel syndrome.

Physical findings include tenderness over the deep peroneal nerve at the dorsum of the foot. A positive Tinel's sign just medial to the dorsalis pedis pulse over the deep peroneal nerve as it passes beneath the fascia is usually present. Active plantar flexion will often reproduce the symptoms of anterior tarsal tunnel syndromes. Weakness of the extensor digitorum

brevis may be present if the lateral branch of the deep peroneal nerve is affected.

TESTING

Electromyography will help distinguish lumbar radiculopathy and diabetic polyneuropathy from anterior tarsal tunnel syndrome. Plain radiographs are indicated for all patients who present with anterior tarsal tunnel syndrome to rule out occult bony pathology. Based on the patient's clinical presentation, additional testing, including complete blood count, uric acid, sedimentation rate, and antinuclear antibody testing, may be indicated. Magnetic resonance imaging of the ankle and foot is indicated if joint instability or a space-occupying lesion is suspected. The injection technique described here will serve as both a diagnostic and therapeutic maneuver.

DIFFERENTIAL DIAGNOSIS

Anterior tarsal tunnel syndrome is often misdiagnosed as arthritis of the ankle joint, lumbar radiculopathy, or diabetic polyneuropathy. Patients with arthritis of the ankle joint will have radiographic evidence of arthritis. Most patients suffering from lumbar radiculopathy will have reflex, motor, and sensory changes associated with back pain, whereas patients with anterior tarsal tunnel syndrome will have no reflex changes and motor deficit. Sensory changes will be limited to the distribution of the distal deep peroneal nerve. Diabetic polyneuropathy will generally present as symmetrical sensory deficit involving the entire foot rather than limited to just the distribution of the deep peroneal nerve. It should be remembered that lumbar radiculopathy and deep peroneal nerve entrapment may coexist as the "double crush" syndrome. Furthermore, because anterior tarsal tunnel syndrome is seen in patients with diabetes, it is not surprising that diabetic polyneuropathy is usually present in diabetic patients with anterior tarsal tunnel syndrome.

TREATMENT

Mild cases of tarsal tunnel syndrome will usually respond to conservative therapy, and surgery should be reserved for more severe cases. Initial treatment of tarsal tunnel syndrome should consist of treatment with simple analgesics, nonsteroidal anti-inflammatory drugs, or cyclooxygenase-2 inhibitors and splinting of the ankle. At a minimum, the splint should be worn at night, but 24 hours a day is ideal. Avoidance of repetitive activities thought to be responsible for the evolution of tarsal tunnel syndrome, such as prolonged squatting or wearing shoes that are too tight, will also help ameliorate the patient's symptoms. If the patient fails to respond to these conservative measures, a next reasonable step is injection of the tarsal tunnel with local anesthetic and steroid.

Tarsal tunnel injection is performed by placing the patient in the supine position with the leg extended. The extensor hallucis longus tendon is identified by having the patient extend his or her big toe against resistance. A point just medial to the tendon at the skin crease of the ankle is identified and prepped with antiseptic solution. A 1½-inch 25-gauge needle is then advanced through this point very slowly toward the tibia until a paresthesia into the web space between the first and second toes is elicited. The patient should be warned to expect a paresthesia and should be told to say "there" immediately on perceiving the paresthesia. Paresthesia will usually be elicited at a depth of ¼ to ½ inch. If a paresthesia is not elicited, the needle is withdrawn and redirected slightly more posteriorly until a paresthesia is obtained. Once paresthesia in the distribution of the deep peroneal nerve is elicited, the needle is withdrawn 1 mm, and the patient is observed to be sure he or she is not experiencing any persistent paresthesia. If no persistent paresthesia is present and after careful aspiration, 6 mL of 1.0% preservative-free lidocaine and 40 mg methylprednisolone are slowly injected. Care must be taken to not advance the needle into the substance of the nerve during the injection and to inject the solution intraneurally. After injection of the solution, pressure is applied to the injection site to decrease the incidence of postblock ecchymosis and hematoma formation.

COMPLICATIONS AND PITFALLS

Failure to adequately treat tarsal tunnel syndrome can result in permanent pain, numbness, and func-

tional disability. This problem can be exacerbated if coexistent reflex sympathetic dystrophy is not aggressively treated with sympathetic neural blockade. The main side effect of deep peroneal nerve block is postblock ecchymosis and hematoma. As mentioned, pressure should be maintained on the injection site postblock to avoid ecchymosis and hematoma formation. Because a paresthesia is elicited with this technique, the potential for needle-induced trauma to the common peroneal nerve remains a possibility. By advancing the needle slowly and then withdrawing the needle slightly away from the nerve, needle-induced trauma to the common peroneal nerve can be avoided.

CLINICAL PEARLS

It should be remembered that the most common cause of pain radiating into the lower extremity is herniated lumbar disc or nerve impingement secondary to degenerative arthritis of the spine, not disorders involving the common or deep peroneal nerve per se. Other pain syndromes that may be confused with deep peroneal nerve entrapment include lesions either above the origin of the common peroneal nerve, such as lesions of the sciatic nerve, or lesions at the point at which the common peroneal nerve winds around the head of the fibula. Electromyography and magnetic resonance imaging of the lumbar spine combined with the clinical history and physical examination will help sort out the etiology of distal lower extremity and foot pain.

The described injection technique is useful in the treatment of anterior tarsal tunnel syndrome. Anterior tarsal tunnel syndrome is characterized by persistent aching of the dorsum of the foot that is sometimes associated with weakness of the toe extensors. This pain is frequently worse at night and may awaken the patient from sleep. It is relieved by moving the affected ankle and toes. Anterior tarsal tunnel syndrome can occur after squatting and leaning forward for long periods of time, such as when planting flowers. Diabetics and others with vulnerable nerve syndrome may be more susceptible to the development of this syndrome. Most patients with anterior tarsal tunnel syndrome can be treated with deep peroneal nerve blocks with local anesthetic and steroid combined with avoidance techniques.

Careful preblock neurological assessment is important to avoid preexisting neurological deficits being later attributed to the deep peroneal nerve block. These assessments are especially important in those patients who have sustained trauma to the ankle or foot or in those patients suffering from diabetic neuropathy in whom deep peroneal nerve blocks are being used for acute pain control.

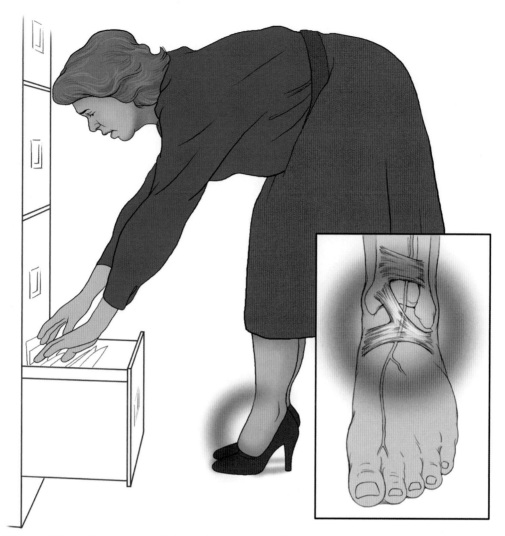

Figure 72–1. Anterior tarsal tunnel syndrome will present as deep, aching pain in the dorsum of the foot, weakness of the extensor digitorum brevis, and numbness in the distribution of the deep peroneal nerve.

73

Posterior Tarsal Tunnel Syndrome

ICD-9 CODE 355.5

THE CLINICAL SYNDROME

Posterior tarsal tunnel syndrome is caused by compression of the posterior tibial nerve as it passes through the posterior tarsal tunnel. The posterior tarsal tunnel is made up of the flexor retinaculum, the bones of the ankle, and the lacunate ligament. In addition to the posterior tibial nerve, the tunnel contains the posterior tibial artery and a number of flexor tendons that are subject to tenosynovitis. The most common cause of compression of the posterior tibial nerve at this anatomic location is trauma to the ankle, including fracture, dislocation, and crush injuries. Thrombophlebitis involving the posterior tibial artery has also been implicated in the evolution of posterior tarsal tunnel syndrome. Patients with rheumatoid arthritis have a higher incidence of posterior tarsal tunnel syndrome than does the general population. Posterior tarsal tunnel syndrome is much more common that anterior tarsal tunnel syndrome.

SIGNS AND SYMPTOMS

Posterior tarsal tunnel syndrome presents in a manner analogous to carpal tunnel syndrome. The patient will complain of pain, numbness, and paresthesias of the sole of the foot. These symptoms may also radiate proximal to the entrapment into the medial ankle (Fig. 73–1). There are medial and lateral plantar divisions of the posterior tibial nerve that provide motor innervation to the intrinsic muscles of the foot. The patient may note weakness of the toe flexors and instability of the foot due to weakness of the lumbrical muscles. Nighttime foot pain analogous to the nocturnal pain of carpal tunnel syndrome is often present.

Physical findings include tenderness over the posterior tibial nerve at the medial malleolus. A positive Tinel's sign just below and behind the medial malleolus over the posterior tibial nerve is usually present. Active inversion of the ankle will often reproduce the symptoms of posterior tarsal tunnel syndromes. Weakness of the flexor digitorum brevis and the lumbrical muscles may be present if the medial and lateral branches of the posterior tibial nerve are affected.

TESTING

Electromyography will help distinguish lumbar radiculopathy and diabetic polyneuropathy from posterior tarsal tunnel syndrome. Plain radiographs are indicated for all patients who present with posterior tarsal tunnel syndrome to rule out occult bony pathology. Based on the patient's clinical presentation, additional testing, including complete blood count, uric acid, sedimentation rate, and antinuclear antibody testing, may be indicated. Magnetic resonance imaging of the ankle and foot is indicated if joint instability or a space-occupying lesion is suspected. The injection technique described here will serve as both a diagnostic and therapeutic maneuver.

DIFFERENTIAL DIAGNOSIS

Posterior tarsal tunnel syndrome is often misdiagnosed as arthritis of the ankle joint, lumbar radiculopathy, or diabetic polyneuropathy. Patients with arthritis of the ankle joint will have radiographic evidence of arthritis. Most patients suffering from a lumbar radiculopathy will have reflex, motor, and sensory changes associated with back pain, whereas patients with posterior tarsal tunnel syndrome will have no reflex changes. Motor and sensory changes will be limited to the distribution of distal posterior tibial nerve. Diabetic polyneuropathy will generally present

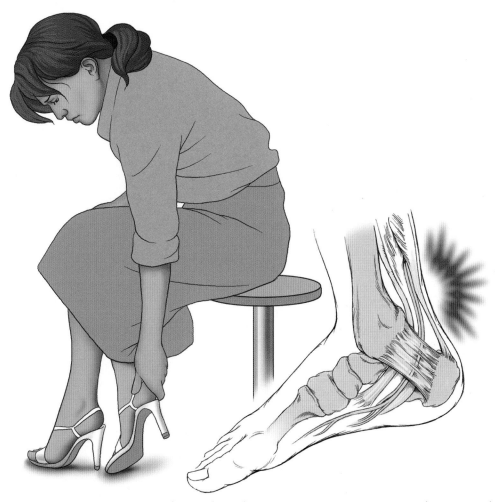

Figure 73–1. Posterior tarsal tunnel syndrome presents in a manner similar to carpal tunnel syndrome and is characterized by pain, numbness, and paresthesias of the sole of the foot.

as symmetrical sensory deficit involving the entire foot rather than limited to just the distribution of the posterior tibial nerve. It should be remembered that lumbar radiculopathy and posterior tibial nerve entrapment may coexist as the "double crush" syndrome. Furthermore, because posterior tarsal tunnel syndrome is seen in patients with diabetes, it is not surprising that diabetic polyneuropathy is usually present in diabetic patients with posterior tarsal tunnel syndrome.

TREATMENT

Mild cases of tarsal tunnel syndrome will usually respond to conservative therapy, and surgery should be reserved for more severe cases. Initial treatment of tarsal tunnel syndrome should consist of treatment with simple analgesics, nonsteroidal anti-inflammatory drugs, or cyclooxygenase-2 inhibitors and splinting of the ankle. At a minimum, the splint should be worn at night, but 24 hours a day is ideal. Avoidance of repetitive activities thought to be responsible for the evolution of tarsal tunnel syndrome will also help ameliorate the patient's symptoms. If the patient fails to respond to these conservative measures, a next reasonable step is injection of the tarsal tunnel with local anesthetic and steroid.

To treat the pain and disability of posterior tarsal tunnel syndrome with injection, the patient is placed in the lateral position with the affected leg in the dependent position and slightly flexed. The posterior tibial artery at this level is then palpated. The area between the medial malleolus and the Achilles tendon is identified and prepped with antiseptic solutions. A 1½-inch 25-gauge needle is inserted at this level and directed anteriorly toward the pulsations of the posterior tibial artery. If the arterial pulsations cannot be identified, the needle is directed toward the posterior superior border of the medial malleolus. The needle is then advanced slowly toward the tibial nerve that lies in the posterior groove of the medial malleolus until a paresthesia in the distribution of the tibial nerve is elicited. The patient should be warned to expect a paresthesia and should be told to say "there" immediately on perceiving the paresthesia. Paresthesia will usually be elicited after the needle is advanced ½ to ¾ inch. If a paresthesia is not elicited, the needle is withdrawn and redirected slightly more cephalad until a paresthesia is obtained.

Once paresthesia in the distribution of the tibial nerve is elicited, the needle is withdrawn 1 mm and the patient is observed to be sure he or she is not experiencing any persistent paresthesia. If no persistent paresthesia is present and after careful aspiration, 6 ml of 1.0% preservative-free lidocaine and 40 mg methylprednisolone are slowly injected. Care must be taken to not advance the needle into the substance of the nerve during the injection and to inject the solution intraneurally. After injection of the solution, pressure is applied to the injection site to decrease the incidence of postblock ecchymosis and hematoma formation.

COMPLICATIONS AND PITFALLS

Failure to adequately treat tarsal tunnel syndrome can result in permanent pain, numbness, and functional disability. This problem can be exacerbated if coexistent reflex sympathetic dystrophy is not aggressively treated with sympathetic neural blockade. The main side effect of the described injection technique is postblock ecchymosis and hematoma. As mentioned, pressure should be maintained on the injection site postblock to avoid ecchymosis and hematoma formation. Because a paresthesia is elicited with this technique, the potential for needle-induced trauma to the nerve remains a possibility. By advancing the needle slowly and then withdrawing the needle slightly away from the nerve, needle-induced trauma to the nerve can be avoided.

CLINICAL PEARLS

It should be remembered that the most common cause of pain radiating into the lower extremity is herniated lumbar disc or nerve impingement secondary to degenerative arthritis of the spine, not disorders involving the tibial, common, or deep peroneal nerve per se. Other pain syndromes that may be confused with posterior tarsal tunnel syndrome include lesions above either the origin of the tibial or common peroneal nerve. Electromyography and magnetic resonance imaging of the lumbar spine combined with the clinical history and physical examination will help sort out the etiology of distal lower extremity and foot pain.

74

Achilles Tendinitis

ICD-9 CODE 727.00

THE CLINICAL SYNDROME

Achilles tendinitis is being seen with increasing frequency in clinical practice as jogging has increased in popularity. The Achilles tendon is susceptible to the development of tendinitis both at its insertion on the calcaneus and at its narrowest part at a point approximately 5 cm above its insertion. The Achilles tendon is subject to repetitive motion that may result in microtrauma, which heals poorly due to the tendon's avascular nature. Running is often implicated as the inciting factor of acute Achilles tendinitis. Tendinitis of the Achilles tendon frequently coexists with bursitis of the associated bursae of the tendon and ankle joint, creating additional pain and functional disability. Calcium deposition around the tendon may occur if the inflammation continues, making subsequent treatment more difficult. Continued trauma to the inflamed tendon may ultimately result in tendon rupture.

SIGNS AND SYMPTOMS

The onset of Achilles tendinitis is usually acute, occurring after overuse or misuse of the ankle joint. Inciting factors may include activities such as running and sudden stopping and starting as when playing tennis. Improper stretching of the gastrocnemius and Achilles tendon before exercise has also been implicated in the development of Achilles tendinitis as well as acute tendon rupture. The pain of Achilles tendinitis is constant and severe and is localized in the posterior ankle (Fig. 74–1). Significant sleep disturbance is often reported. The patient may attempt to splint the inflamed Achilles tendon by adopting a flatfooted gait to avoid plantar flexing the affected tendon. Patients with Achilles tendinitis will exhibit pain with resisted plantar flexion of the foot. A creaking or grating sensation may be palpated when passively plantar flexing the foot. As mentioned, the chronically inflamed Achilles tendon may suddenly rupture with stress or during vigorous injection procedures into the tendon itself.

TESTING

Plain radiographs are indicated for all patients who present with posterior ankle pain. Based on the patient's clinical presentation, additional testing, including complete blood count, sedimentation rate, and antinuclear antibody testing, may be indicated. Magnetic resonance imaging of the ankle is indicated if joint instability is suspected. Radionuclide bone scanning is useful to identify stress fractures of the tibia not seen on plain radiographs. The following injection technique will serve as both a diagnostic and therapeutic maneuver.

DIFFERENTIAL DIAGNOSIS

Achilles tendinitis is generally easily identified on clinical grounds. Because a bursa is located between the Achilles tendon and the base of the tibia and the upper posterior calcaneus, coexistent bursitis may confuse the diagnosis. Stress fractures of the ankle may also mimic Achilles tendinitis and may be identified on plain radiographs or radionuclide bone scanning.

TREATMENT

Initial treatment of the pain and functional disability associated with Achilles tendinitis should include a combination of the nonsteroidal anti-inflammatory drugs or cyclooxygenase-2 inhibitors and physical therapy. The local application of heat and cold may also be beneficial. Avoidance of repetitive activities responsible for the evolution of the tendinitis, such as jogging, should be encouraged. For patients who do not respond to these treatment modalities, the following injection technique with local anesthetic and steroid may be a reasonable next step.

Injection for Achilles tendinitis is carried out by placing the patient in the prone position with the affected foot hanging off the end of the table. The foot is gently dorsiflexed to facilitate identification of the margin of the tendon to aid in avoiding injection directly into the tendon. The tender points at the tendinous insertion and/or at its narrowest part approximately 5 cm above the insertion are identified and marked with a sterile marker.

Proper preparation with antiseptic solution of the skin overlying these points is then carried out. A sterile syringe containing 2.0 mL of 0.25% preservative-free bupivacaine and 40 mg methylprednisolone is attached to a 1½-inch 25-gauge needle using strict aseptic technique. With strict aseptic technique, the previously marked points are palpated. The needle is then carefully advanced at this point along the tendon through the skin and subcutaneous tissues, with care being taken not to enter the substance of the tendon. The contents of the syringe are then gently injected while slowly withdrawing the needle. There should be minimal resistance to injection. If there is significant resistance to injection, the needle tip is probably in the substance of the Achilles tendon and should be withdrawn slightly until the injection proceeds without significant resistance. The needle is then removed, and a sterile pressure dressing and ice pack are placed at the injection site.

COMPLICATIONS AND PITFALLS

The possibility of trauma to the Achilles tendon from the injection itself remains ever-present. Tendons that are highly inflamed or previously damaged are subject to rupture if they are directly injected. This complication can be greatly decreased if the clinician uses gentle technique and stops injecting immediately if significant resistance to injection is encountered. Approximately 25% of patients will complain of a transient increase in pain after this injection technique and should be warned of such.

CLINICAL PEARLS

The Achilles tendon is the thickest and strongest tendon in the body, yet is also very susceptible to rupture. The common tendon of the gastrocnemius muscle, the Achilles tendon, begins at mid-calf and continues downward to attach to the posterior calcaneus, where it may become inflamed. The Achilles tendon narrows during this downward course, becoming most narrow approximately 5 cm above its calcaneal insertion. It is this most narrow point at which tendinitis may also occur. This injection technique is extremely effective in the treatment of pain secondary to the aforementioned causes of posterior ankle pain. Coexistent bursitis and arthritis may also contribute to posterior ankle pain and may require additional treatment with a more localized injection of local anesthetic and methylprednisolone acetate.

The described technique is a safe procedure if careful attention is paid to the clinically relevant anatomy in the areas to be injected. The use of physical modalities including local heat as well as gentle range of motion exercises should be introduced several days after the patient undergoes this injection technique for ankle pain. Vigorous exercises should be avoided because they will exacerbate the patient's symptomatology. Simple analgesics and nonsteroidal anti-inflammatory drugs may be used concurrently with this injection technique.

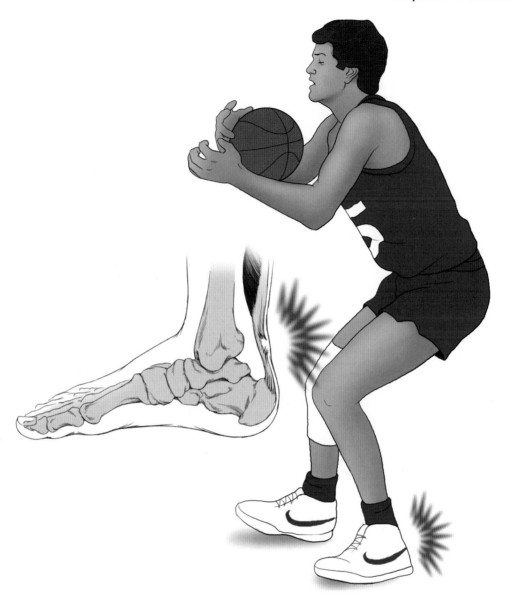

Figure 74–1. The pain of achilles tendinitis is constant and severe and is localized to the posterior ankle.

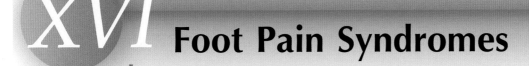

XVI Foot Pain Syndromes

75

Arthritis Pain of the Toes

ICD-9 CODE 715.97

THE CLINICAL SYNDROME

The toe joint is susceptible to the development of arthritis from a variety of conditions that have in common the ability to damage the joint cartilage. Osteoarthritis of the joint is the most common form of arthritis that results in toe joint pain. However, rheumatoid arthritis and post-traumatic arthritis are also common causes of toe pain secondary to arthritis. Less common causes of arthritis-induced toe pain include the collagen vascular diseases, infection, and Lyme disease. Acute infectious arthritis will usually be accompanied by significant systemic symptoms, including fever and malaise, and should be easily recognized by the astute clinician and treated appropriately with culture and antibiotics rather than with injection therapy. The collagen vascular diseases will generally present as a polyarthropathy rather than a monoarthropathy limited to the toe joint, although toe pain secondary to collagen vascular disease responds exceedingly well to the intra-articular injection technique described here.

SIGNS AND SYMPTOMS

The majority of patients presenting with toe joint pain secondary to osteoarthritis and post-traumatic arthritis pain will present with the complaint of pain that is localized to the affected joint of the foot. The great toe is most commonly affected (Fig. 75–1). Activity, especially flexion of the toe joints, makes the pain worse, with rest and heat providing some relief. The pain is constant and characterized as aching in nature. The pain may interfere with sleep. Some patients will complain of a grating or popping sensation with use of the joint and crepitus may be present on physical examination. In addition to the pain, patients suffering from arthritis of the toe joint will often experience a gradual decrease in functional ability with decreasing toe range of motion, making simple everyday tasks such as walking, standing on tiptoes, and climbing stairs quite difficult.

TESTING

Plain radiographs are indicated for all patients who present with toe joint pain. Based on the patient's clinical presentation, additional testing, including complete blood count, sedimentation rate, and antinuclear antibody testing, may be indicated. Magnetic resonance imaging of the toe is indicated if joint instability, occult mass, or tumor is suspected.

DIFFERENTIAL DIAGNOSIS

Entrapment neuropathies such as tarsal tunnel syndrome may also confuse the diagnosis, as may bursitis and tendinitis of the foot, both of which may coexist with arthritis of the toes. Primary and metastatic tumors of the ankle and foot may also present in a manner analogous to arthritis of the ankle, as can occult fractures of the tarsals and metatarsals, as well as fractures of the sesamoid bones of the foot.

TREATMENT

Initial treatment of the pain and functional disability associated with arthritis of the toes should include a combination of the nonsteroidal anti-inflammatory drugs or cyclooxygenase-2 inhibitors and physical therapy. The local application of heat and cold may also be beneficial. Avoidance of repetitive activities that aggravate the patient's symptomatology, as well as short-term immobilization of the joints of the toes, may also provide relief. For patients who do not respond to these treatment modalities, an intra-articular injection of the affected joints with local anesthetic and steroid may be a reasonable next step.

To perform intra-articular injection of the toes, the patient is placed in the supine position, and the skin overlying the affected toe joint is properly prepared with antiseptic solution. A sterile syringe containing 1.5 mL of 0.25% preservative-free bupivacaine and 40 mg methylprednisolone is attached to a ⅝-inch 25-gauge needle using strict aseptic technique. With strict aseptic technique, the affected toe is distracted to open the joint space. The joint space is then identified. At this point, the needle is carefully advanced perpendicular to the joint space just next to the extensor tendons through the skin and subcutaneous tissues through the joint capsule into the joint. If bone is encountered, the needle is withdrawn into the subcutaneous tissues and redirected superiorly. After entering the joint space, the contents of the syringe are gently injected. There should be little resistance to injection. If resistance is encountered, the needle is probably in a ligament or tendon and should be advanced slightly into the joint space until the injection proceeds without significant resistance. The needle is then removed, and a sterile pressure dressing and ice pack are placed at the injection site.

SIDE EFFECTS AND COMPLICATIONS

Failure to identify primary or metastatic tumor of the ankle or foot that is responsible for the patient's pain may yield disastrous results. The major complication of intra-articular injection of the toes is infection. This complication should be exceedingly rare if strict aseptic technique is followed. Approximately 25% of patients will complain of a transient increase in pain after intra-articular injection of the ankle joint and should be warned of such.

CLINICAL PEARLS

Coexistent bursitis and tendinitis may also contribute to arthritis pain of the toes and may require additional treatment with more localized injection of local anesthetic and methylprednisolone acetate. The injection technique is extremely effective in the treatment of pain secondary to the aforementioned causes of arthritis of the joints of the toes. This technique is a safe procedure if careful attention is paid to the clinically relevant anatomy in the areas to be injected. The use of physical modalities including local heat as well as gentle range of motion exercises should be introduced several days after the patient undergoes this injection technique for arthritis pain. Vigorous exercises should be avoided because they will exacerbate the patient's symptomatology.

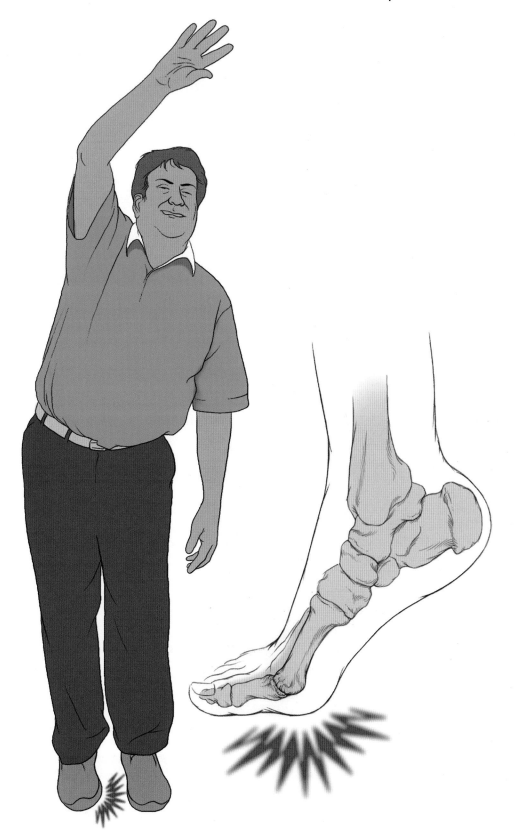

Figure 75–1. Arthritis affecting the joints of the toe will often present as pain made worse with weight-bearing activity.

76

Bunion Pain

ICD-9 CODE 727.1

THE CLINICAL SYNDROME

One of the most common causes of foot pain encountered in clinical practice is the bunion. The term *bunion* refers to a constellation of symptoms that includes soft tissue swelling over the first metatarsophalangeal joint associated with abnormal angulation of the joint resulting in a prominent first metatarsal head with associated overlapping of the first and second toes (Fig. 76–1). This deformity is referred to as the hallux valgus deformity and occurs more commonly in females. The first metatarsophalangeal joint may ultimately sublux, and the overlapping of the first and second toes will worsen. The development of an inflamed adventitious bursa may accompany bunion formation. The most common cause of bunion formation is the wearing of narrow-toed shoes. High heels may exacerbate the problem.

SIGNS AND SYMPTOMS

The majority of patients presenting with bunion will present with the complaint of pain that is localized to the affected first metatarsophalangeal joint and the inability to get shoes to fit. Walking makes the pain worse, with rest and heat providing some relief. The pain is constant and characterized as aching in nature. The pain may interfere with sleep. Some patients will complain of a grating or popping sensation with use of the joint, and crepitus may be present on physical examination. In addition to the pain, patients suffering with bunion develop the characteristic hallux valgus deformity, which consists of a prominent first metatarsal head and improper angulation of the joint with overlapping first and second toes.

DIFFERENTIAL DIAGNOSIS

The diagnosis of bunion is usually obvious on clinical grounds alone. Complicating the care of the patient suffering from a typical bunion deformity is the fact that bursitis and tendinitis of the foot and ankle frequently coexist with the bunion pain. Furthermore, stress fractures of the metatarsals, phalanges, and/or sesamoid bones may also confuse the clinical diagnosis and require specific treatment.

TESTING

Plain radiographs are indicated for all patients who present with bunion pain (Fig. 76–2). Based on the patient's clinical presentation, additional testing, including complete blood count, sedimentation rate, and antinuclear antibody testing, may be indicated. Magnetic resonance imaging of the toe is indicated if joint instability, occult mass, or tumor is suspected.

TREATMENT

Initial treatment of the pain and functional disability associated with bunion deformity should include a combination of the nonsteroidal anti-inflammatory drugs or cyclooxygenase-2 inhibitors and physical therapy. The local application of heat and cold may also be beneficial. Avoidance of repetitive activities that aggravate the patient's symptomatology, as well as avoidance of narrow-toed or high-heeled shoes, combined with short-term immobilization of the affected toes may also provide relief. For patients who do not respond to these treatment modalities, the following injection technique with local anesthetic and steroid may be a reasonable next step.

To inject the bunion deformity, the patient is placed in the supine position, and the skin overlying the bunion is properly prepared with antiseptic solution.

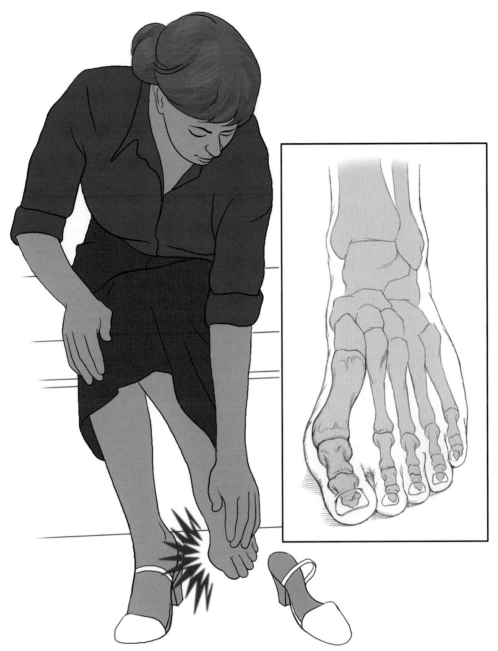

Figure 76–1. Narrow-toed shoes are frequently implicated in the development of bunion deformity of the foot.

A sterile syringe containing 1.5 mL of 0.25% preservative-free bupivacaine and 40 mg methylprednisolone is attached to a ⅝-inch 25-gauge needle using strict aseptic technique. With strict aseptic technique, the bunion is identified, and at this point, the needle is carefully advanced against the first metatarsal head. The needle is then withdrawn slightly out of the periosteum, and the contents of the syringe are gently injected. There should be little resistance to injection. If resistance is encountered, the needle is probably in a ligament or tendon and should be advanced or withdrawn slightly until the injection proceeds without significant resistance. The needle is then removed, and a sterile pressure dressing and ice pack are placed at the injection site.

SIDE EFFECTS AND COMPLICATIONS

Failure to identify primary or metastatic tumor of the foot that is responsible for the patient's pain may yield disastrous results. The major complication of the described injection technique is infection. This complication should be exceedingly rare if strict aseptic technique is followed. Approximately 25% of patients will complain of a transient increase in pain after this technique and should be warned of such.

CLINICAL PEARLS

Coexistent bursitis and tendinitis may also contribute to foot pain and may require additional treatment with more localized injection of local anesthetic and methylprednisolone acetate. The described injection technique is extremely effective in the treatment of pain secondary to bunion deformity. This technique is a safe procedure if careful attention is paid to the clinically relevant anatomy in the areas to be injected. The use of physical modalities including local heat as well as gentle range of motion exercises should be introduced several days after the patient undergoes this injection technique. Narrow-toed and high-heeled shoes should be avoided because they will exacerbate the patient's symptomatology.

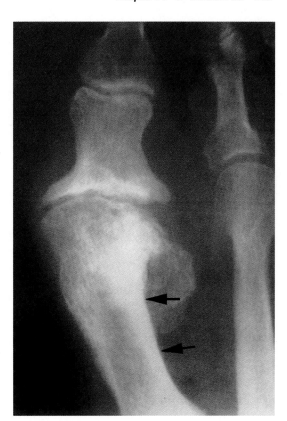

Figure 76–2. Osteoarthritis of the first metatarsophalangeal joint in a patient with a hallux valgus deformity. The sesamoids are lateral to the metatarsal head. There is narrowing of the joint space with subchondral bone and osteophyte formation. There is marked thickening of the lateral cortex of the metatarsal shaft (*arrows*). (From Brower AC, Flemming DJ: Arthritis in Black and White, 2nd ed. Philadelphia, WB Saunders, 1997, p 280.)

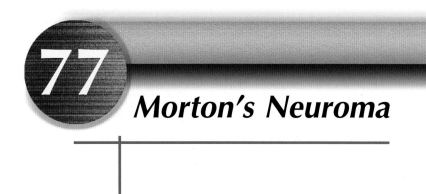

77

Morton's Neuroma

THE CLINICAL SYNDROME

Morton's neuroma is one of the most common pain syndromes affecting the forefoot. Morton's neuroma is characterized by tenderness and burning pain in the plantar surface of the forefoot with associated painful paresthesias into the affected two toes. This pain syndrome is thought to be caused by perineural fibrosis of the interdigital nerves. Although the nerves between the third and fourth toes are affected most commonly, the second and third toes and, rarely, the fourth and fifth toes can be affected (Fig. 77–1). The patient often feels like he or she is walking with a stone in the shoe. The pain of Morton's neuroma worsens with prolonged standing or walking for long distances and is exacerbated by improperly fitting or padded shoes. As with bunion, bunionette, and hammertoe deformities, Morton's neuroma is most often associated with the wearing of tight, narrow-toed shoes.

SIGNS AND SYMPTOMS

On physical examination, pain can be reproduced by firmly squeezing the two metatarsal heads together with one hand while placing firm pressure on the interdigital space with the other. In contradistinction to metatarsalgia, in which the tender area remains over the metatarsal heads, with Morton's neuroma, the tender area will be localized to only the plantar surface of the affected interspace with paresthesias radiating into the two affected toes. The patient with Morton's neuroma will often exhibit an antalgic gait in an effort to reduce weight bearing during walking.

DIFFERENTIAL DIAGNOSIS

Fractures of the sesamoid bones of the foot are often confused with the pain of Morton's neuroma. Although the pain of such fractures is also localized to the plantar surface of the foot, they are less neuritic in character than the pain of Morton's neuroma. Tendinitis and bursitis of the foot as well as stress fractures of the foot can also mimic the pain of Morton's neuroma.

TESTING

Plain radiographs are indicated for all patients who present with Morton's neuroma to rule out fractures and identify sesamoid bones that may have become inflamed. Based on the patient's clinical presentation, additional testing, including complete blood count, sedimentation rate, and antinuclear antibody testing, may be indicated. Magnetic resonance imaging of the metatarsal bones is indicated if joint instability, occult mass, or tumor is suspected. Radionuclide bone scanning may be useful in identifying stress fractures of the metatarsal bones or sesamoid bones that may be missed on plain radiographs of the foot.

TREATMENT

Initial treatment of the pain and functional disability associated with Morton's neuroma should include a combination of the nonsteroidal anti-inflammatory drugs or cyclooxygenase-2 inhibitors and physical therapy. The local application of heat and cold may also be beneficial. Avoidance of repetitive activities that aggravate the patient's symptomatology, as well as avoidance of narrow-toed or high-heeled shoes, combined with short-term immobilization of the affected foot may also provide relief. For patients who

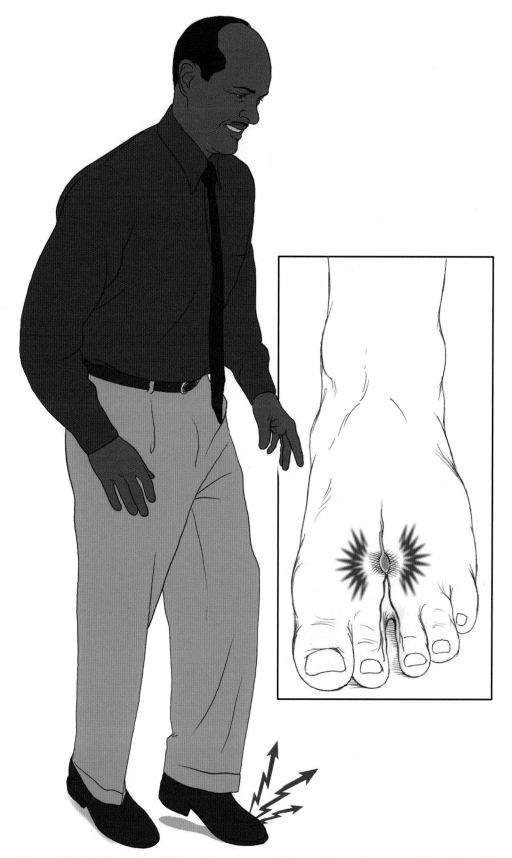

Figure 77–1. The pain of Morton's neuroma is frequently made worse with prolonged standing or walking.

do not respond to these treatment modalities, the following injection technique with local anesthetic and steroid may be a reasonable next step.

To inject Morton's neuroma, the patient is placed in a supine position with a pillow placed under the knee to slightly flex the leg. A total of 3 mL non–epinephrine-containing local anesthetic and 40 mg methylprednisolone is drawn up in a 12-ml sterile syringe. The affected interdigital space is identified, and the dorsal surface of the foot at this point is marked with a sterile marker. After preparation of the skin with antiseptic solution, at a point proximal to the metatarsal head, a 1½-inch 25-gauge needle is inserted between the two metatarsal bones in the area to be blocked (Fig. 77–2). While the clinician is slowly injecting, the needle is advanced from the dorsal surface of the foot toward the palmar surface. The plantar digital nerve is situated on the dorsal side of the flexor retinaculum, and thus the needle will have to be advanced almost to the palmar surface of the foot. The needle is removed, and pressure is placed on the injection site to avoid hematoma formation.

SIDE EFFECTS AND COMPLICATIONS

Failure to identify primary or metastatic tumor of the foot that is responsible for the patient's pain may yield disastrous results. The major complication of the described injection technique is infection. This complication should be exceedingly rare if strict aseptic technique is followed. Because of the confined nature of the soft tissue surrounding the metatarsals and digits, the potential for mechanical compression of the blood supply after injection of the solution must be considered. The clinician must avoid rapidly injecting large volumes of solution into these confined spaces, or vascular insufficiency and gangrene may occur. Furthermore, epinephrine-containing solutions must always be avoided to avoid ischemia and possible gangrene.

Approximately 25% of patients will complain of a transient increase in pain after this technique and should be warned of such.

CLINICAL PEARLS

Coexistent bursitis and tendinitis may also contribute to foot pain and may require additional treatment with more localized injection of local anesthetic and methylprednisolone acetate. The described injection technique is extremely effective in the treatment of pain secondary to Morton's neuroma. This technique is a safe procedure if careful attention is paid to the clinically relevant anatomy in the areas to be injected. The use of physical modalities including local heat as well as gentle range of motion exercises should be introduced several days after the patient undergoes this injection technique. Although the described injection technique will provide palliation of the pain of Morton's neuroma, the patient will often also require shoe orthoses and shoes with a wider toe box to help remove pressure from the affected interdigital nerves.

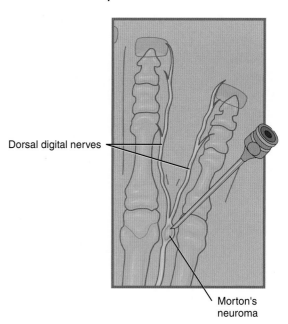

Figure 77–2. Proper needle placement for injection of Morton's neuroma. (From Waldman SD: Atlas of Pain Management Injection Techniques. Philadelphia, WB Saunders, 2000, p 363.)

78

Plantar Fasciitis

ICD-9 CODE 728.71

THE CLINICAL SYNDROME

Plantar fasciitis is characterized by pain and tenderness over the plantar surface of the calcaneus. Occurring twice as commonly in women, plantar fasciitis is thought to be caused by an inflammation of the plantar fascia. This inflammation can occur alone or can be part of a systemic inflammatory condition such as rheumatoid arthritis, Reiter's syndrome, or gout. Obesity also seems to predispose to the development of plantar fasciitis, as does going barefoot or wearing house slippers for prolonged periods (Fig. 78–1). High-impact aerobic exercise has also been implicated.

SIGNS AND SYMPTOMS

The pain of plantar fasciitis is most severe on first walking after non–weight bearing and is made worse by prolonged standing or walking. Characteristic radiographic changes are lacking in plantar fasciitis, but radionuclide bone scanning may show increased uptake at the point of attachment of the plantar fascia to the medial calcaneal tuberosity.

On physical examination, the patient will exhibit point tenderness over the plantar medial calcaneal tuberosity. The patient may also experience tenderness along the plantar fascia as it moves anteriorly. Pain will be increased by dorsiflexing the toes, which pulls the plantar fascia taunt, and then palpating along the fascial from the heel to the forefoot.

DIFFERENTIAL DIAGNOSIS

The pain of plantar fasciitis can often be confused with the pain of Morton's neuroma or sesamoiditis. The characteristic pain on dorsiflexion of the toes associated with plantar fasciitis should help distinguish these painful conditions of the foot. Stress fractures of the metatarsals or sesamoid bones, bursitis, and tendinitis may also confuse the clinical picture.

TESTING

Plain radiographs are indicated for all patients who present with pain thought to be emanating from plantar fasciitis to rule out occult bony pathology and tumor. Based on the patient's clinical presentation, additional testing, including complete blood count, prostate specific antigen, sedimentation rate, and antinuclear antibody testing, may be indicated. Magnetic resonance imaging of the foot is indicated if occult mass or tumor is suspected. Radionuclide bone scanning may be useful to rule out stress fractures not seen on plain radiographs. The following injection technique will serve as both a diagnostic and therapeutic maneuver.

TREATMENT

Initial treatment of the pain and functional disability associated with plantar fasciitis should include a combination of the nonsteroidal anti-inflammatory drugs or cyclooxygenase-2 inhibitors and physical therapy. The local application of heat and cold may also be beneficial. Avoidance of repetitive activities that aggravate the patient's symptomatology, as well as avoidance of walking barefoot or with shoes that do not provide good support, combined with short-term immobilization of the affected foot may also provide relief. For patients who do not respond to these treatment modalities, the following injection technique with local anesthetic and steroid may be a reasonable next step.

To inject plantar fasciitis, the patient is placed in the supine position. The medial aspect of the heel is

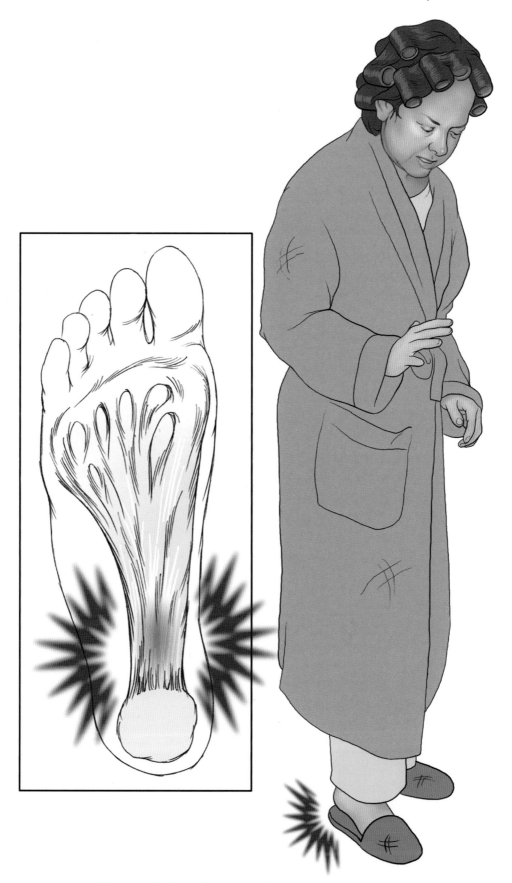

Figure 78–1. The pain of plantar fasciitis is often localized to the hindfoot and can cause significant functional disability.

identified by palpation. Proper preparation with antiseptic solution of the skin overlying this point is then carried out. A syringe containing 2.0 mL of 0.25% preservative-free bupivacaine and 40 mg methylprednisolone is attached to a 1½-inch 25-gauge needle. The needle is then carefully advanced through the previously identified point at a right angle to the skin directly toward the center of the medial aspect of the calcaneus. The needle is advanced very slowly until the needle impinges on bone. The needle is then withdrawn slightly out of the periosteum, and the contents of the syringe are then gently injected as the needle is slowly withdrawn. There should be slight resistance to injection given the closed nature of the heel.

COMPLICATIONS AND PITFALLS

Many patients will complain of a transient increase in pain after the injection. This side effect can be minimized by injecting gently and slowly. Infection, although rare, may occur if careful attention to sterile technique is not followed.

CLINICAL PEARLS

The use of physical modalities including local heat as well as gentle stretching exercises should be introduced several days after the patient undergoes this injection technique. Vigorous exercises should be avoided because they will exacerbate the patient's symptomatology. Heel pads or molded orthotic devices may also be of value. Simple analgesics, nonsteroidal anti-inflammatory drugs, and antimyotonic agents such as tizanidine may be used concurrently with this injection technique.

This injection technique is extremely effective in the treatment of plantar fasciitis. This technique is a safe procedure if careful attention is paid to the clinically relevant anatomy in the areas to be injected. Care must be taken to use sterile technique to avoid infection and to use universal precautions to avoid risk to the operator. Most side effects of this injection technique are related to needle-induced trauma to the injection site and underlying tissues.

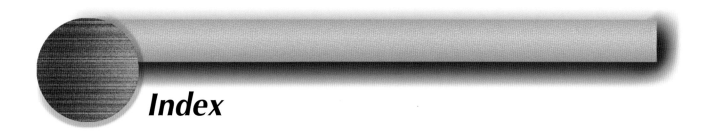

Index

Note: Page numbers followed by the letter f refer to figures; those followed by the letter t refer to tables.

Abdominal/groin pain syndrome(s)
  acute pancreatitis in, 185–187
  chronic pancreatitis in, 188–191
  genitofemoral neuralgia in, 196–199
  ilioinguinal neuralgia in, 192–195
Abductor pollicis longus tendon, inflammation and swelling of, 122. *See also* De Quervain's tenosynovitis.
Abortive therapy
  for migraine headaches, 9, 11
  for tension-type headaches, 14
Achilles tendinitis
  signs and symptoms of, 291, 293f
  treatment of, 291–292
Acromioclavicular joint pain
  differential diagnosis of, 76
  signs and symptoms of, 76, 77f
  treatment of, 76, 78, 79f
Adjuvant analgesics
  for herpes zoster infection
    of thoracic dermatomes, 174
    of trigeminal nerve, 6
  for phantom limb pain, 240
  for postherpetic neuralgia, 178
Adson's test, 59, 60f
Aluminum sulfate, topical, for herpes zoster lesions, 6–7, 174
Amitriptyline
  for diabetic truncal neuropathy, 154
  for post-thoracotomy pain, 166
  for tension-type headaches, 14
Amputation, phantom limb pain following, 238, 239f. *See also* Phantom limb pain.
Analgesic(s)
  for compressed thoracic vertebral fractures, 182
  for diabetic truncal neuropathy, 156
  for herpes zoster infection
    of thoracic dermatomes, 172, 174
    of trigeminal nerve, 6
  for Pancoast's tumor, 64
  for pancreatitis, 186, 190
  for phantom limb pain, 240
  for postherpetic neuralgia, 178
Analgesic rebound headache, 11
  differential diagnosis of, 21
  drugs implicated in, 19t
  signs and symptoms of, 19, 20f
  treatment of, 21
Analgesic rebound phenomenon, associated with migraine headache, 8
Anesthetics, local, blockade with. *See* Depot-steroid/local anesthetic blockade; Methylprednisolone/local anesthetic blockade.
Ankle, arthritis of, 275–276, 277f
Ankle pain syndrome(s)
  Achilles tendinitis in, 291–293

Ankle pain syndrome(s) *(Continued)*
  arthritis in, 275–277
  deltoid ligament strain in, 282–284
  midtarsal joint pain in, 278–281
  tarsal tunnel syndrome in
    anterior, 285–287
    posterior, 288–290
Antiarrhythmic agents, for diabetic truncal neuropathy, 156
Anticonvulsants. *See also* specific agent, e.g., Gabapentin.
  for diabetic truncal neuropathy, 154, 156
Antidepressants. *See also* specific agent, e.g., Nortriptyline.
  for atypical facial pain, 38
  for diabetic truncal neuropathy, 156
  for herpes zoster infection
    of thoracic dermatomes, 174
    of trigeminal nerve, 6
  for intercostal neuralgia, 150
  for phantom limb pain, 240
  for postherpetic neuralgia, 178
  for post-thoracotomy pain, 166
  for tension-type headaches, 14–15
Antiviral agents, for herpes zoster infection
  of thoracic dermatomes, 174
  of trigeminal nerve, 6
Arachnoiditis
  clinical features of, 209t
  differential diagnosis of, 210
  signs and symptoms of, 209, 211f
  treatment of, 210
Arnold-Chiari malformation, vs. tension-type headache, 14
Arthritis
  degenerative. *See* Degenerative arthritis.
  gouty, of elbow, 109
  of ankle, 275–276, 277f
  of carpometacarpal joint, 118, 125–126, 127f
  of hip, 231–232, 233f
  of knee, 247, 248f–249f, 250
  of midtarsal joint, 278, 279f, 280, 281f
  of toe, 297–298, 299f
  of wrist, 115–116, 117f
Aspiration
  of Baker's cyst, 268
  of ganglion cyst, 138
Atypical facial pain, 37f
  differential diagnosis of, 38
  signs and symptoms of, 36
  treatment of, 38
  vs. reflex sympathetic dystrophy, 41t
  vs. trigeminal neuralgia, 36t
Auditory aura, associated with migraine headache, 8
Aura, associated with migraine headache, 8–9

Baclofen
  for brachial plexopathy, 61
  for Pancoast's tumor, 64
  for thoracic outlet syndrome, 68
  for trigeminal neuralgia, 32
Baker's cyst, of knee, 266, 267f, 268
Beta-blocking agents, for migraine headaches, 11
Bicipital tendinitis
  signs and symptoms of, 84, 85f, 87f
  treatment of, 84, 86
Biofeedback, for tension-type headaches, 15
Blood sugar, control of, in diabetic truncal neuropathy, 154
Brace, for compression fractures of thoracic vertebrae, 182
Brachial plexopathy
  differential diagnosis of, 59, 61
  signs and symptoms of, 59, 60f
  treatment of, 61–62
Brachial plexus, local tumor infiltration into, 63. *See also* Pancoast's tumor.
Brachial plexus block
  for Pancoast's tumor, 64, 66
  for plexopathy, 61
  for thoracic outlet syndrome, 68, 70
Brachial plexus pain syndrome(s). *See* Neck/brachial plexus pain syndrome(s).
Bunion
  signs and symptoms of, 300, 301f
  treatment of, 300, 302
Bupivacaine, in nerve blocks. *See* Methylprednisolone/local anesthetic blockade.
Bursal sac, calcification of, 82, 90
Bursitis
  infrapatellar
    deep, 263–264, 265f
    superficial, 260, 261f, 262
  ischiogluteal, 223–225, 225f
  olecranon, 109–110, 111f
  pes anserine, 269–270, 271f
  prepatellar, 257–258, 259f
  subdeltoid, 80, 81f, 82, 83f
  suprapatellar, 254, 255f, 256
  trochanteric, 242, 243f, 244

Calcification, of bursal sac, 82, 90
Capsaicin, topical
  for phantom limb pain, 240–241
  for postherpetic neuralgia, 178
Carbamazepine
  for brachial plexopathy, 61
  for herpes zoster infection
    of thoracic dermatomes, 174
    of trigeminal nerve, 6